Healing
Our Bloodlines

The 8 Realizations of
Generational Liberation

G. K. HUNTER

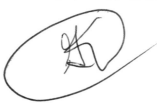

A Kindred House Media Book

Published by Kindred House Media LLC
P. O. Box 893603
Mililani, HI 96789

ISBN: 978-1-7340092-0-0 Print
ISBN: 978-1-7340092-1-7 eBook

Library of Congress Control Number:

Cover Photography: G. K. Hunter
Cover Design and Layout: Jana Rade
Illustrations: G. K. Hunter
Editor: Linda Fookwe

Table of Contents

Foreword

It is indeed an honor to write this Foreword to Healing Our Bloodlines. After working many decades in the arena of generational healing I have become keenly aware that this may perhaps be the initial task facing humanity if we are to continue living on our earth. I have found that most, if not all, of the symptoms that we treat in many of our health settings have their genesis in trauma, also known as 'Injury where blood doesn't flow' by Indigenous ways of knowing. The injury where blood doesn't flow becomes part of the bloodlines that carry the injury into subsequent generations.

G.K. Hunter, takes the theoretical notion of bloodline lineage trauma and gives us a path to healing the bloodline. He gives us a map on which we can set off on a journey of healing that is practical and gives us hope that this journey can be completed. I am grateful that he includes compassion as one of the gates towards the attainment of healing. There are many practitioners of various healing arts that although being very smart, technical and expert diagnosticians are lacking in the most important aspect of healing the human soul; that is compassion.

I believe that compassion is the 'wormhole' that leads into liberation. Liberation in the larger sense means more than being free of symptoms. Hunter's understanding is that liberation entails a greater soul task involving forgiveness and shared peace. Forgiveness along with compassion are the sine que non of healing the collective world soul. Through the process described by Hunter, by healing families, we will create a critical mass of energy that will facilitate the healing of the collective soul wounding. Hunter gives us a way to transform this intergenerational violence that has taken a seat in the human heart into peace that can be found by entering the wormhole of forgiveness and compassion.

Thank you, George for taking on this most sacred task.

Teoshpaye ta Woapeya Wicsasa aka Eduardo Duran PhD

Preface

When I first decided to hang my shingle as an Intuitive Healer, I didn't know that I would be working with survivors of the Holocaust. They found me. They became my inspiration for an approach to healing that directly addresses the cyclic pain that gets passed down through multiple generations of every family lineage. What started off as unconventional endeavors to help the children and grandchildren of Holocaust survivors find relief soon blossomed into an approach to generational healing for people from all cultural backgrounds. Bloodline Healing was born.

While I felt the calling to become a Healer ever since I was a child, I wasn't sure how I would express this healer-ship. Would I become part of the clergy, a therapist, or a physician of some kind? Would I sacrifice the prestige of these established vocations for something more alternative, something complementary to conventional therapeutic care? My decision to become an Intuitive Healer, a vocation that would leave most high school guidance counselors scratching their heads in confusion, was the first step in developing a back door to the conventional healing process.

Before I could be a clear messenger for a path to generational healing, I first had to be honest with myself about who I was. I am a rule breaker, a sacred witness, and a guide for other world changers who seek more authentic lives. I had to break free from the cyclic pain that was repeatedly inflicted in each new generation. In my family, alcoholism and drug addiction were all too common. We were all born into the pain of various forms of emotional and physical abuse, then we were taught to hide the secret abuse when in public. We all found our ways to numb this inherited pain, typically by working too much, then drinking too much. But my family taught me how to see the good in people, even during the most painful moments. To their credit, they always saw my goodness, even when they were in pain. In my lifetime, I have faced many of the inherited cycles of pain that have been in my family for several generations. I've shared that inspiration with other family members, becoming a Catalyst for the changes they were making in their lives. When one family member can do it, others believe that perhaps they can change their lives for the better as well.

I made the decision to become a full-time Healer a few years after graduating with my pre-medical bachelor's degree from Cornell University. At the time, I was planning on attending medical school. In the hopes of obtaining a letter of recommendation from a famous physician, I started working at Memorial Sloan Kettering Cancer Center as a research associate for the Integrative Medicine Department. This new department was studying reiki, massage, and acupuncture to see if these modalities could reduce pain in terminally ill cancer patients. I was responsible for coordinating the different practitioners who would administer treatment, explaining the studies to participating clients, and managing the clinical data. It was there that I first met Aviva Shira Bernat, MD, an attending physician in the Pain and Palliative Care Department. She helped me find patients for my studies.

Dr. Bernat was a young, open-minded physician who was intrigued by the various intuitive-based healing trainings that I had done. One weekend, I did a practice healing session on her that combined many of the methods that I learned from my teachers, along with some of my own techniques. She was so moved by the experience that she referred many clients to me. As she put it, "Even the taxi driver noticed my glow after my first session with you." That was high praise coming from an overworked New York City cabby. This influx of clients prompted me to open a part-time private practice in Manhattan and ignited my passion to creatively share my intuitive gifts.

It wasn't long after starting my healing practice that I abandoned my plans of going to medical school completely. I quit my job at Memorial and rolled the dice to see if I could make it as a full-time Healer in NYC.

When Dr. Bernat moved to Los Angeles to be with her family, she invited me to fly out to LA to offer healing sessions to people in her California-based community. That's when I first started working with the original survivors of the Holocaust, their children, and their grandchildren. These second and third generation survivors had already been in therapy for many years as they had inherited the historic pain from the original survivors within their families. Their pain was often hidden, as public attention focused on the original survivors who had experienced and survived the concentration camps. The pain still felt by the original survivors often eclipsed the deeply inherited anxiety, anger, and grief that were empathetically felt by the later generations. Many of my second and third generation clients had grown up safely in the United States and lived comfortable middle-class lives. They'd benefited from sound educations from well-known universities and had access to many years of therapy. Yet their therapists told them that they still suffered from extreme anxiety and depression.

These Holocaust survivors became my indirect teachers. I began to see the invisible burdens that they carried. These burdens were the unexpressed emotions and expectations of their families, compounded by all their own personal feelings about the atrocities that their relatives had endured.

I felt a moral obligation to find a fresh way to help them reach past all that collective hurt and grief that they held onto on behalf of their families. I wanted them to find the peace of being alive, and the passion of having a life that was not defined by the emotional scars that their families carried.

But in order to help them, beyond the conventional therapies they had already undergone, we would need to explore an unknown path together. I didn't have a manual on how to help people in this situation. This is the guidebook that I wish I could have taken with me when I first visited Dr. Bernat's community in Los Angeles.

Initially, I thought the work that I was doing would become a method specifically for a niche population of Jewish Holocaust survivors. But these early clients were the extreme cases who mapped the way for me. Their stories illustrated the movement of the painful, unfinished stories from the older generations onto the younger generations. I began noticing this same dynamic with my other clients, from various cultural backgrounds, and my work organically expanded into a system of releasing inherited family pain for all people.

I further developed this generational healing approach with a team of practitioners, who had graduated from the school I founded, the Bluestone Institute for the Healing Arts, where they learned Intuitive Healing and energy work. Dr. Bernat incorporated energy healing and intuitive work into her practice as a physician. Her biological sister, Dina Bernat-Kunin, and her adopted sister, Jessica Gelson, were already therapists. They, too, went on to incorporate the intuitive healing work into their private practices. I affectionately called them "the Three Sisters." We were eventually joined by Ann Molitor, a group facilitator who specialized in women's empowerment. Soon, we began holding Bloodline Healing workshops for people of all backgrounds.

There are countless people who contributed to this work. While I may be the architect who combined all the pieces, there are so many who each contributed their gifts and moments of wisdom to make this work possible. I am eternally grateful to the clients, colleagues, and special helpers who supported this work each step of the way.

The stories featured in this book are the authentic experiences of people that I've had the honor to help. Some of their personal details were altered for the sake of preserving their confidentiality. While some clients were on medications prescribed by their physician, no hallucinogenic drugs or herbs were used in any of the sessions or workshops. Thank you to all those people who willingly offered their inspirational stories so that we may learn from their ordeals and triumphs. You have given a gift to the future generations of humanity that could never be quantified, yet the residual impact can be felt.

Introduction

Every family has unfinished stories. We are born into them. These stories contain the unmet longings of the generations gone before us. They carry old mistakes never corrected, the feuds that were never resolved, and the thefts and debts that were never repaid. They also hold the dreams of our parents, and their parents - visions and ambitions that were never fully realized.

I call this collective mass of unfinished
family business the Invisible Burden.

We often don't realize just how much these Invisible Burdens impact on our current lives, albeit from behind the scenes. They weigh on us. When elders pass away, the burdens that they carried only *seem* to disappear, and for a while they are forgotten, like a shoe box of old photos in a dusty attic.

But these unfinished family stories don't resolve themselves; they merely sink below the surface of our conscious awareness submerged into the depths of our collective family histories where they remain hidden. The stories hibernate and fester, until someone new is born into the family to once again bear the load. Then the unfinished business rears and rises up from our blood to replay itself in the next generation of our lineage. These unresolved stories repeat themselves until someone in the bloodline wakes up and finishes the story.

Summer 1957, Brooklyn, New York

My father, George Ralph Hunter, was only five years old when he became ensnared by one of those family stories. My paternal grandfather, George Francis Hunter, took my father to the ocean. My father didn't yet know how to swim. So, my grandfather tried to show him how to swim by simply throwing him headlong into the water. The crash course shocked my father, and he flailed his arms in the overhead water, crying out for help. What began as a rough initiation became a swim for his life.

My grandpa George was not a cruel man. He was an orphan, toughened up by the hardships of his early life. He worked two labor jobs and even moonlighted as a pub boxer for extra money on the side. His working man fists were big as melons, and his palms were as rough as sandpaper. Grandpa learned to fend for himself early on. Calluses on his hand bore testimony to his hard work, and the thick skin he wore to protect his caring heart bore testimony to the many betrayals he'd encountered throughout his life. He was a Native American boy who was born in a cornfield in Upstate New York shortly after his family left the reservation (a sovereign Indigenous territory belonging to one or more tribes within the borders of the U.S. or Canada). We grew up knowing that we were Mohawk, but my grandfather rarely shared much with us about his culture. Every time we asked him questions about our family's origins, he got that far away look in his eyes, like we asked him to recall something very painful, but he didn't want to show it. It made me wonder if there was a falling-out between our family and our community. I had to learn about our culture from other Iroquois elders, a reconnection that brought healing to our family. Efforts to verify which reservation our family came from has been stalled for decades due to a genealogical document hunt that remains another unfinished story in my lineage. As a result, we are not enrolled in a tribe, and thus are not citizens of any indigenous nation. I've heard many times in my life that we are not "real Native Americans" because we grew up off the reservation, because of our light appearance, and because my grandfather married outside of his race, breaking cultural customs. However, these facts didn't stop the beatings and ridicule that my grandfather endured for his appearance. He faced his pain alone, without the validation or support of a Native community.

Grandpa George was taunted when he left the farmlands of Ulster County, NY to live in the city streets of Brooklyn. He never had the chance to go to school. He never ran off like his father did. Grandpa stayed and provided for his family. Providing for the family is how he showed his love to us. My grandfather's abuse was not just a family story that was passed down through the generations by an unreliable narrator. I personally witnessed a dinner plate thrown at my grandfather's head as he was cursed for being a "dirty Indian" in the 1980's. Fortunately, his boxing skills stayed with him even in his elder years, and he was able to evade the assault.

My grandfather had a rougher childhood than my father. At 5 years old, my grandpa stepped in as a main provider to his family's income, working as a farmhand, because his dad had abandoned his family. My father, at that age, was able to enjoy a leisurely stroll with his father along the Brooklyn shoreline. My father surely enjoyed that moment of his childhood, that peaceful walk in the summer heat at Coney Island; a calm moment just before the spontaneous swimming lesson would rock his world.

There, on the shores of Brooklyn, my young father continued to flail in the deep, salty water. He splashed and gasped and swallowed. His father chuckled, the way a hard man does when he knows he is toughening up his son through a rough game. Maybe this was how grandpa was taught to swim. Perhaps he was just passing on what was normal to him. My thick-skinned grandfather hadn't yet realized that something was wrong. He couldn't see that my father wasn't learning to swim; my young father was drowning.

Finally, a deeper fatherly instinct kicked in as Grandpa pulled my father out of the water. But the damage had been done. The surprise had broken my father's heart. It scarred him. He felt abandoned by his father, and he never fully recovered from that day. After the shocking experience, my dad never had a heart-to-heart talk with his father about the deep pain that was inflicted on him that day. After nearly drowning, my dad needed to cry in his father's arms. He needed to ask his dad "why did you do that?" and to hear "you're safe now." My father's brush with death made him hyper vigilant about safety. For the rest of his life, he had a crippling aversion to the ocean.

Because they never talked about what had happened, and because my father never sought therapeutic help for what he went through, the story of nearly drowning was never resolved. It became an unfinished family story that sank back down into the Hunter bloodline, waiting for its chance to resurface again. I became the next holder of that painful and frightening family story.

INTRODUCTION

As the eldest son of my family, I was named George Christopher Hunter, after my father and my grandfather. My very name seemed to tie me to an incident that happened before I was even born. That unfinished story of my father nearly drowning seemed to hover over all who were named George Hunter, like an unseen cloud, until it finally resurfaced again. This time, it would be reenacted by my younger brother Sean and I.

Summer, 1992, Jones Beach, New York

Hurricane Andrew, a Category 5 hurricane with gust winds upwards of 175 mph, pummeled the Caribbean and the Southeastern states of the U.S. in mid-August of 1992. The storm hit Florida, then shredded its way up the east coast, destroying 63,000 homes and claiming the lives of 65 people. It was the costliest hurricane to date in U. S. history, until Hurricane Katrina devastated the Gulf of Mexico a little over a decade later. [1]

While the people of Florida and the Caribbean were picking up the shingles of their shattered houses, I was a carefree 15-year-old enjoying a summertime beach day with my mother and younger brother at Jones Beach. Though Hurricane Andrew never made it to Jones Beach, which was about 900 miles up the coast, the waves had become charged by the mammoth storm. The shimmering sun and the calls of the greedy seagulls masked the true danger that the super-powered waves posed to oblivious swimmers. The incoming waves were larger than normal, but once the swimmers made it past the shore break they appeared to be cushioned from the pounding surf. Few realized that the actual danger wasn't the incoming waves. The real threat was the unseen undertow, the pull of the ocean after the wave has already crashed on the shore.

---

1   Encylopedia Britannica; https://www.britannica.com/event/Hurricane-Andrew

My father didn't come with us to the beach anymore. The memory of his near-drowning ran too deep. While we were at the beach, he sat in his bedroom next to a humming air conditioner to escape the heat. He spent his time listening to the talk radio news, undoubtedly hearing about the aftermath of Hurricane Andrew. So, in my father's stead, it became my job to look after my younger brother Sean, just 10 years old at the time.

I walked down to the shore to check on Sean, and I can still clearly remember the sound of the thunderous punch as the ocean plowed its giant knuckles into the compacted wet sand. In between the sounds of the pounding surf, lifeguard whistles pierced the air as they corralled the swimmers back to shore. I squinted through the ocean spray, scanning the sea for Sean. When I spotted him, I was gripped by his panicked eyes. The undertow had him.

As the water sucked him deeper out to sea, I saw him mouth my name, *George.* But I couldn't hear him over the whistle blows and crashing waves. The lifeguards were overwhelmed, diving into the water like frantic dolphins, trying to rescue the scores of people who had been tricked by the seemingly calm ocean on a hot summer's day. The magnetic pull of guilt tugged on me before I even moved a muscle. I felt a sense of responsibility for my brother's well-being, especially because I couldn't call upon my father for help, and the lifeguards were overwhelmed in their rescue attempts. As the next waves slammed onto my feet, I feared for my own life. I feared for my brother's life. I was scared that he would slip through the cracks because the lifeguards couldn't cope. My brother flailed in the seas, growing smaller by the minute as he was pulled further out. His cry for help pulled me forward as my knees chopped through the surface of the hard water. I dived beneath the next waves just before it released its thunder crack onto the shore. I popped up on the other side of the crash zone as the physical undertow of the ocean sucked me into its thirsty embrace. I pumped my limbs until I felt the fierce embrace of my brother.

After calming him down, I put my arm around him and pulled Sean towards the shore. My little brother kicked fiercely as we both stroked through the undertow. But the shore was not coming any closer. It was gradually drifting away. Now the undertow had us both.

There is an eerie thickness in the air when death is near. I experienced it as a sinking realization that this could be it, that this might be the end of our lives. It's a powerless sensation when that ache from the other side starts to set in, a strangely familiar silence that will pull you from your life and bring you elsewhere against your will. Despite feeling a dark chill that I might soon drown, I kept my brother calm. I was proud of myself for not staying safely on the shore and leaving my brother alone. Even if it meant that we might both perish, at least he wouldn't die alone.

As we treaded waters in the cold, dark sea, I wondered if my 5-year-old father had felt the same way when his father had thrown him into the sea so many years ago. Did he, too, feel abandoned by his father, as I now did? Would my father have faced his fear of the ocean if he had seen Sean get sucked out to sea? While the finer details of our situations were different, the repeating theme of drowning was remarkably similar. Both near-drowning events were clear examples of fatherly abandonment.

My trance-like near death experience was broken by a young lifeguard with curly blond hair. He shoved a buoy with a lifeline into my hands. The three of us swam back to safety as the rescuers pulled the buoy rope, hauling us to shore.

We could kiss the sand when we reached the shore. As we panted on dry land, I was overwhelmed with profound love for, and loyalty to, my brother. Our mother weaved through the crowded beach to embrace us, grateful that we were still alive. She had felt that grip in her gut, a mother's instinct that told her that her boys were in trouble.

On that day at Jones Beach, I felt like I was fulfilling a role on behalf of my father. If he had been at the beach that day, he would have come face-to-face with his fear of drowning that had stemmed from his experience in Brooklyn. He would have felt the pull to save his youngest son from drowning. He would have been forced to choose between staying safely on the shore and swimming out to save his son. Instead, by hiding in his room while we were at the beach, he had relinquished the story for his oldest son to complete. The unfinished story of my father almost drowning in Brooklyn began with my grandpa George unwittingly putting his son in peril. That story found a resolution when I helped my brother avoid peril. My thick-skinned grandfather didn't realize the terror and abandonment that he had caused my father. When I swam out to my panicked brother, I was truly with him. I calmed him down for long enough so that the overtaxed lifeguards could find us. The anxiety and abandonment that began the unfinished family story ended with the reassurance that my brother was not alone, a feeling that could only be experienced by my direct presence and the lifeguard coming to his aid. By not facing his fear of the ocean and avoiding the family beach day, my father was perpetuating that story of male abandonment that was exemplified by his botched swimming lesson in Brooklyn.

By swimming out to my brother, I became the George Hunter of the lineage who finally ended the sense of fatherly abandonment. A sense so often felt by sons from their fathers at the moments they most need them.

My brush with death at Jones Beach initiated me as a Catalyst for change in my lineage.

I am not the only Catalyst out there. More and more people are waking up each day. They are the people who are facing the unfinished stories in their lineages and finding ways to free themselves of them. Over the past 15 years, while serving as a Healer and workshop facilitator, I have witnessed thousands of people embrace their own personal awakenings; those watershed moments where they released the old family stories in exchange for a new, chosen path. These are the people who are able to see the bigger pictures of their families' experiences. These Catalysts discover the courage to speak up and end the cycles of violence and to stop the madness that most family members just learn to tolerate. By living an authentic life, they model for the younger generations how healthy relationships are formed and how the sweetness of life can be savored. These Catalysts are the unsung family heroes who never get a medal for their sacrifices, and rarely hear a thank you. But they don't do it for recognition. They stand for the truth, honesty, and personal freedom. They interrupt repetitive abuses, they witness courageous triumphs, and they share their innate gifts with the world, transforming it into a better place to live. They liberate themselves and illuminate a path for other family members to follow.

A Catalyst is someone who follows their Inner Voice of Truth, a deeper voice inside which tells us how to be free of the stories that no longer suit us. It is the song that leads us to living our most authentic life. It is the voice that guides us to being free. When we listen to it, our Inner Voice of Truth becomes our personal source of inner guidance, that wisdom which leads us to live our truest and most satisfying lives.

Too often, Catalysts feel lonely. They face the challenges of their family's stories with little to no support, fueled by pure courage and the sheer will to be free of their inherited suffering. They step out into the unknown, not even sure if they are walking a genuine path of personal transformation.

Imagine how comforting and reassuring it would be if guidelines existed to steer us through this process? This became my goal as I documented the breakthroughs experienced by my clients. They became my unexpected teachers. Each offered some kind of clue into this rich, transformative journey that we must all face at some point in our self-discovery. The experiences expressed by clients from very different cultural backgrounds showed me the common threads that ultimately wove together to reveal principles to the generational healing process. Finally, writing about my immersion into this work birthed the 8 Realizations that make up the Path of the Catalyst. By embodying each one of these Realizations, you reclaim a corresponding Birthright, the reward for doing the brave work featured in each step of this path.

This book will guide you to identify the 8 Realizations that lead you to personal liberation from painful family lineages. These Realizations were distilled from thousands of real-life private sessions and dozens of workshop experiences. Each Realization comes with personal exercises and an actual success story, to help you walk your own path of self-discovery. By the end of this book, you will have a clearer sense of your identity, which will no longer be defined by the story of your family. With this freedom comes the space to discover your passions, your purpose, and an unbreakable bond with your Inner Voice of Truth.

Unfinished Family Stories

Being born into unfinished family stories means that we do not have a choice about whether or not we take them on. As children, we are completely dependent upon our families. We are like sponges who soak in the love, the grit, and all the expectations, both cultural and other, that our families feed us. Being a part of a family is integral to our sense of belonging and formation of our identities, but it also obliges us to follow the family flow and to take on certain unresolved stories that our elders may pass onto us.

The more aware we become of these inherited family stories, the more choice we have in how we carry them. Some, who possess a high level of self-awareness, may choose whether or not to participate in the family story at all. Most, however, will be living out the stories given to them by elders. The work is to identify which stories truly belong to *us* and which stories are we carrying on behalf of *someone else.* By leaving the stories that don't fit who we are, and by claiming the power to write our own life stories, we will be able live the most empowered and fulfilling life possible.

Before we can liberate ourselves from the residual impact of family history, we must first acknowledge that we, as individuals, still carry "something" on behalf of our elders. But how do we recognize when we are carrying an unfinished family story?

The Script

Unfinished stories come with a script. And the script will feature repetitive cycles that stand out to us. These are the spoken phrases and the behaviors that happen over and over again within the family. Some scripts are simple routines, like family traditions during holidays, and aren't harmful at all. Think of the annual Thanksgiving holiday celebrated in the United States and Canada, where a turkey is traditionally served with predictable side dishes. Before the meal, someone will say some words about gratitude. If you recorded this annual speech, then listened to each year in a sequence, you will probably hear similar phrases and themes being repeated. They may even have been said by the same person each year. These repetitive elements are an example of a script. Here is an example of phrases that would likely be repeated every year.

> *Today, I am grateful for this family, for my friends,*
> *and for all the people in my life that I love. I'm*
> *grateful for this food that we are about to eat. I'm*
> *thankful for this life that I have been given.*

This common example poses no harm to the family members and can be enjoyed as a family tradition. There is nothing wrong with this script. However, there are elements of the scripted family story that are harder to identify and can be harmful to one or more individuals in a family.

Scenario

Every year at Thanksgiving, your uncle and aunt, Henry and Sylvia join your family for lunch. And every year he drinks too much alcohol. He starts off the holiday with cracking jokes and being the life and soul of the party. Then during dinner, after the words of gratitude have already been shared, he reaches that tipping point as he finishes his fourth drink. Without fail, he starts to speak his mind - without any filters. He will start a politically-charged conversation that stirs up racial issues, and will launch into a judgmental rant that feels cathartic to him... but socially awkward for everyone else at the table.

Each year, your father tells him to stop. He never does. With the beautifully cooked meal ruined, your mother, who spent all day preparing it, finds an excuse to go into the kitchen to cry. Your Aunt Sylvia always goes to the kitchen to "help" your mother. Your aunt consoles your mother because she knows how Henry behaves when he's drunk. The rest of table eats dessert under a blanket of polite silence while trying not to notice your mother's tear-smeared mascara.

When the party is over, your father always says not to invite Henry next year because he always ruins Thanksgiving. Your mother agrees with him, but always changes her mind the day before the holiday because Henry has nowhere else to go. "After all, he's family," she concludes. Your dad stays out of it. When Uncle Henry comes for Thanksgiving the next year, you roll your eyes and mutter to your cousin, "This is why I don't invite my friends over for Thanksgiving."

If you recorded Uncle Henry's antics every year, then watched them back to back, you would almost be able to predict how many drinks he will have before he starts spewing the same toxic conversation that he initiates year after year. Nothing changes. Uncle Henry ruining Thanksgiving becomes a scripted part of your family's tradition, and so too does everybody's predictable response to his behavior... including you rolling your eyes. Obviously, this repetitive script is emotionally stirring and harmful to many within the family.

When you reflect on your own family's behavior and dynamics, you may recall similar circumstances where people repeat the same conversations, have the same fights, and react in predictable ways. During these moments, people are not consciously aware of what they are doing, rather they are living unconsciously according to a script. They are so entrenched in their characters, with such a limited awareness of how they impact others, that they repeat the same behavior over and over again without actually outgrowing the script. Unless they change how they are behaving, they will blindly follow the script and continue to hurt the people around them who are also somehow tied to the script.

While not every script is harmful, many family scripts inflict emotional and sometimes even physical damage to specific family members. Without first *recognizing* the abusive scripts, an intervention to stop the abuse is not possible. This can be difficult, because repetitive abuse becomes familiar (from the word family), and thus people get used to the abuse, even expecting it to happen. Becoming numb to the abuse leads to enduring it. This is an act of *surrendering to the script* and letting the unresolved family story take over your life during the moments that the drama unfolds. In these moments, your life is not your own. You become a vessel for the story to play itself out through you and through the other members of the family who are participating in the script. When this takeover happens, you are not in your power, and you must endure the harm that comes with your role in the family play.

Scripts like Uncle Henry ruining Thanksgiving every year is an obvious form of an unresolved familiar story that people can see coming. Because Henry has a reputation for his agonizing rants, the other participants at Thanksgiving dinner can mentally prepare themselves for that tipping point after the fourth drink, and the abrasive verbal onslaught that follows. But other forms of scripts are more insidious and known only to the abuser and the victim. Painful scripts like child abuse from a babysitter is a deeper form of script, in that no responsible adults are aware of the abuse. Whereas Uncle Henry's rants are overt, free for anyone to hear and witness, covert scripts are carried in painful silence. This hidden pain becomes an unhealthy part of the script.

The more we relive these painful cycles of scripted events and repeat the same fights and struggles over and over again, the more fatigued we will feel from re-enacting these scripted stories. This Fatigue is your friend. When you start saying to yourself, "I'm so tired of this," or "here we go again (sigh)," you are experiencing the early indications that you're stuck in the repetitive script of a family story. It means that on some deeper level, you no longer want to be subservient to the family script and wish to live a freer form of life.

> This is the start of your personal awakening,
> an inner will to break free from the scripts
> you've been burdened with and the first step
> towards living an unbridled way of life.

27

The problem of living by the repetitive scripts of your inherited family stories is that the script often does not include a resolution – what you've inherited from your ancestors is unresolved. Without a finale, without a clear ending, the unfinished family stories find new generations of participants to recruit, ensnaring them into unsavory scripts, and repeating the same painful play over and over again. This dynamic happens until the participant either breaks free from the script entirely by choosing to live their own life, or they make different choices to their predecessors and find a way to end the story.

A common example of finishing an inherited story can be seen in families who have several generations of divorces. For instance, the child of an alcoholic who had a parent with no sense of accountability will choose a partner who doesn't have a rampant addiction and always takes ownership for their actions. By choosing a partner who differs from the pattern, the script is changed enough to sustain a long-term partnership and the cycle of separation is broken.

An example of someone leaving a script would be your mother kicking Uncle Henry out of the house on Thanksgiving and not inviting him back the next year. By setting the boundary that he can't come to the family event until he gets help and makes a change, she has left the scripted fiasco of a ruined Thanksgiving dinner. Henry will continue to carry the script, alone, until he hits rock bottom and decides to make a change in his life.

Many of the family stories that we inherit have remained unresolved over the years, and hence they get repeated. It is only when a family member, a role-player in the script itself, reaches a sufficient state of awareness that a conclusion can be written to the conflict. In other words, you stop living by the script and you start writing *your own* script. To do so, you need to build enough awareness of the repeating lines of the script. Ask yourself, "Am I the first member of my family to say these lines of the script?" When you find yourself sounding like your parents or grandparents, and become aware of the familiar echoes spoken before, you'll be able to identify that these thoughts are not your own; rather, they are part of a script that was drilled into you.

That moment where you watch the scripts of your family repeat, as if you are an audience member in a theater, you are separating from the script in an empowering way. But becoming consciously aware of the script is merely the beginning of an important healing process that can lead to unburdening the family stories that don't fit the person you are becoming. In many meditative practices, you watch your thoughts as a way of separating your attachment to them. The thoughts float through your mind and you witness them passing through without fixating on any one thought. Similarly, in generational healing, you begin your practice by watching the repetition of unhealthy family scripts, but without getting sucked into them. By being detached, you begin to reclaim your inner space that the family story has taken up inside of your mind and heart.

This direct practice creates the inner space needed to explore how the script is stuck to you on a deeper, more emotional level. This meditative practice separates your brain from the script so that your conscious mind can look inwards at your body, your heart, your guts, and your hips. Doing so enables you to find those deeper emotional blocks that keep you ensnared into the script.

Once we become aware of the script at work in our minds, how do we release it from the body completely? To release the emotional glue that keeps these scripts attached to our thinking minds, we must feel our pain. Feeling and releasing pain loosens the emotional glue that keeps us attached to the scripted family story.

We All Carry Family Pain

We all carry the unexpressed pain of our ancestors. Most of us conduct our lives blissfully unaware of how the lives of people who are no longer physically present in our lives still play a role in steering our fate. Even for those who do not believe in spiritual contact with deceased loved ones, the legacies of our ancestors shape who we are expected to be by our families. While our intellectual awareness may forget the stories of our family trees, our places in our families and communities were forged before we arrived in our mothers' wombs. Have you been named after an ancestor who shoes you may be expected to fill? These expectations may not ever have been verbalized to you, but you may have felt the weight of these expectations subconsciously. If only these family expectations were spelled out in a handbook, we would at the very least have clear instructions on how to live these which have been partially predetermined for us.

Of course, we are not referring to completely reliving the lives of our ancestors who grew up in different times. We are only reliving the stories that never resolved the hidden pains that they endured. The cries they never shared, the regrets they never fully faced, and the struggles that never lead to satisfying conclusions don't just disappear when their bodies return to the earth. The stories about what they never got to receive or experience in life are inherited by the next generations.

Ask any child of an immigrant what their parents had to sacrifice for their sakes, and they can quickly list the hardships their parents had endured to provide their families with better opportunities. They can share in detail the laments of their parents having to leave the comforts of their homelands, all the wonderful traditional foods they miss, and all the sadness they endure from moving to a place where they struggle to fit in. Then ask that child how they feel about this situation. More often than not, they'll share the gratitude but also the guilt they feel for what their parents had to give up for them. That child of an immigrant will share the conflicting feelings of shame and pride they feel about being 'different' to others in the society they've been born into. Some may also feel a deep sense of responsibility for integrating their parents into this new society by translating for them and educating them on the nuances of the social norms. This, in turn, also leads to their own social awkwardness as they grapple with carving out their own social identities growing up. They may also feel pressurized into earning notable achievements because of all the sacrifices made for the sake of their education and well-being. These pressures often lead to feelings of deep resentment as they are trapped by so many expectations that were forged by the sacrifices their parents made for them. They felt pressure to make their parents proud. The pain of the immigrant parents is not just their own. It is shared by their children and grandchildren and permeates everyday life.

But what if your ancestors have been in the same place for many generations and you inherited wealth? Surely you are off the hook when it comes to inheriting family pain? Ask anyone who has inherited a family business how they feel about it. No matter how well they are provided for by their family, they will have plenty of emotions about what they are expected to be and how their life path has been tied into what their grandparents and great-grandparents created for them. Deep inside, they nurture a longing to be free to live a life of their own choosing. This yearning is often coupled with a deep rage about feeling trapped, about being obligated to live a life that was crafted for them before they were even born. Their lives were partially mapped out for them before they were even witnessed for who they are as unique individuals.

Examples of how our lives have been at least partially pre-planned are so numerous, that we have just accepted this as a "normal" part of life. Pre-arranged marriages still happen. Being the next soldier in a military family with a long line of service still occurs. Inheriting land from your family who happen to be multigenerational farmers comes with expectations of its continued existence. If you are the first child to go college in your family, you better make it good by becoming a doctor or a lawyer. Being born a woman comes with the expectations of settling down and starting a family, whereas male children are often encouraged to 'sow their wild oats' before finding a suitable wife. Even an orphan was not the first orphan in their lineage. If you look far enough back in the family tree, you may be surprised just how similar the life you are living is to an ancestor who walked the earth before you.

Many people agree to live the scripted life that their families have created for them. By accepting the family script, you receive a role in the family, a hometown, and a predictable daily life. However, along with this agreement, you are obliged to take on the pain of your family connected to the script. For instance, there may be benefits to being the pastor's child in your community, but when he secretly gets drunk, you will receive the pain of his emotional and physical abuse when he lashes out. Or to gain your parents approval, you have to choose a mate who fits the checklist of what your parents recognize as a good partner. You may be more attracted to someone that they don't approve of, so you're forced into the dilemma of having to choose a mate who is better for you, or who fits their expectations for you. Both instances will leave you with emotional anguish: either your parents' unhappy reaction, or your feelings of regret for not running away with the love of your life. Just because we behave according to the script, doesn't mean we will be free of the inherited pain.

The pain follows the script.

Our Bodies Hold the Pain

We inherit our bodies from our ancestors. From them, we also inherit the familiar scripts. It's our physical bodies that hold the emotional anguish of our unfinished family stories. The very tensions that arise from the conflict between living the life our family needs us to live, versus living the free life that we yearn to experience, are held in our chests, our stomachs, our necks, and our heads. The mental stress becomes physical tension. That tension, when held long enough becomes physical pain that originates from this emotional anguish.

The body is honest. It can't lie. Our bodies remember everything that we have been through and everything that we have inherited from our upbringing. The body holds the unresolved stories, like frozen memories. We are not consciously aware of the pain from these memories because we are conditioned to avoid pain. Rather than face it, we numb it, and we remain distracted from feeling our bodies. This historic hurt is avoided because we believe that if we open up and feel it, it will break through and interrupt the surface of our daily lives.

Ironically, the complete opposite is true. By harboring this inheritance inside our bodies and distracting ourselves from feeling it, the hurt builds up inside. When a crisis hits, all that stored up pain spills to the surface and overwhelms us. Addressing the stored up hurt in advance gives us the option to gradually unpack the painful memories at a more manageable pace. But without awareness of the hurt that we are carrying inside, we cannot do it.

If you have done extensive yoga or meditative practices, you already recognize that focusing attention on the present moment brings you in touch with what you are feeling, and not just what your mind is thinking. If you have any doubt that you are carrying residual pain, go on a week--long silent retreat. By fasting from technology and turning off your cell phone, you will be able to create the space you need to catch up with yourself. Without the distractions and numbing agents, the pain tucked away inside will begin to surface. You may perceive it as physical hurt, or you may start crying without knowing why. Memories could surface that you might have buried in the recesses of your mind. This natural process happens when we stop being "busy" and just "be" with ourselves. This practice will allow you to see which physical pains are connected to which emotional memories. Only through first-hand experience can you fully recognize the connection between unexpressed emotions from unresolved memories and the physical sensations, such as tension and pain, that are held in the body.

Unconventional Eyes

One of the benefits of being an odd child who spent a lot of time in solitude was that I developed my own way of seeing the world. We all do this to some extent; however, my connection to my intuitive senses was never broken as I matured into adulthood. This is rare. Most people disown their intuition to conform to an intellectually based society, and then learn to listen to that voice of intuition again after a series of hard life circumstances. This recovery of these perceptive abilities can be a long, hard road back to what was freely available to us in our youth. Since I didn't lose contact with my intuitive abilities, my intellectual mind developed around my intuitive core, rather than in opposition to it.

This inner harmony was not easy to establish. However, having a rational mind that works cooperatively to validate my intuitive impressions gave me unconventional eyes. My unique lens helps me to see pieces of information that most people ignore or throw away. If I could give you a pair of goggles to show you how I see the world, you'd see wind streams pushing clouds of information between people. These clouds would light up and change colors based on the moods of the people talking to each other.

If two people were talking and I witnessed their hips light up, turning amber or a smoldering cherry color, I knew that they were sexually attracted to each other. When someone's body turned a cold blue or became very dim, I knew that they were scared and withdrawing. People having an intellectually stimulating conversation would have bright white and yellow shimmers around their heads. A singer who shared a passionate ballad would have a waterfall of purples, greens, pinks, and gold running down their bodies representing a flood of inspiration. When two people expressed love for each other, their hearts beamed forth green, or pink, or sometimes orange towards each other, and the rest of their bodies would light up from the exchange. These colorful clouds don't lie. They make the unseen become visible.

When I viewed my clients with my unconventional eyes, I gathered additional information that would help me uncover what exactly my clients were holding onto inside their bodies. This is important because so many factors in modern societies lead us away from the memories that we hold in our bodies. Social pressures tell us to ignore the painful exchanges in these memories held inside our bodies. Having keen sight helped me to stay focused on what was really being held inside as each client struggled with their denial of what happened to them. The art of using this keen intuitive perception was to feel out what the client was ready to face at the right time. Staying focused on the cloud of hurt that my clients were holding was essential to helping them uncover the unfinished family stories that were causing them anguish.

Clouds of Hurt

One of the ways in which I honed my intuitive abilities to see the energy exchanges between people was to watch my parents fight. They taught me how much words can hurt. When they spat judgments at each other, the harm of the words wasn't just the demeaning ideas that went from one brain to another. It is also a transfer of energy that is sent with those words, and that stays with one long after the fight is over. It creates a lingering feeling which is held inside the body and that doesn't seem to go away, no matter how many years have passed, until the memory of the unresolved conflict is addressed.

I remember showing my mother how to see the clouds of feelings around someone's body one night. She wanted to see what I saw. I guided her by helping her shift into a semi-meditative state to open up her perceptive abilities. It was only the two of us in the room and the closed door made my father, who was in the next room, feel excluded and neglected. The private lesson wasn't meant to be a hurtful exclusion. Closing the door simply made it easier to focus without hearing the noise of the TV coming from the next room. But to my father, this was an offense. He spat angry guilt trips through the wall, scolding my mother for leaving him alone in his room. His words penetrated the wooden door and I could see a dark cloud of smooth tentacles creep into the room. They were trying to grab my mother by her shoulders and neck. Not quite solid in appearance, the inky tendrils, airy and gaseous, were faded black with tinges of sickly green. Dad had found a way to include himself in our little experiment. His intrusion was unplanned, of course, like an envious octopus that was creeping up on its prey.

But the tentacles were only the beginning of his manipulation. My mother's gut looked like a stream of taffy was being pulled out of her torso. With heavy need, my father was pulling at the emotional bond between their stomachs. It made my mother slouch forward, like the wind had been knocked out of her. The impact of the emotional battle had made her physical body contort.

But my mother wasn't a meek, emotionally battered wife who would just endure this normally invisible assault. I saw a bright flash of red come up from her chest. She instinctively lifted her arm up to protect herself from the cloud of dark tendrils coming her way. She couldn't see them, but she could feel their invasive presence, much in the same way you can sense when someone is staring at you from behind. The red flash in her heart expanded briefly before contracting again, as if she was loading up a harpoon gun. The angry energy in her heart then shot through her hand as she chopped at the floating tendrils in the air. The chop sent a red dart into the air, through the closed door, and struck my father in the next room. As she chopped the air, she screamed "enough!" at my father.

Those black, smothering clouds of tendrils that had been pulling on my mother, jolted back as the red dart hit its mark. The taffy at her stomach pulled off as well, leaving my mother's body clear of the covert abuse. Her defense had worked. My father recoiled and remained silent throughout the rest of the exercise.

These clouds of pain communicate so much about what is actually happening behind the scenes in our conflicts. The clouds take many shapes, some very defined, like the dart my mother threw. Others are more gooey and gaseous, like the possessive, octopus-like tendrils of my father. My father, because of the story of his own abandonment, wanted to ensure that he was given all the attention from my mother that he felt was lacking in his childhood. My mother wanted to have control of her own energy, seeking the free will to exchange with others as she needed to do in order to grow. I could see this dynamic very clearly because I could see the clouds of hurt.

This example of the pain clouds between my parents is not unique to my family. Every family has their subtle ways of sharing pain. For some who are abandoned and have little interaction with their family, you can see hard shields, like giant eggshells that encapsulate them and keep them from having any meaningful exchange with other family members. It leads to a starvation, and over time, I can see this neglect in the form of a painful, dark void in the chest and torso. It looks like stark nothingness that always comes with a low self-esteem. Children raised in such a walled off family can often inflict pain on themselves, either physically to their bodies or verbally in their minds, just to be able to feel something. They often develop feelings of worthlessness, because they are not getting attention from their families. All too often, these children grew up with similar abandonment to their parents, and their parents display that same vacant darkness in their chests. Even in these more subtle scenarios, there is still a transfer of pain in the form of neglect.

Pain clouds are as real as our ability to feel their impact. Their movement between each generation of the family helps us to recognize when we have taken on pain that is not uniquely our own. If we were all trained to see these invisible transfers of pain, we would be faced with witnessing them daily: at the office during passive aggressive arguments, when the children scream with glee in playgrounds, husbands and wives bickering in hushed tones behind closed bedroom doors, irate drivers stuck in traffic jams and young people making their voices heard in civil protests. If everyone was able to see these interactions in that level of detail, the realization of just how much we actually affect each other would be shocking. But even if you can't see these clouds, you can increase your awareness to be able to feel them when they transfer from one person to another.

Our Emotional Body

The ability to see clouds of hurt is not just phenomenon that is unique to specially trained Intuitive practitioners. Science has begun to validate that our bodies are able to detect and react to what we are feeling emotionally.

An innovative study titled "Bodily Maps of Emotions" (2013), which was published in the Proceedings of the National Academy of Sciences (PNAS), gives us a glimpse into how our bodies hold and express emotions. In this study, the researchers asked 701 people from either Western Europe or Eastern Asia to view emotionally evocative photos, movies, and words. Then they asked them to draw before and after snapshots of how their bodies felt using a unique multicolored topographical method. Basically, the study subjects were asked to use different colors drawn on different areas of their bodies to make body maps that describe what they were feeling emotionally while viewing the photos, movies and words. The researchers then sorted the body maps and found that regardless of cultural background, the body consistently communicated an emotional response for each kind of emotion such as fear, anger, happiness... etc. The resulting body maps showed what each emotional response looked like in the body.

To see a full color rendition of the Bodily Maps showing different emotional states, please visit https://gkhunter.com/research/.

The "clouds of hurt" phenomenon that I had been witnessing in my client sessions for years very closely resembled the body maps from this study. Somatic based therapies and Energy Healing are now being validated by science. This study indicates that our physical body has specific responses to our emotional states. For instance, the emotional state described as Love had the brightest colors in the heart area that communicated a sensation of warmth throughout most of the body. Depression was in stark contrast to Love, having no coloring or sensation in the chest area, and a cool sensation throughout the rest of the body. Because participants from distinct cultures had consistent body responses, it suggests that our physical bodies have some sort of programming that responds to our emotional state, and that is not inherited from our culture. This evidence suggests that the body's intelligence is universal amongst humans.

This study makes the emotions that we carry inside visible. This visual evidence of a mind-body connection can impact how we approach the healing process because the presence of feelings in a particular spot, like for instance the heart area, can indicate the location of an emotional wound. This means that our body has a physical site where a wound is located, and these images might be the first snapshots as to what emotional wounds look like in a scientific study.

A classic example of how our bodies carry emotional pain in a localized spot is when we experience heartbreak. There are many ways for us to experience heartbreak, for instance when someone lies to us and we feel betrayed. Even though the person hasn't physically harmed you, it is possible for you to feel physical tension, heat, and pressure in your body that can even cause physical pain. Where do we often feel heartbreak? We feel that wound in our hearts as anxiety, "butterflies" in our chest, sharp twinges of pain, and we might even have physical palpitations and feel sick to our stomachs as we learn about the details of the betrayal. This physical response is so common among people that we even created the word "heartbreak" to describe the feeling of our chests being physically being ripped open, when we are let down, betrayed or losing someone. Even though our ribcage has not been physically torn, the emotional body inside of us is being ripped open by the hurtful act, creating a wound that can only be detected when we shift into a more concentrated state and focus on the painful area of our body.

You need not be a trained Healer or therapist to detect when your heart is breaking. You can feel it. If you take the time to dialogue with your body, like the Body Dialogue exercise (which will be explained later), you may be surprised by how much information, visual or otherwise, you can receive from the wound. All that is required is the willingness to tend to the wound and the endurance to feel every feeling that comes out of the wound when you pay attention to it.

Now, let's take a look at a client session that I did early on when developing the work to learn more about how we carry pain on behalf of our lineage.

41

The Scream of Geraldine: *Second Generation Holocaust Survivor*

Geraldine arrived in her Sunday comfy clothes. She still had bed head, a sign of her busy life that prioritized getting things done over her weekend appearance. Sunday was when hardworking Jewish mothers caught their breath after a long week that often ended with hosting Friday night Shabbat dinner.

I made a heart connection with Geraldine, a special compassionate bond that creates a safe bubble around the client. As this connection grows stronger, it feels like a pipeline that is opening up between my chest and theirs. As that pipe opens up, I can empathically feel what the client is going through. Before I see the clouds of hurt, I feel them first. In this moment, it's as if I have stepped inside of my client's body and feel what they are feeling inside my own body. Before connecting with Geraldine, I felt calm and curious about her story. Once the connection had been forged, my feelings switched from mine to hers. My head felt damp and foggy, like I had to work very hard to focus on one thought at a time. My chest felt cold and my gut felt hot, almost irritated. It felt a bit harder to breathe, as If I was carrying a dark, burlap cloak over my head. My neck began to hurt, as if I was carrying a heavy backpack. These sensations made me wonder, "what has Geraldine been through?"

As the connection deepened, I switched senses from feeling what Geraldine was going through, to visualizing her clouds of hurt. This shift feels like I'm popping through a gelatin mold, a slight push through the thick air in front of me, until I pop through to the other side of the gelatin mold. Once the shift was complete, I stared at the outline of Geraldine's body and a movie began playing in my head. Flickers of red crawled up her torso and stopped at her neck. As I watched the red clouds move up her body, I felt angry. It was Geraldine's red-hot anger that was stifled inside of her belly. This was a clue.

"You look so angry," I finally admitted to Geraldine after visually reading her body.

"I look angry?" Geraldine responded with worry and surprise. She didn't deny my statement. After a brief pause, she asked, "How can you see that?"

I explained to her how my intuitive senses worked and shared with her my intention to help her release whatever she was ready to release today. Then I asked her to share the story that was connected to this feeling of anger.

Geraldine shared how both of her parents had survived the Jewish concentration camp, Auschwitz, during World War II. Her parents grew up in the same town of Warsaw, the sweet little village that eventually became the Jewish Ghettos in Poland during the war. Jews were confined there, made to wear the Star of David, and their lives became a trial of daily survival. As teens, both her parents were transported with family members from the Warsaw ghettos to Auschwitz after it was converted from a work camp into a killing camp.

The more we spoke about her family's past, the more I could feel that heat radiating from her body. The sheer empathy of the moment made me break into a light sweat. Deep in the pit of her gut, near her belly button, I saw a dark coal with red cracks. The rage about what happened to her parents had been living inside of her. Even though she had not personally survived the camps and had grown up safely in America, Geraldine still carried a sense of outrage about what had happened to her parents. Growing up, she had heard her father's stories about how the Nazis had treated them. As he vented his anger to his daughter, she was ingesting it, keeping it inside of her intestines. As painful as this was for her, she did it to comfort her father, to be a good daughter to someone who had endured atrocity. But there weren't many opportunities in her American life to let go of all the anger that she had ingested. After all, it was her parents who had endured the concentration camps directly, not her. But that didn't mean that her family history didn't deeply impact her daily life. She lived with the rage every day.

I asked Geraldine to feel that dark rock in the pit of her stomach.

"It feels tight, like it's hard to breathe," she responded. I could see the red in her stomach growing brighter, a sign that an emotional release was about to happen. With her permission, I moved to sit next to her and pressed my fingers into her gut with a gradually increasing pressure.

"It hurts," she said.

"Just breathe," I said. The heat I saw earlier in her gut was breaching. My fingertips got red hot as I held them firmly into her abdomen. The pit of her gut raged hotter, revealing a deep tenderness in her belly.

"I hate this feeling. I'm tired of this!" she blurted.

"Tired of what?" I challenged her, continuing to press the pressure point in her stomach.

"I'm tired of living like this! I'm tired of holding this pain...tired of hearing about Auschwitz from my parents and my community. I'm so sick of people looking at me like the child of Holocaust survivors. I am so much more than that! I'm angry that I have to live with this," she said.

"Who are you angry at?"

"My father! Everything is always about him. Everything is about his anger, about how he hates the Nazis, about how he is mad at God for letting this happen to our family. I can't breathe around him. Everything is about his burning need. I feel like his personal nurse. I just want to be my own person," she said. "I can't breathe around him!"

Searing, salty drops fell from Geraldine's eyes and rolled down to her chin. Her parents were marked by numbered tattoos, so their scars were visible. Her mark of wounding was invisible - shielded as she was by her American upbringing, quality education and career as a successful cantor (a Jewish religious singer). By all accounts, she *should* be happy. Most people would be surprised by her anger.

My hand made sweeping movements across her belly, like I was playing a cello, tugging away at the painful dark crust around the molten red core that I saw in her belly. After I finished cleaning it out of her, the fire in her belly transformed into a white-hot ball with red edges. White flare pushed through her heart and left her breath, as if white gas was escaping from her mouth. This was the emotional release.

"I feel so guilty for feeling this way," Geraldine said. "How do you tell your father that you hate him? He survived Auschwitz! No pain in my life can compare to that. I mean, I don't really hate him. I hate what he had to carry, what he still carries today. I hate those heavy feelings that I have to carry with him. And he doesn't see it. Our relationship is all about him. Our whole lives were built around his rage. I know he loves me, but I feel like I have to take in all his rage just to get some of the warmth from his heart. It's not fair! It's not fair to me."

More tears fell. Geraldine heaved loudly, as if giving birth to the dark feelings that were exiting her body. The white heat pushed out dark pieces of shrapnel through her skin. The dark pieces symbolized the edges of her grief, the sadness of not being allowed to share what she was feeling with her parents. She wiped her dripping nose and then wailed again in low tones. These low wailings were only the first rumbles of the volcano she held inside.

"I feel like I need to scream. I feel like I am carrying this scream inside of me that's not mine," she said.

"Whose scream is it?"

"I feel like it's the scream that my family didn't get a chance to make. It's my dad's cousins and siblings, the ones he couldn't save. They all died at Auschwitz and no one heard their screams when it happened."

"Let it out Geraldine," I said as I held her tighter. "Release the scream that you are holding on behalf of your family."

"I'm too scared." She tried to shout, but her throat closed up. She coughed, almost dry heaving, as if choking on a chicken bone. The skin of her throat became a rich red, but the sound would not come out. "I'm not ready. I can't do it. I'm too scared and embarrassed to scream in front of you."

With encouragement, she tried again. Out came a gut-wrenching scream that pushed through her tight raspy vocal chords. The flames in her stomach moved up to her chest. The shout continued, then cut again like a police siren that suddenly lost power. Breathing heavily, she attempted another sonic blast, but it was interrupted by another coughing fit. This time, her coughing sounded more like she was having an asthma attack. There was a wheeze, a gritty drag of air against her breastbone. Her face turned a deep crimson. I held her firmly and reassured her that it had to come out.

With another moan that sounded like labor pains, she held her lower belly as if the rage had impregnated her. This deep feeling had only begun to come to the surface. Her body moved like a mime swatting flies. Her face was still flushed. The air around her became a sick green. The scream remained caught in her throat, her vocal chords gripping fearfully, preventing the full release. The bags under her eyes grew more pronounced, as if her skull was trying to swallow her eyeballs. Panting, she leaned forward and put her head on her knees. I rubbed her back firmly like a midwife.

Moments later, her sweaty face emerged from her fit. Some of the heat had released. She felt relief, as if something festering and painful had left her body. There was more, but this release had made the burden which she carried in her guts clear. It had begun the important exodus from her body.

"Great work, Geraldine. This was an important step," I said.

"You don't think I'm a bad person for what I just said about my father, do you?"

"No, I think you're courageous. It's clear to me that you really love your father. You clearly want a healthier relationship with him. But there needs to be more space for your feelings in order to have a more honest exchange."

"I really do love my family. I really do care about my ancestors. When I was beginning to scream, I felt like I was expressing what they never had a chance to say. It's not just my pain. I carry their pain, too."

The Pain Contest

You need not have survived the Holocaust to carry pain on behalf of your family. In fact, one of the key blocks that I encounter with clients is that they compare their pain to what other people have endured. They minimize their own suffering, saying that other people go through worse things than them, so they shouldn't complain. They believe that they shouldn't get attention for what they have been through. I call this the Pain Contest.

The Pain Contest is when everyone shares what they have been through in the past, and the most dramatic story is the person who wins everybody's attention in the conversation. It is based on the scarcity mentality that there is only a little bit of attention to go around, so if you don't have something super urgent or very important to share, you should be silent. In general, the most painful stories are seen as the most urgent matter in these unspoken moments.

The problem with the Pain Contest is that it becomes an excuse not to do the inner work. Sharing the pain of what you have been through and talking about the pain of what your family has been through are necessary parts of the healing process. But years of facilitating this work has taught me that there is room for everyone's pain. It's not a competition, nor is it helpful to harbor your pain inside because you don't think it's big enough to be important.

I once had a Japanese-American workshop participant named Yuki who thought that her pain was not enough to warrant being at the Bloodline Workshop. Both of her parents came to the United States shortly before World War II. Before enrolling, she inquired about what kind of people typically came to our workshops. I shared that the work began with Holocaust survivors and had evolved to be open to people of all backgrounds. Though the workshops were multicultural in nature, there were still a fair amount of second and third-generation Holocaust survivors who typically came to the workshops. The reason Yuki asked me these questions was that she was worried that her family, who had been relocated to the Japanese internment camps during World War II, was not a painful enough issue to warrant her attending one 0f our workshops. She was comparing her family's pain to the families who had survived the Holocaust, and she had deemed her pain not great enough to receive attention at the workshop. She really wanted to come to the workshop, however she saw her pain as less than that of the children of the Holocaust survivors, and she didn't want to take up the time of other people who needed help more than what she thought she did. In her mind, she had lost the Pain Contest, and the right thing to do was to graciously bow out of enrolling in the workshop.

I first expressed to Yuki how astounded I was to hear that she regarded her family's pain of being shamed and held captive in an internment camp as being too insignificant to be shared at a workshop that was designed to heal ancestral pain. I then reassured her that there was room for everybody's pain and grief to be released. It's not odd that she expressed these concerns, because our society is constantly telling us that we haven't got time for the pain. Just kill the pain and move on. This narrative is heard on a daily basis through television commercials, company bereavement policies, and cultural attitudes. Yuki's Japanese background had its own rules around when she was allowed to express pain. The message she received growing up was that it was almost never a good time for someone so young in the family to share their tears. But by dispelling the Pain Contest and assuring her that there was room for her pain, she was able to make it to the workshop and do some very meaningful work.

But what if you were born in a rich nation, with light skin, and you are not aware of the historic details of your family story? If you came from a privileged upbringing or you inherited millions of dollars, does this mean that you are free of these family stories? It is true that minority groups have suffered more historic wounding when you look at the last thousand years of history. It's true that women, people with darker skin, and people of certain religious backgrounds have been brutalized more consistently than people with lighter skin and people of wealth. Denying this painful history as a whole would also deny the residual scars that they still carry from the past. However, money can't buy you out of the healing process and the wounds that you inherit won't go away because you were born a man of lighter skin. Your pain is also real. If you look back in your lineage, you may find a great-grandmother who was shamed for being Irish and who had tried to escape the potato famine. You may find an Italian grandfather who was put in an internment camp during World

49

War II when Mussolini joined the Axis Powers. Even in the absence of a significant historic event, families around the world carry pain. The death of a patriarch or matriarch could have rocked your family so hard that it appeared to break apart. Remember, there is room for everybody's pain and the cooperative healing process works best when everyone gets their turn to share their hurt.

Generational Pain Rank

The Pain Contest plays out in individual families as a seniority-based system that assigns every family member a Generational Pain Rank. Of course, this ranking system is not spoken aloud to everyone directly, and you won't find a ranking roster hanging on the fridge. This largely unspoken dynamic is learned based on how the younger generation is taught the family rules by the words and reactions of the older generations.

While every family and culture will have their own nuances, the broad strokes of the ranking system can be summed up largely in the following way. Older family members receive higher seniority and priority of attention than younger family members, especially if they have control over a large inheritance. Females tend to be given a lower priority than males in most cultures (not all). The elders, who are seen as the matriarchs or patriarchs, will have higher influence than their siblings and cousins within the same generation. Often the matriarch or patriarch is the eldest child, although if they don't want the job, it is possible for a younger sibling to fulfill the role, but it often happens without title so their rank is not as high as it could be. People can use their illnesses, newly-found wealth and fame, job titles and achievements, or even simply producing a lot of kids for the continuation of the lineage, as ways to move up the priority ladder of the ranking system. But these broad strokes tend to be the starting points.

I call it a Generational Pain Rank because those who are more senior in the family line will have their pain heard before lower ranking members. This is significant because people can use their pain to gain influence over members of the family. For instance, an elder may use the fact that they are hospitalized as an occasion to test the love of younger family members, who may be beneficiaries of their large inheritance. The ones who show up maintain their inheritance status, while those who are too busy to visit their poor sick grandma in the hospital can be put on notice that the will could be rewritten.

The youngest sibling in the family is the last one to the party. Before their arrival a whole power structure and responsibility system had already been constructed. They didn't get a say in how the power structure was arranged and they will often feel that it isn't fair. They endure wearing hand-me-down clothing and often carry less responsibility than the older children who may help raise them. But this reduced responsibility often means less influence over the family. In order to get the attention for their struggles, they will need to amplify their emotional expressions, learning how to use their illnesses, financial struggles, and achievements to push to the front of the line of the siblings who got there before them. Because the youngest child must work to get more attention in this way, they can be often labeled as a "cry baby" or "drama queen", which are forms of shaming that limits how seriously their emotional expressions are taken by the rest of the family.

These supposedly endearing terms are common examples of how the older siblings and more senior generations "pull rank" over the more emotionally expressive baby of the family. Pulling rank means that the more senior members of the family reassert their power over other relationships by convincing the other family members that their painful individual story is more important than the stories held by anybody else.

The darker side of the Generation Pain Rank system becomes a serious problem, however, when it takes on a more sinister form. When physical abuse or sexual assault of a minor takes place within a family unit by a more senior member of the family, the younger member will often feel pressure to keep the abuse secret. Disclosing the secret could result in a full out family war erupting, often with the perpetrator getting the benefit of the doubt purely because of seniority, and victim doubted and shamed for being a "liar." The ranking system tends to protect the senior members as they pass on their pain to the younger generations.

Generational Dumping

We are taught that time heals all wounds. This is not always true. Time may be an important ingredient in the healing process, but without consciously understanding the stories we carry, we are merely containing the past, not transcending it.

That accumulated past can be likened to a septic tank hidden inside our bodies. We attempt to distance ourselves from it by residing in our heads and becoming numb to our inner pain. We would be able to successfully ignore it if our inner load did not seep to the surface and manifest itself as inexplicable bodily pains and masked depression.

Our wounded pasts, if left unaddressed, can pour into our loved ones of the next generation. To break free of the abusive cycles of dumping, we need to empty the septic tank.

Catalysts are the people who are able to help us break free. Their inspiration, their emotional friction, and their willingness to express themselves influence others around them. They activate people into their healing process. Instead of children living their own lives, they begin to take on the responsibilities and expectations that originally belonged to the older generations. Because the older generations tend to hold seniority, the dumping typically happens from the older generations down to the younger generations.

It was at my retreat house, on a small Native American pueblo in New Mexico, where I first saw the bigger picture of how our older generations pass on both their love and pain onto our youth. After returning from a work trip to Los Angeles, I was sitting on my back porch, staring at the unobstructed view of St. Peter's dome, the sacred rounded peak of the Jemez Mountain range. There are a few miles of scrub cedar trees between my porch and the foothills of the range. The morning dew evaporated from the cedar into the hot sun, releasing the glorious scent of cedar into the air and cleansing the troubled minds of whoever could smell it. Beyond the cedar-filled foothills, a range of plateaus that looked like carved teeth jutted out. Behind the plateaus were the smooth peaks of the Jemez Mountains, which sat on top of the horizon against a pale blue sky. At sunset, that triple-layered range would dance with tangerine and salmon hues, before fading to deeper magenta and finally resting in purple tombs for the night.

As the sun rose on my back porch, I sipped my dark roast black coffee. My daily meditation was to stare at the mountain range and attempt to be as still as St. Peter's dome. As I stared at the three levels of green foothills, toothy plateaus, and the peaks at the top, my eyes went soft. Like a daydream, I saw the faces of my clients. These faces landed in generational layers on the horizon, with the grandparent generations appearing at the mountaintops, the parent generations on the plateaus, and the children on the bottom of the foothills. Each generation had its own layer. The older generations poured down a stream to the generations beneath them, as if they held pitchers of water that poured into the cups of the younger generations. That water represented the love, the knowledge, and the very life force that the older generations are meant to pour into the cups of the next generation. Some of these flows were more robust and ample in certain lineages. Other families were bare and thin. Many of these downward flows were muddy, as if the love that was being passed onto the next generation was a cocktail of nurture and anxiety, much like Geraldine's experience of her father.

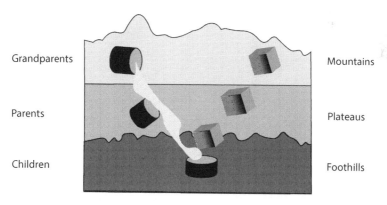

Figure 1. Diagram of Generational Dumping

This vision represented in figure 1 revealed a pattern of Generational Dumping which was emerging among so many of my clients. Often the grandparents survived harder times than the parents and children. But the older generations didn't have the therapeutic resources to release all those emotions they kept inside about the upbringings they endured. They packaged the emotions up inside which made them feel emotionally distant from their children. These emotions merged together into a collective heaviness that became the burdens they carried. When the older generations scolded or vented to the younger generations, they passed on these painful burdens onto their children.

On the left side of diagram 1, you see the flow of nurture and support, like milk flowing down from the older generations to the younger generations. This was the beneficial inheritance that reaffirmed the capability and lovability of the children of the family. On the right side, the burdens are passed down as well from the older generations to the younger generations. These represent a collection of unexpressed pain and unfinished stories that became the burdens of the younger generations if the work was not complete by their predecessors.

The most aware people of the family tree sought help to ensure that they didn't make the same mistakes as their parents had made. But even those who possess this self-awareness can inflict generational pain onto the next generation.

The parent generation in the plateaus endured the pain inflicted on them by the grandparent generation. They too struggled to ask for help and although more therapeutic resources were available to them, many of them felt shame in asking for help with such personal matters. There was a stigma attached to seeking therapy and sharing emotions, so they too eventually inflicted what they were going through onto their children. In the foothills of my vision I witnessed how they poured both love and pain to the next generation.

That cocktail of love and pain mixed together looked like muddy water falling down each layer of the generations. As the children drank the love, they also took in the emotional pain of their parents. This cycle continued as the children on the bottom layer, symbolized by the cedar foothills, moved up to the middle plateaus when their grandparents died and they themselves had children. They eventually became the grandparents at the top of the mountains. The cyclic pain that is passed on through families continued.

When you begin to see the prevalence of Generational Dumping, it may leave you feeling overwhelmed or possibly even hopeless about breaking free from this powerful mechanism. You may feel that it's unfair for the older generations to dump their stuff on the younger members of the family. Or, upon closer introspection, you may just simply feel overwhelmed by the enormity of your own family's unfinished history.

The unconscious act of dumping emotional burdens from elders to children is dependent upon people either denying that the dumping is happening or going through extensive efforts to keep the abuse secret. The abuse cannot continue in the same way as more and more members of the family become aware of the dumping.

Challenging this entrenched system of Generational Dumping is fraught with both family and community punishment and censure. Many cultures around the world still reinforce a system of seniority within families. A younger child complaining aloud in a public setting about a family issue would be regarded as 'disloyal.' Indeed, phrases such as: *Know your place. Your parents have been through so much already. Don't bring shame to your family* - probably have a familiar echo for many. In this way, the younger generation has learned to shut up, and often, to suffer in silence.

In the case of Holocaust survivors, the first generation survivors didn't only have an elevated status of seniority just because of age. They also gained influence because they had endured the most pain. The only ones who seemed to trump the pain of the first generation were those family members who had perished in the concentration camps. The closer someone had come to perishing, the higher their pain rank seemed to be. The greater the amount of pain carried by an individual, the more right they had to be heard on the emotional stage. In many cases, being a survivor gave them the authority to dominate conversations. It gave them the right to absorb all the attention and support for themselves. To be good, supportive and deserving children and grandchildren, the second and third generations of these survivors silently endured the invisible dumping and draining which was a pervasive presence in their daily lives.

This pain-based identity eclipsed the voices of the second and third generations and silenced them from expressing their own truths. The children and grandchildren unconsciously learned to devalue their heartfelt expressions, after being repetitively trumped by their battle-scarred elders. There simply was no room for them to express how they felt, and they were left with feelings of being unimportant and unworthy.

The teenager being bullied at school, the young woman being sexually harassed at her first office job, the new mom feeling overwhelmed by the demands of her young family and husband, the father feeling weighed down with the responsibility of financial support to his elderly parents - these are all very real issues which deserve attention. But against the backdrop of ancestors who had suffered, sacrificed and survived so much, these concerns are buried and hidden and, in our minds, labeled as "petty."

Whether you're a fifth generation descendent of Irish immigrants who had survived the potato famine during the 1800's, a sixth generation descendent of an African slave, or a third generation descendent of a Chinese family that survived the persecution of the Cultural Revolution, you will be able to trace Generational Dumping and draining within your family. It's not your family's fault for having endured these historic hardships. But it is the responsibility of every family to recognize the residual impacts that unhealed wounds can happen on the next generation.

Humanity's Plight: All This Historic Pain and No Place for It to Go

Think not forever of yourselves, O chiefs, nor of your own generation. Think of continuing generations of our families, think of our grandchildren and of those yet unborn.

—The Peacemaker, Founder of the Iroquois Confederacy[2]

Geraldine showed me something much more than the plight faced by many second generation Holocaust Survivors. She was shedding light on the current state of humanity. I needed to see a severe case of historic pain in order to recognize the Generational Dumping that every family endures. Each family holds a piece of humanity's pain, which means every family member has experienced the dumping in some way.

But what does this Generational Dumping look like? Unless physical bruises are left on the body of a physically assaulted family member, it's hard to even envision how pain is passed from the older generations to the younger generations.

In the case of Geraldine, I used my intuitive sight to further delve into how she took on her father's pain. I witnessed her father puke a stream of the fear, disdain, and rage that he felt about the Nazis onto Geraldine. To an outside advisor, it just seemed like a father venting his feelings to his daughter. It may have been an intense experience to listen to, but no overt harm was seen to be done to Geraldine. Nor did her father intentionally try to hurt his daughter. He was just caught up in a rageful, lamentable moment as he remembered what the Nazis did to him and his kin.

---

2   Wallace, P. (1946) *White Roots of Peace*. Santa Fe, NM. Clear Light Publishers

But if you put those intuitive goggles back on, you would see those heavy streams flowing from his mouth into Geraldine's chest and stomach areas. They were black, with sickly olive-colored veins and flashes of bright red, as they oozed from his body and were absorbed into Geraldine's heart and abdomen. She endured it because she believed it was her job to take care of him emotionally. It was her way of sharing the load with him. Geraldine continued to participate in this subtle form of abuse, because she was convinced that her father was not strong enough to handle it on his own. So, she remained a recipient of his angst and did not interrupt his angry monologues.

Amid all that muck that he regurgitated during his disturbed monologues, I could see another stream. It was a delicate sheen of pink that came from his heart and surrounded her. This was love. He clearly loved his daughter, but he seemed to be unaware of the emotional dumping that polluted that love, just like the muddy waters I had seen in the visions from my back porch. Though he did not direct his outbursts or judgments *towards* Geraldine, she still felt obliged to *receive* what he shared. She feared saying "No" to him. Setting a boundary with her father was forbidden because his pain rank, as a Holocaust Survivor, was so high, and it was highly unlikely that she would receive any validation from family or friends of the family who were aware of the wounds he carried. She didn't interrupt him because she didn't want to hurt his feelings, nor did she want him to pull his love away from her.

After studying the dumping that Geraldine endured, I began seeing that same dynamic with so many others who had nothing to do with the Holocaust. It happens to everyone in every family, regardless of ethnicity, religion, or place of origin.

Now that we have traced how our families pass on both their best traditions and these painful, unfinished scripts to the next generation, what do we do about it? We need a vision of liberation from these hurtful cycles. We need a path to walk, some tools to bring with us, and support along the way. How do we break free from the unconscious cycles of wounding that have been in our families for generations?

Modern Day Liberation

You don't need to break free from every script in your life to be free. You need only break free from the most painful and restricting scripts that prevent you from walking your most authentic path. While we are constantly receiving validation for carrying scripts and playing certain roles in our communities, it is our Inner Voice of Truth that holds the final authority when choosing which scripts to keep and which scripts to let go of. Without shifting the scripts of our lives, worldwide slavery would still be an acceptable practice. Without shifting the scripts throughout the world, women would still not have the right to vote. All of us are born into the residual pain of our families.

I grew up in a family that was plagued by alcoholism on both sides. Emotional and physical abuse occurred, but it was kept secret which enabled the abuse to continue. We were expected to keep those secrets out of loyalty to the family. We all endured the abuse, in one form or another, so we accepted that this was just part of belonging to a family.

Those who did not become alcoholics found other ways to distance themselves from the pain of our family's past. Instead of drinking or using drugs, I became reclusive, and spent most of my childhood alone making art, journaling, and running cross country. While I did endure the abuse that had been in my family for generations, I had created enough distance to observe my family through a detached lens. It was as if I was watching a movie that was teaching me the fundamentals of the healing work that I was born to do.

Even through the rough times within the family, there were many redeeming moments of love and care for each other. My first home was the small three-bedroom house of my grandparents, which we shared with ten other people. It was hard to get a moment alone in the only bathroom of the house. Loud fights in a crowded house were just a part of our everyday lives. Everyone knew what it was like to be poor, all of us faced hard times, and everyone had a couch to sleep on during financial struggles. But we suffered together, and everyone always had a roof over their heads and a plate of food on the table.

When I chose to leave home in search of a different way of life, I broke many unspoken rules.

Don't leave your family, especially during hard times. Don't be happy when your loved ones are suffering. Live your life based on obligations. Passion is a luxury, so don't chase it.

But something inside of me told me to leave this way of life. Doing so gave me the space to finally discover my own way of living life.

While I've had numerous profound spiritual experiences and deep moments of inner peace, I don't claim to have obtained the enlightenment taught by the Buddha. What I can claim is that I have walked my own path, outside of the footsteps of my ancestors. My path has been parallel to many of the great luminaries that lived before us, yet even then, my footsteps in the sand have been my own. I believe that each one of us eventually reaches a point where we press our own footprints in the sand, making a mark that is beyond the greatest elders of our family tree and even outside of the known steps of the luminaries that brought us religion, civil rights, and great art.

By having the courage to walk my own path, what I embody now is a free life that is directed by my own Inner Voice of Truth. I make my life decisions based on my authentic passions, knowing that sharing my exuberance with the world will serve it so much more than jumping from one obligation to the next. My service to the world comes from a unified purpose to help future generations to release the historic pain that demands that they live their lives from a place of guilt, shame, and fear rather than from a deep calling and inspiration. I still experience emotional hurt and physical pain; however, this suffering no longer comes from the cyclic anguish of my family in the throes of survival. I no longer self-inflict ridicule or push my body beyond what it is telling me it can do. My discomfort comes from enduring the misguided reactions of the vast majority of people who still live in angst and who spill that angst onto me at the coffee shop, in traffic, and standing in line at the bank. I no longer do the spilling of pain onto others.

This free life has given me a profound sense of fulfillment and daily gratitude. Most importantly, with the awareness that I have worked so hard to glean, I have choice. I chose my relationships based on truth, I follow my inspiration when choosing work projects, and I decide how to make the celebration of my life a part of each day. This recipe ensures that simple joy is a part of my daily life.

Two Paths to Freedom

There are two major ways to grow beyond the familiar scripts of our upbringing: the passive and active approaches. The passive approach is to follow the script and wait for a crisis to hit. In this crisis-based approach, the crisis brings us to our limits and forces us to choose another way because the script is too restrictive to maintain under the extenuating circumstances. In short, we reach our breaking point and we are forced to change in an unplanned way.

The passive approach seeks as many moments of immediate comfort as possible in the short term, but ultimately delays the pain and fears that are inevitable. By being passive, you will be rewarded by receiving validation for playing your role in the family and you will be able to weather the storms until you find your next escape.

Most people you meet follow this passive approach because it's usually the more predictable path, except when an unexpected crisis hits. By delaying the pain and fears, they build up inside until a crisis cracks open their pent-up emotions. The effects of this are almost always overwhelming, and the participants are usually unprepared and caught off-guard by the emotional expressions triggered by the crisis. This passive approach has a much slower pace of emotional maturation, and because of this, tends to stifle the manifestation of your heart's desires. But this approach comes with a momentary illusion of control which most people find temporarily comforting and reassuring as they are able to plod along a predictable, albeit, externally controlled path.

The other path is the active approach, which starts with admitting what you truly want out of your life. Once you have a clear dream to follow, the work becomes making the changes so that you can manifest that life. I call this active approach the Path of the Catalyst. It requires courage as you break away from the unhealthy scripts to make room for your new life. It is more empowering in that you face your emotions directly. As the pain is cleared from your mind and body, you create new space for a better life. You actively comb through each script that you have inherited and carefully assess which scripts are healthy and which ones are holding you back from the life you long to live. You will sacrifice family approval by leaving the painful scripts, but you will gain true autonomy over your life. This means choosing a partner who truly fits you, creating authentic and nourishing friendships based on your true identity, and fulfilling your work in the world in a way that is passionate and purposeful.

Crisis

The majority of humankind is dependent upon crisis in order to grow. Most people are just getting through the day, so they don't devote the time and space to unpack their emotions in order to discover what unresolved stories are left over from their upbringing. The scripts of our lives don't leave a lot of room for crying or taking a break from our daily routines in order to understand what we are going through.

Crisis interrupts the family scripts. It creates a gap in our normal routine and shakes the emotions inside of us up so that we can get at them. We need crisis as an excuse to break from the normal expectations of paying bills, raising kids, and showing up to community events. We need a catastrophe to break the spell, to miss work, and make space for what we are feeling. Often, crisis leads us towards discovering what we really want out of life, including our true purpose.

Another reason that we do not take inventory of our inherited hurts is that we do not have enough support to go through it. If nearly everyone you know has been conditioned to numb or to escape their pain, then where will you receive a truly present listener? Everyone is filled with pain, the septic tanks we have learned to maintain instead of ridding our bodies of them. When crisis strikes, the septic tank overflows in dramatic ways. Someone with a full septic tank doesn't have the internal room to listen to another person's emotions, while in that state. It is far more likely that they will dominate the conversation with their own worries and venting.

A community of people who are going through personal transformation with you is not enough on its own. We also need guidance. The biggest reason why we do not face the ancestral inheritance we have been given is because we're not sure where it will lead us. That scares us. That is why I wrote this book, to assure people that there is a way out of inherited family suffering. It starts with personal liberation, which eventually sends healing ripple effects to other members of the family. By choosing our most authentic life, we become a Catalyst for change in our families and our communities.

Becoming a Catalyst

A waterfall begins from only one drop of water...Look what comes from that...a line from the movie "The Power of One" Bryce Courtenay (novel), Robert Mark Kamen (screenplay) 1992.

Who are you to break away and live your own life? Who gave you permission to do so?

The Catalyst is the empowered individual who courageously answers these questions. "I am me. I'm allowed to be. I give myself permission to live my own life."

These responses could immediately be judged as being selfish. But being who you are is not a crime, nor is embracing your identity an offense to a family who expects you to live by its script. Your existence and the essence of your inner identity came first. The family script came second. Discovering who you are as you mature is your right. When the script interrupts this process, it is the script that is creating the offense. It is the generational abuse that interrupts the respect of who you are deep inside, not the other way around.

Evolving to become the greatest expression of who you are will challenge the generational ranking system. By not following a script, you are breaking a family rule. By expressing who you are in ways that trigger disapproval from your elders, you challenge the seniority of the elders who still protect or inflict that abuse on the younger generations. This unconscious system of power, put in place before you were born, before you could even have a say in the matter, already puts people doing their inner work in a compromising position. This conflict plays out when you are expected to behave in a certain way, but something inside of you wants to go in a different direction.

These conflicts play out in every family, even "good" families. Very often, when I point out a script that might not work for a client or workshop participant, they will defend their families by saying "I come from a good family." This is another script that clients from all different cultural backgrounds and countries of origin repeat almost verbatim. When facing the generational abuse and the seniority system of your family, it's important that you realize that you are not putting your family on trial for its "crimes." If a legitimate crime was committed, like sexual abuse for instance, then those individuals are beholden to the legal system for their crimes. But when it comes to the inner work, it is about evaluating which scripts in your family don't fit the person you are today.

In the past, you may have tolerated abuses that have happened in your family for generations. Today, you may not be able to endure those repeating abuses anymore. You are not a "bad" person for standing up for yourself. So too, your family, in its entirety, is not a "bad" group of people. But if an abuse is being inflicted, there are individuals in your family who are doing something wrong. At some point, as you awaken, you will need to face this disrespectful behavior and decide whether or not you will continue to participate in this script and endure the harm that comes with it.

Many people need a crisis of some form to bring them to their limits before they start actively walking the Path of the Catalyst. I call this the catalyzing event, that extenuating circumstance that finally gives you the motivation to break free from the unwanted abuse or subtle form of disrespect. In this moment, you stop asking your abusers for permission to tell them to stop abusing you. It's that turning point moment where you realize that the validation from people who are colluding with disrespectful behavior is not worth enduring more disrespect. The crisis of a catalyzing event is typically so overwhelming that it breaks your fearful hold on your past illusions so that you can see your family through new eyes. You will recognize that not everyone in your family has integrity and that not every member in the family is treated in the same way.

If you are the first in your family to break free among its living members, then you will be a trailblazer who gets very little validation for your efforts. But this lack of validation doesn't mean that breaking free from the abusive scripts is wrong. What matters is what is right for you. By having self-respect, you will easily see which family members also have respect for you and the choice you are making.

You are not the first Catalyst in the long history of your family tree. You might be fortunate enough to have another member of your family also break free before you, or in some cases, at the same time as you. But even if you don't have someone in your bloodline that understands why you are choosing to walk your own path, there are many people out there from other families who are also doing this brave work.

By becoming a Catalyst, you become a leader without a title among your family and your community. Because the role of the Catalyst is not written into your family's scripts, being a Catalyst won't necessarily give you a position of influence in your family structure, because people who live by the script do not have a role to assign to you. You are off the script, off the map of what they know, so most people won't be sure what to make of you. You may be labeled as being different, odd, or strange because they can't figure out how to include you in their script. This can bring up fear in others because it means that you are unpredictable. When fear comes up with people who live heavily scripted lives, they may even attempt to shame you, meaning they give you a demeaning label such as problem child, crazy, selfish, or freak. These are just further attempts to give you some kind of role that they can understand, a way to put you in a box so they have an excuse to distance themselves from interacting with you in a meaningful way. These labels are so prevalent that every single Catalyst has had to face being misunderstood when they choose to leave the script. The great Catalyst Nina Simone sang it best, "I'm just a soul whose intentions are good, oh Lord, please don't let me be misunderstood."

Becoming who you are isn't being about being selfish, rather it's about claiming your right to self-care. By taking care of yourself, you are stronger, more nourished, and better equipped to help other people. Catalysts are notoriously known for self-neglect, often giving so much of themselves that they feel depleted. They can even get sick because they don't care enough for their own well-being. They don't realize that they're on the selfless end of the spectrum, and being "selfish" actually brings them back to the middle, to that balance point between being completely selfless and the other extreme of being completely narcissistic.

Budding Catalysts feel so alone initially when they start breaking away from the script that they hesitate to ask for help. Asking for help is a necessary part of the healing process. It requires humility to recognize that you can't do it all on your own and the courage to risk rejection when asking for help. It is a very vulnerable act to ask someone to hold you when you are feeling strong emotions. By seeing the courage to be vulnerable as a strength, and not as a weakness, and by choosing open-hearted people as your supporters, you create the most direct path to personal healing.

As emerging Catalysts do their inner work, they often find that they will "rub people the wrong way," even if they haven't spoken a word or made a facial expression. The more they do the work, the less they resonate with the socially acceptable scripts that no longer fit who they are becoming. It creates a dissonance that people living heavily scripted lives can feel, but they can't intellectually recognize, nor can they put it into words. The shift of vibration will feel uncomfortable to them, even threatening to their way of life. Longtime friends may accuse them of changing in a disapproving tone of voice. "You've changed!" they chide, with no further explanation of why change and growth is a negative occurrence. Why else would we be alive if not to change and grow?

It can be disheartening when new Catalysts first learn that disapproving family members and friends have expressed their judgments of their growth behind their backs. But these family members might not be able to fully explain why they are disturbed by your newly-found self-awareness. They only know that they don't like it, that it makes them uncomfortable, so they attempt to give you a new role in their script. They may even campaign to other people that you know to endorse the new role, seeking validation for the subtle abandonment that they feel for you leaving the script without their permission.

When you leave the script, family members may neglect to invite you to certain events, even though no outward conflict has been expressed in an argument, even though you have done nothing wrong. You may

71

even doubt yourself at these moments, turning on yourself as if *you* are the problem rather than seeing that this immature behavior is just the current state of humanity. Catalysts seem to repel the people who are most resistant to doing the work on themselves. While this can be initially hurtful, it is a necessary part of the long-term liberation process.

Trusting this shedding process of the unsupportive people in your life becomes easier when you start feeling relief that these toxic people are no longer all up in your space. You may even ask yourself why you waited so long to release the high maintenance relationships in your life that gave you little in return, especially if they were emotionally or physically abusive relationships. After repelling the people who have judged you harshly for evolving, you will experience all your juicy energy returning to your body. That shiny life force becomes a beacon for attracting the right people into your life. When you create space for new people to arrive, it is only a matter of time before you will make new friends. I see this happen all the time at workshops and retreats. People stay in touch after sharing powerful moments together and find a new support in their life.

Your newly-emerging vibe is beneficial in that it attracts support but it also triggers others in a necessary way. Before unsupportive people pull away from you, there is usually an interaction between both of you that triggers an important frozen memory. This trigger may give you both something to examine in greater depth, which is essentially a gift to you both. Touching on this conflict may lead to them being plagued by nagging memories or issues, which could nudge them towards eventually asking for help themselves. The triggered memory is a gift in disguise to both of you, and each of you will unwrap that gift when you have the courage and support to release your emotions and discover the insight that was borne from the conflict.

The Catalyst is the living representation of the next step for healing in a family. When the Catalysts become versed in speaking their truth, even in awkward family conflicts, they greatly enhance their impact on the families and help carve a path for the future generations to follow. It gives other family members permission to be who they are and to speak their own truth.

As a Catalyst, you are the vessel for change in your family and community. It may not be initially understood or praised. The change you represent will most likely be fought and you may feel like you are being unfairly punished for healing yourself and sincerely trying to share that bounty with other loved ones. It will feel unfair. Double standards will become glaringly obvious. The very abuses that have been handed down through the generations will also become clear in a way that you could not have realized when you were nestled in the bear hug of your family story. This separation is necessary for you to truly witness yourself as distinct from who your family needed you to be.

The Voice of Truth Will Set You Free

Before you break the scripts and challenge the roles that have been given to you by your family, there is a voice inside of you that speaks up. This voice may not be the loudest voice at first; however, it stands out in that it doesn't follow the script of the usual thoughts flowing through your mind. This voice has a different tone, and when it speaks, it makes your whole body ring like a bell. What this voice speaks, it just *feels* right. This sensation tells you that whatever is being said is true.

This is your Inner Voice of Truth. It's the voice that starts the whole liberation process by saying things that don't fit into the script. When a child speaks their Inner Voice of Truth early on, the adults in the family may or may not recognize that they are speaking from a place of truth. They may laugh it off as a crazy thing that kids say. They may even get upset that a less senior member of the family had the audacity to say what many adults have been secretly feeling inside for years. Because the Inner Voice of Truth is not beholden to the script, adults of the family may not validate the voice, or worse, attack the child for speaking it.

Most people in modern Western Societies are taught to divorce themselves from their Inner Voice of Truth and to follow the rationale and opinions of elders, teachers, coaches, and community leaders. We all have an Inner Voice of Truth, but not everyone is supported when they express it. The Civil Rights Movement in America was based on the truth that all human beings are created equal. But people were ridiculed and even killed for speaking this universal truth. Similarly, on a family level, the Inner Voice of Truth may not be immediately received or welcomed.

There is a constant internal tension between the emerging Inner Voice of Truth and the scripted lines that our brains recite over and over again. Which voice do we listen to? What voice makes the decisions in our lives?

Eventually this inner conflict reaches a climax. We hit some kind of crisis point, a catalyzing event that makes us choose which voice to follow. This breaking point could be the death of an important person in your life. Their parting irrevocably interrupts the script of you daily life, creating an opportunity to experience your life in an unscripted way. In a similar way, when we leave a romantic relationship, or the other person breaks up with us, it creates space around the scripts we used to play out with that person. It's an opportunity to hear the Inner Voice of Truth more intimately because the script has been momentarily weakened. If we listen to our truth, we have an opportunity to shake the script completely rather than repeat the same old script... with another person in a new relationship.

Our Inner Voice of Truth longs for us to walk the unknown path. It is the voice of our essence, the thing that defines us as unique humans, who are all on our own journeys. The Inner Voice of Truth guides us through our decisions that lead us to become the person we long to be. We long to transform into a greater expression of ourselves, yet we also fear it.

Envision our lives for a moment as us all being actors on a stage. When we, as actors, are reciting our lines, we are all entrenched in the script. When the director yells "Cut," it can be likened to our Inner Voices of Truth breaking through the script. Once the director yells "Cut" and we are forced to break on set, we have to shed our characters and decide what we are going to do next. Do we get lunch? Do we go back to our trailers? That break is when the Inner Voice of Truth starts speaking to us most clearly, because routine is interrupted, and a special inner space is created. As crisis interrupts our family script just long enough for our Inner Voice of Truth to come to the surface, we have a chance to make a choice which may be different to what is expected by our families. We have an opportunity to write the next chapter of our own lives firsthand rather than hypnotically following the script that was handed to us by our ancestors.

Spiritual growth is rooted in hearing our Inner Voice of Truth. We each have a deep yearning for what it will tell us, for its guidance as we transform into who we wish to become. Who we wish to be is already buried inside of us, but we need those life-changing moments to arouse the deepest voice inside of us. With practice, we learn to trust that voice above all the other voices in our heads and which are all clamoring for our attention. The evolving Catalyst learns to distinguish their Inner Voice of Truth from the choir of mind noise. They make decisions based on that inner guidance rather than re-enacting the same mistakes of their ancestors. These are the people who co-create authentic friendships and honest partnerships. Our reward for bravely following our Inner Voice of Truth is wholeness. We become full expressions of who we are. That wholeness comes with the daily experience of fulfillment, gratitude, and the peace shared with people who we mutually love and respect.

Preparing for Your Journey

After working with a few thousand clients in personal sessions and workshops, I've distilled their collective experiences into 8 Realizations. By working the exercise in each Realization, you can greatly accelerate your liberation from the painful scripts you inherited. By building awareness through each Realization, you reclaim the power of choice. With this new awareness, you can choose whether you will bring a family story to resolution or if you will release that story because it no longer fits who you are today. Rather than living out a script based on obligation, you can choose to bring a family story to resolution by finding a way to complete what your ancestor started. Or, you can choose to inform your family members that you will no longer take responsibility for the story that you've been holding all these years. The more you exercise these choices based on the guidance provided by your Inner Voice of Truth, the more liberated your daily life will become.

The three ingredients you need to walk the Path of the Catalyst in a sustainable way are courage, support, and guidance. You can build your bravery gradually by building confidence with each breakthrough you make. Asking for help takes courage. Each time you ask for help and receive it, your courage will build a little bit more.

Support in the beginning can be difficult to build, especially if you are struggling to hear who your Inner Voice of Truth is guiding you to, to ask for help. If you've already built a support network from previous self-improvement efforts, start there and see who will be able help you through the next steps of your healing process. By working through the Realizations, you will send out an increasingly clear signal to those who have also picked up this book and need support. You can help each other.

While you are learning to hear the guidance from your Inner Voice of Truth, the 8 Realizations will be your companion on the Path of the Catalyst. Think of the structured exercises and the step-by-step wisdom of these Realizations as the handrails on a new trail as you leave the scripts that no longer serve you.

Program Buddy

As you enter into the path of the Catalyst, I strongly recommend that you have a friend who can share in the experience alongside of you. This Program Buddy is important for a couple of reasons. Firstly, having someone to witness you while you go through this transformational process will help you to catch up with all the changes that will happen, both internally and in your external life circumstances. You can be witnesses to each other. It is also very affirming to be walking the path with someone else because it reinforces that you are not alone in this journey.

The Program Buddy need not be present for each and every exercise in the upcoming Realizations. You can do the exercises on your own and then debrief with each other afterwards by phone or in person. You can also make a commitment to do each and every exercise together, putting down a regular meeting time on the calendar as a way of establishing a dedicated time to do your inner work. If you are fortunate enough to have several supportive people in your life already, consider forming a Catalyst Support Group, with a set time to either do the exercises together or share about your personal experiences after you have done them on your own.

For those who feel like they are trapped inside a zombie movie and as if you are the only person who is awakening in your current community, there is hope. Just sitting with each of these Realizations will begin to activate you in ways you could not predict. Once enough of the burdens start shaking loose, many people experience that they gravitate towards other people who are just emerging from their communities. New friends will enter into your life. While you are waiting for these people to arrive, your journal will be your Program Buddy.

It is possible to have several shifts happen without immediately understanding all the changes that have taken place. The writing of your experiences while walking this path will help you integrate these changes. It is also possible to share what you have written later on with new-found friends, a mentor, or a counselor to help you further understand who you are becoming.

Even if you do not have someone to share with when you start this program, know that there are others like you out there who are reading this book at the same time as you. It is only a matter of time before you bump into one of them. Remember, you are not alone.

Let's take a snapshot of your current support network by completing a Community Map. This tool will help you determine who is in your corner and which longtime relationships may be shifting in a way that you can feel, but haven't yet named. Community Maps can be repeated periodically to track the movement of the supporters in your life as you work each Realization.

Exercise: Community Map

Think of yourself standing in a room full of all your supporters, like a big birthday party. Now imagine that the floor has a small circle in the middle of the room where you are standing. Outside of this small circle are three more circles, each circle bigger than the last. Now imagine there is a camera on the ceiling overhead looking down at you directly under it, like a satellite camera. From the ceiling camera viewpoint, it will look like you are standing in the bullseye of a dartboard. The Community Map is an aerial view of all the supporters in the room who are standing around you. The closer that a supporter is standing to you, the more trusted and emotionally available that supporter is to you. The further away the people are, such as the people standing outside the third circle at the edges of the wall, the less available these people are to support you in your inner work.

Each of us has a certain number of close-by, key spots in our support network which are crucial to us feeling stabilized and loved. The number of spots will vary from person to person. A social butterfly may have many close friends that they confide in on a regular basis. Others may be more solitary and only have one best friend, or only handful of close people.

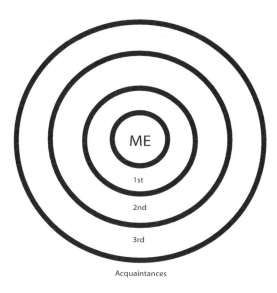

Figure 2. Preview of the Community Map

A Community Map is a snapshot of those spots. It gives us a sense of who we can rely on when sharing intimate information, who consistently supports us, as well as those people we thought would be there but who are not actually available to support us.

Each one of those circles is assigned a tier number. The first tier contains the people we trust the most and are the people that we feel the most unconditional support from. When we need them, they make themselves available. They know our secrets and keep them confidential.

The second tier also contains important supports for us, but we may not tell them everything about what is going on because there may be a judgment or some other relationship limitation that prevents us from opening up fully to them. Nonetheless, these are people we interact with often, or old friends that we're able to pick up where we left off, no matter how much time has passed. They know who we are more so than the average person, but you might not share every private thought or new endeavor with them, or at least not immediately.

The third tier represents the people who we may share birthday parties with or socialize together with at weddings, but the nature of the exchange is not necessarily deep. They know who you are, they care about you, but they don't know your secrets. They may be friends from high school who are fun to go out to dinner with, or maybe they are co-workers who you don't really share much personal information with. They are important because they round out the container of community around us, furthering the number of people who know us and care for our well-being. They are crucial to the mass of people who celebrate who you are and who you are becoming.

It is also possible to have empty spots in the tiers of your support map that have not been filled yet. Some people prefer to have less people who are really close instead of a larger rotation of supporters for comfort reasons. I have met others who have no-one in their first tier because their lives feel simpler without the intrusion of other people's drama – these are usually people who have been wounded in the past and have given up hope that someone could actually meet their needs. Others may have decided that their needs are not important, because they were so devalued growing up.

Every human being does have core emotional needs. This map is meant to be read on the availability of support and access to care. It is not a love contest, where the friends and relatives closest to the center of the map win, and everybody on the edges of the map royally suck. It is about the availability of their support and how much you trust them with your secrets.

This map is for your eyes only. After completing it, I don't recommend sending an email to the people who appeared on your Community Map to give them an update on where on the map they landed.

Dear Ashely,

I regret to inform you that you are no longer in the first tier of my support network. You never call anymore, and it makes me feel like you are more of a floater between the second and third tier of my Community Map. Perhaps we can re-establish you in the first tier at my next birthday party, but we'll see about that. No promises.

The process of filling the spots of our support map enhances our transition from survival more to a state of truly thriving. The more we are surrounded by the right people, the more celebration, validation, empathy, and compassion we feel in our own lives. In short, the more we are known, the less we feel alone. These are our sacred mirrors who clearly reflect back to us the Essence of our being.

Instructions

- Starting from the center, recognize the center point labeled "Me" as your primary relationship with yourself, such as when you meditate.
- Now turn your attention to the first tier just outside of the center "Me" point.
- Ask yourself, who are the people who I can tell anything to without censoring what I say? Who are the people I trust the most?
- As names arise, instinctively write their names inside the first tier. It is ok to put their names across the border of the first and second tier if you feel like someone is almost there in the first tier. Trust where your subconscious mind tells your hand to go.

- Now turn your attention to the second tier. Ask yourself, who are the people who will always support me, but don't know everything about me? These people may know some of your secrets, but you don't share everything with them. These are very important people in your life, though you may partially censor what you tell them.
- Now turn your attention to the third tier. Ask yourself, who are the people in my life whose birthday party I would definitely attend, yet I don't necessarily need to see them every week to feel supported? These could be co-workers, friends made through your shared interests like art classes or hiking groups, old classmates, or family members. Trust the names that bubble up.
- The rest of the people who fall outside of the main circles are acquaintances, such as neighbors or friends of friends who would help you if they saw you on the side of the road with a flat tire. They may also be new friends who you've just met, but are still building trust with, so they may later move closer into to the center of your support map. Take a moment to write down any names that are significant to you.

Now that you have completed the Community Map, take a look at it, starting from the center and moving your way outwards. You are going to do a gut check on what you have written. The gut check is a way to access our body-based intelligence, which is more closely related to our subconscious, intuitive mind. The gut check keeps us honest. It helps us recognize when a Head Override has happened, meaning the brain has told us where a family member, partner, or friend "should be." A common example is that people will put their partner or parent in their first tier because they think that is what a loyal spouse or child would do. But the gut knows the truth. It knows when a recent conflict has created a rift in the relationship. Remember that the community map is a snapshot, a photograph of one day, and it's not necessarily a predictor for the rest of your life. It is an honest accounting of the **current state** of your relationships, which can fluctuate from time to time.

To perform the gut check, you will need to locate your solar plexus. It is the soft belly area underneath your ribs where your diaphragm (breathing muscle) drops into when you do a belly breath. Place a hand on that space between your belly button and your breastbone (sternum). Next, read each name out loud a few times, one name at a time. As you speak a name, feel your solar plexus. What is the sensation of your gut? Does it get tight? Does it feel open or bright? Is there pain or discomfort of any kind?

The gut will tell you if that person belongs in the spot using the language of sensation. If it feels heavy, cramped, tight, or dull, those are negative responses which tell you that a person is not in the right place on the map. Bright, open, flowing, and relaxed responses in the gut are affirmative responses, saying that the person is where they need to be.

Go through each name, one by one, and on a separate piece of paper, write down the basic response that you noted. If at any moment, you get a negative response and want to try moving the name to another part of the map, cross out the old spot and try a new one, rechecking the new position with the gut.

When you look at your complete Community Map, did the position of any of your supporters surprise you? Did someone end up in the second or third tier when you expected them to be in the first tier? Did you put anyone in a closer position at first, because you had a certain image of the relationship in your mind, but after doing a gut check, you moved them further away from you?

You may also recognize that new friends, or old friends that you haven't spoken to in a while, are gravitating inwards to the center of the map, indicating a change in your supporters. To help you interpret what your map is saying to you, ask yourself these focus questions and write a response for each one.

Focus Questions:

1. Did the position of anyone in your support network surprise you? If so, were you surprised that they were on the outer edges of the map or the inner circle?

2. Did you find that you had to move anyone from their original position to another place on the map? What does this move tell you about what is happening in that relationship?

3. Is anyone missing from the map? Why did you either forget them or choose to not put them on the map?

4. Do you desire more support from anyone on the map? If so, write a request to that person saying, "I need _____" and fill in the blank of what you would like to receive from them.

5. If you were to change your support map, how would that look? Would you add more people or have less people around you? Would there be more people closer to the center or more people further away, indicating the need for personal space?

By reflecting on these questions, you can get a deeper sense of the relationship shifts that are already taking place. Once you realize the shifts that need to happen in your support network, make a wish for yourself, aloud, that supports that shift. Write that wish down and put it in a visible place. It represents your intention that will direct you through your personal transformation.

We will be using this Community Map again in later processes, so be sure to save it.

Community Map Worksheet

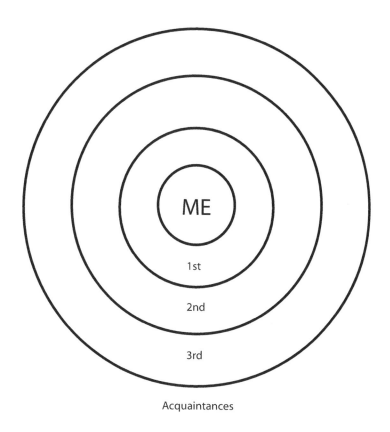

Figure 3. Community Map Worksheet

Coming to the Shore: A vision of Humanity's Healing

There is a vision that I return to often when I ponder the plight of humanity. We seem to make the same mistakes over and over again. Even when we have solutions to our repeating problems, we often don't implement them. When we speak to each other, we only partially listen to each other. It's as if humanity is currently caught in some hidden trap. I asked Life to show me that trap. What came next was a vision of humanity's current state of survival and the path to living together in peace.

This vision represents the big picture view of the Path of the Catalyst. It is a way to take enough steps backwards, to understand both your personal healing journey and also how it relates to the rest of the world. To help you digest this vision gradually, I share a piece of this vision at the beginning of each of the 8 Realizations before we delve into the practical details of making your personal liberation a daily reality.

It happens initially between two people, one standing on the shore and one who is treading water out to sea. When they see each other, the simple act of helping each other ensues. This represents a crucial part of the healing process when one person helps another person. At times, you may read it and feel like you are the one on the shore. Other times, you might feel like you are the one in the water. We all start off being out at sea treading water, because that is the current state of humanity. By doing the work, we get to be on the shore, thriving instead of just surviving.

The vision provides the overview of humanity's healing in the form of a metaphor. Here is the vision in its entirety.

The crack of the water against the sand sprayed salt into the air. I stood at the shoreline, smelling the sea breeze and pondering the plight of humanity. As the waves splashed their rhythmic sound, my eyes went soft. A vision came to me. In the vision, I stood alone at the shore, watching thousands of the people treading water in the cold ocean. Some flailed their arms, struggling for their lives, and others were calmer, their heads still above water. Each of them was entranced in a perpetual state of survival mode.

The sobering realization sunk in. I could not save them all. There just weren't enough people on the shore yet to do it.

"Why don't they just swim to the safety of the shore?" I asked myself. Many of them would most likely make it if they only tried. I yelled out to them, waving my arms as if directing an airplane to land. A few swimmers stared at me like zombies, while others shouted in panic, reaching out their hands, imploring me to save them.

A fire rose up inside me, a combination of frustration that people would not heed my advice to swim ashore and a passionate heroic flame that sought to drag every last one them to the safety. "I have to do something," I finally decided.

Diving through the waves, I reached the first group of desperate swimmers. I tried to calm them, but I quickly became the next victim as they pulled me underwater. There was no shaking them from their panic-stricken state. Pulling away, I made my way to a calmer man who seemed indifferent about the whole situation. Could he not see the people in panic beside him? Was he enjoying a dip in the ocean? He didn't appear to be enjoying himself. He wore an apathetic stare. His eyes were hollow, opaque. Feeling secure that he would not dunk me under the water's surface, I grabbed hold and lumbered his dead weight to shore. Arriving on terra firma, he stood, legs wobbly, as if his feet were not used to the gritty ground below. I collapsed, heaving with exhaustion. But at least I was able to help one of them. I needed to rest before I tried again.

Without warning, he walked back into the water like a deranged, balding Frankenstein monster. The man slowly swam out to where I had rescued him from and resumed his stationary treadmill among his kin.

Confused, I again scanned the sea of people, searching for a clue to explain this calamity. What appeared to be a woman with short hair, the person furthest out from land, finally dipped her head beneath the water. She never returned to the surface. The whole scene twisted my guts into a knot.

My eyes met those of another woman, who appeared to be observing me as well. I was an oddity to her, a strange outsider who had the gall to stand on dry land. She began to stroke toward me. On an impulse, I heaved my knees through the white caps, meeting her halfway. She clenched my hand with both of hers, and I towed her to shore. Dropping to her knees in the sand, she tried to speak, but no words came out. Her lungs heaved. As I stared at the recovering woman, I realized that she represented many of the clients who had come to see me. Some of those clients were men, many more of them women, seeking a way out of that collective survival mode of their daily lives. They were the people doing the deep inner work, those making courageous choices to leave the familiar   enough to recognize that help was there, then they too had a chance of reaching the shore.

Many woke up, trying to convince their family and friends to come with them. No matter how hard they tried, they couldn't wake the others up. Guilt kept so many tied to the same fate as their family. It's not that they didn't realize that they had a chance to live. It's that they would rather die than feel the guilt of leaving them and the shame of being disowned. "Don't leave us," the families would cry. So many turned back to be with their drowning kin. It was heartbreaking to the lines of rescuers.

"It's not fair," said a woman next to me in the lifeline. She had tried to get her parents and sibling to come with her. But they remained, nearly killing her as she wrestled her way ashore. It took her nearly being drowned by her family to realize that they had betrayed her first. They would rather she died loyal to the family than to live. "Why can't they all come with us?" she asked me, her eyes sick with guilt.

"They're not ready," I responded. "Our families are clinging to the familiar. They are holding onto what they know, even if it's hostile and unhealthy. They're more scared of the unknown than they're afraid of drowning."

Leaving the Script

Feeling trapped in a life that does not fulfill you is not a bad sign. It's an indication that you are aware that something is restricting you from growing. You may be aware of the growing pressure of expectations from others, or you may feel that you are carrying feelings and responsibilities that are not your own. In conflict situations with loved ones, you'll possibly be able to predict what they will say next because the same angry lines and sob stories get repeated each time. It feels as if you are trapped inside a bad movie that is not your story.

When you can no longer live by the script of that horrid movie, is when change begins to happen in your life.

Very often, we need a crisis to serve as an excuse to make a change. It can be the death of someone special in your life or the end of a relationship that serves as the occasion to make a major life change. Sometimes the crisis comes with a decision you make, like leaving the family home to attend college in another state, which upsets the family and creates a crisis for the whole family. In either case, the function of crisis is to disrupt the script.

When a crisis occurs, there is a socially acceptable period of time, outside of your normal routine, that one is allowed to feel your emotions and to reflect on your life. When someone close to you dies, you are typically permitted to take time off from work to attend the funeral, to grieve, and to recover. This is a special time, or more accurately, a special space that you can enter into that feels like a bubble outside the normal functions of your daily life. You can see your life from the outside looking in to see what is most important to you as an individual.

Most people will keep busy during a crisis to avoid the important steps of feeling emotions and considering personal needs. The busier you stay during a legitimate crisis, the deeper your attachment to the script. If you are checking work emails instead of crying at grandma's casket, you are clinging to the familiar comfort of the script. When people return to work immediately after a parent or sibling dies, it's not because they are feeling strong; it's because they feel so emotionally overwhelmed that they need a routine to distract them from the unexpressed grief until they have the courage and support to face it.

When we stop participating in the expected scripts of life, it can feel as if we are breaking the rules. Even when there is a culturally acceptable reason, for example the death of a loved one, to slow down the pace of life and to allow ourselves space to feel the emotions of grief, the period is limited to what is deemed acceptable by society. We often go back to work and our daily routines before finishing the first chunk of grief that needs to pass through. Taking out more time to let the natural pace of the inner process ensue can come with repercussions or even negative consequences at your job.

This is not to say that every script in life is bad. Having traditions, holidays, and a structured work week moves life forward. A healthy script frames phases of our lives to help us focus on particular facets in life, like raising kids or beginning a long-term relationship. It is when the scripts of our lives ask us to live other people's part in the movie that the friction between us and the script emerges.

It is possible to dump our responsibilities and roles in the family onto other people. In many societies, the oldest child is expected to help the parents out with raising their siblings. The eldest may also be given certain inheritance rights or authority that the other children are not given. But those privileges come at a cost. They are expected to carry certain responsibilities. Very often, the parents will even dump the responsibility for the day-to-day raising of the siblings onto the eldest, making them the surrogate parent. This transfer of responsibility can feel like a heavy burden to the child who must grow up too fast for the sake of giving their parents relief.

This script, in which the eldest child is assigned the role of becoming the emotional parent of the family, is very common in many cultures across the world. The thought of even asking someone in that eldest child role: "Does this expectation work for you?" can be regarded as being disrespectful. The expectation from the parents is often accompanied by an angry push that the child be grateful for what they have been given and that they should fulfill the responsibility without complaint. But many of these burdened children hit a breaking point, which is usually seen when they start their own families. When they once again have to fulfill the role and take care of their own children, is when they begin to rebel against the expectations that they were burdened with during childhood.

Sometimes the eldest child, in order to escape the trap of being the back-up parent to their siblings, will dump that responsibility onto a younger sibling. In this case, the burden is dumped from parents to eldest child, and from eldest child to a middle child or the youngest child. It becomes like a game of hot potato, where you throw the burden to the next person so that you are not left holding it. The person left with the burdensome role is the one who becomes trapped in a script that their parents should have taken on.

There is a Japanese saying, "出る杭は打たれる。" One way to translate this into English is "the raised nail gets hammered down." It means that you will remain safe if you blend in with everybody else, meaning *if you follow the socially acceptable script.* But the individual who stands out, the person who breaks the script and follows an inner impulse to live life differently, will be ridiculed and punished by their community. When we step out of the script, we break an often-unspoken rule to never leave the expected behaviors we are taught.

I call those raised nails, the Catalysts. They are the people who change our families, and our societies, in ways that empower all of us, even when they initially face disapproval in doing so.

Becoming the Catalyst

To become a Catalyst, we must leave the unhealthy patterns of our upbringing. We must free ourselves from those unfinished family stories which we are expected to uphold. By unburdening these stories, we free ourselves from a scripted life and make room for the life we long to live.

Most people are conditioned to believe that living a fulfilling, unscripted life is somehow selfish. We fear what people will think of us if we break ranks and follow our own dreams. But it is more precise to say that when we leave the script, we disappoint people who were expecting us to behave in a certain way. This can make us feel guilty, as if we are abandoning them for the sake of living our own life.

But, leaving the script is a choice. It takes courage and a clear understanding of our inner longings. When we leave the expected behavior of how we were raised, we give permission to others to do the same. Because everyone has the option of leaving the script, a Catalyst who blazes their own trail is not really abandoning their loved ones, because those same loved ones have a choice to either stay in their daily routine or to live a different life. Following your own life is not abandoning others because they too have the power of choice. Just because they chose to stay in what feels familiar to them doesn't mean that you made the choice for them.

When we break free, we stop being predictable. That scares people. When we move away to find true love, or to get an education, or when we shift our priorities towards our newborn children, we disrupt a predictable routine for the sake of something new. To those still trapped in the familiar script, it feels as if we, the Catalysts, are going to a place that they can't follow. It makes them want to grab hold of us to keep us near. When that doesn't work, they lash out as us or pull away from us. These are desperate manipulations which seek to cripple us emotionally (and sometimes physically) so that we don't have the strength to leave. We can even be disowned by the family, like a dishonorable discharge from the military, because we broke ranks and followed what felt true to us. There is no end to the creative ways employed by people who are still caught in the inherited angst of the family can punish those who break free.

But despite all the risk of punishment, something from the depths of our being is always calling to us. It is the voice inside that wants to yell "cut!" to the bad movie we are living. It makes us want to look more closely at the script we were given and so that we can choose which pages are no longer working in our lives. This voice beckons us to become the author of our own story. It is our Inner Voice of Truth, and it is here to guide us in our transformation.

The Inner Voice of Truth

Our most enlightened forebearers left us clues about how to find our Inner Voice of Truth. Gandhi said, "Everyone who wills can hear the inner voice. It is within everyone." Famed poet Rainer Maria Rilke said, "The only journey is the one within." But perhaps a more recent teaching encapsulates the work that we all must do, regardless of our culture or religion. It comes from Tech Guru Steve Jobs ,who said, "Your time is limited, so don't waste it living someone else's life...Don't let the noise of other's opinions drown out your own inner voice. And most importantly, have the courage to follow your heart and intuition. They somehow already know what you truly want to become. Everything else is secondary."

So often, we follow in the footsteps of our ancestors in a way that does not connect us to our inner wisdom. We often follow blindly, hoping that by doing so, we will arrive at a temple where all the answers reside. Sometimes, we make good decisions about which ancestor to follow, which brings us further along the known trail than following an ancestor that was trapped in addiction or a cycle of chronic abuse. We stay on these known paths because it gives us a familiar comfort.

But even when we follow the path of the most enlightened being who came before us, whether they were our direct kin or not, there will come times when the clues they left behind are lacking. War, extinction, and natural disasters have destroyed libraries and oral traditions for millennia. So, there will come a point in the road when the footsteps of our predecessors have taken us as far as they can. Their tracks erode away in the dust or lead us in another direction that doesn't feel like a part of our own path.

The voice inside that tells us when we are veering off our path, that intuition that speaks up and tells us something is wrong, is the way our Inner Voice of Truth first grabs our attention. This is the voice that tells us when someone is lying to us. It's the voice that tells us when a new lover will be with us for life.

The path of a Catalyst asks us to embrace and follow our Inner Voice of Truth. This work is not solely a process of adding more wisdom or knowledge to your brain. Simply ingesting the brilliance of others through writing, art, and music is not the complete process. Of course, being inspired by the true expressions of others nourishes and encourages us to create and grow. But unlike the process of academic learning, which often adds vast quantities of information, the work of a Catalyst is often about stripping away what we no longer need. Rather than pile more voices of experts and teachers into our already busy brains, we must release whatever emotional pain and charged thoughts we cling to in order to clear a path to our truth. We bare ourselves. We surrender the repetitive script of what we should be doing with our lives and open up to a more fluid way of life.

Those who chose to live bravely from their Inner Voice of Truth are the Catalysts that create the world they wish to see. Catalysts are the ones who follow their own path, often inspiring others in the process.

The ultimate goal of the Path of the Catalyst is to hear and live by our Inner Voice of Truth. To get there, we must first untangle ourselves from the painful cycles of familiar abuse and self-defeating behaviors. The 8 realizations are the steps that help us release who we thought we were in order to reclaim the birthrights that reconnect us to that Inner Voice.

Think of your Inner Voice as the wisest conscience you have ever heard. When we hear it clearly, even through the emotionally charged mind noise in our heads, we have a chance to actualize it. It informs our most important decisions and helps us to recognize the truth spoken by other people. It is the ultimate authority of what is right and wrong, of what we must say, and it is our most true worthy guide on what we must change. You can think of it as a tactile and verbal beacon leading us back to our inner sense of self.

But for most of humanity, listening to all of the conflicting thoughts and voices in our busy minds is much like listening to competing radio stations filling the air while cars are trapped in a traffic jam. The unity of thought just isn't there. These voices of worries, frustration, inspiration, and humor all jumble together, so that the inner voice of our conscience is not immediately accessible to us. It resides below, as a softer utterance that doesn't compete with all the shouting voices, but our ability to hear it can be eclipsed.

The goal is to be able to *hear* that Inner Voice, regardless of our outer circumstances. When times get tough, it is easy to cling to the opinions of others. The familiar ways our families pull us back in. In these hard moments we may even question our self-worth, as if to ask ourselves "Who am I to want more out of my life?"

We are worth it. We deserve liberation. Clearing the path for our life makes falling in love more robust, food taste richer, and breeds a steady gratitude in our hearts. It puts us in daily contact with our truth. Living in truth benefits everybody.

Breaking free is not about selfish escape from our family responsibilities. In fact, liberation is the truest service to our families, especially when it clears a path for our children so that they do not need to endure what we went through. If we can't do it for ourselves, many take those initial brave steps for the sake of their children, nieces, nephews, and grandchildren. That necessary separation from the unhealthy scripts either happens by our own choice, or it happens to us through crisis and the uncontrollable loss of loved ones. When we see the cyclic nature of hurt, those repetitive waves that touch every generation, a fiery determination arises. It is the fire that says *No More!* We do this not only for our own well-being but also for the good of all those generations who come next.

Make no mistake. Liberation requires more than passive waiting. It insists that we consciously break free from the norm. Either way, the path to claiming our own lives begins with recognizing the burdens holding us back.

Becoming who we are is a rite of passage for which our societies have no script. That is why we must leave the script and follow that Inner Voice that already knows who we are becoming.

8 Realizations Bring Us 8 Birthrights

As I helped people to recognize the true weight of their inheritance, some common themes began to emerge among their stories. When a few hundred people from different cultural backgrounds expressed similar struggles, I took notes. When a few thousand people shared similar breakthroughs in the work, I compiled those notes into these 8 Realizations. These powerful insights greatly enhance our ability to claim our Inner Voice of Truth. Once we build enough trust with that voice, we will no longer need validation from other people in the same way. Our choices in life become clear and we no longer allow ourselves to get pulled off our paths by the demands or manipulations of others.

Each of the 8 Realizations leads to a reward called a birthright. Birthrights are the elements that every human being needs in order to have a complete and authentic life. Every human being deserves to receive these birthrights, which is why identifying the abusive generational scripts that interrupt your right to receive them, is so crucial. We need these parts of our humanity for personal healing to happen, which leads to the collective healing of humanity when we help each other. By claiming our birthrights, we affirm our worthiness to be *all of who we are.*

Picture each birthright as a pearl of inner wisdom that we collect from the ocean of our family struggles. As we walk this path, we collect a string of pearls, returning us to a sense of wholeness. By knowing all of ourselves, we are best able to resolve conflict and to build cooperatively.

Here are the 8 Realizations with their corresponding birthrights that we recover when we walk the Path of the Catalyst.

Step	Realization	Birthright
1	**Survival Mode** Humanity currently resides in a state of **survival mode**.	**Recognition** Recognizing our current state of being brings us emotional and physical relief. That relief helps us to step out of survival mode and widens the tunnel vision so that we can **Recogni**ze the need for genuine help.
2	**Invisible Burdens** We all carry **Invisible Burdens**, the unfinished stories, that we inherit from our families	**Awareness** Perceiving our inherited burdens directly awakens new **Awareness**. With **Awareness**, we are able to distinguish our own experiences, and separate them from the stories we are expected to live by our families. Unaddressed burdens, however, will keep us in survival mode.

3	Unburdening	Choice
	Unburdening is the process of releasing the painful stories of our ancestors.	Unburdening clears the path, making the birthright of **Choice** possible. Without separating ourselves from the burdens and their scripts, we are not capable of fully exercising our free will. **Awareness** makes choices outside of our inherited script possible, thus steering our lives in a new direction.
4	**Empathy and Compassion** **Wounds are pathways to empathy and compassion.**	Empathy Expressing our pain cleanses our wounds and inspires the exchange of **Empathy** and **Compassion**. Empathy reminds us that we are not alone in our pain. Emotional expression with Empathy, generates Compassion.
5	**Inner Fire and Passion** We all have an **Inner Fire** that ignites our **Passion**	Passion Claiming our Inner Fire leads to the birthright of **Passion**, the fuel that leads to the fulfillment of our purpose. It cleanses our wounds, energizes our gifts, and inspires us to speak our truth.

6	**Innate Gifts and Purpose** We all have **Innate Gifts** that give us **Purpose**	**Purpose** Innate Gifts are our natural talents and abilities that we are meant to share with our communities. Courageously sharing our innate gifts leads to the birthright of **Purpose.**
7	**Inner Voice and Truth** Hearing and Speaking our **Inner Voice of Truth** is the deepest source of our identity.	**Truth** Being in touch with our Inner Voice of Truth connects us to an innate stream of wisdom, our ultimate source of guidance and authority and leads us to recognize and live by **Truth** to ourselves.
8	**Forgiveness** **Forgiveness** frees us to live our most authentic life and makes Shared Peace possible.	**Shared Peace** By forgiving others and ourselves, we fully accept and release what happened in the past and we allow **Shared Peace** to happen with other forgivers.

Table 1. The 8 Realizations & The 8 Birthrights

When each member of a community has access to these birthrights, the community resides in a state of shared peace. Everyone has enough. That *enough-ness* breeds trust and respect. Each member of the community is recognized, so they are seen and heard. That reflection gives them a greater sense of awareness of themselves and their relationships. With that greater awareness, the individual has the ability to perceive the options open to them as to how they could be living their lives, which in turn opens up the power of choice. Empathy establishes heart-to-heart connections between community members, creating meaningful bonds that are mutually supportive. Empathy creates a space where it is safe for emotions to flow in a way that uncovers our innate gifts. As these gifts are witnessed as unique to the individual, it allows that community member to find a sense of purpose. The gifts inform their vocation, whether it be as a doctor, a shoemaker, or an artist. Sharing those gifts ignites passion, which not only creates personal satisfaction, but it also inspires others to share their own gifts. In this way, the exchange benefits the whole community.

Having all these elements in place helps each member of the community to discover their own sense of truth. These birthrights nourish each community member in a way that alleviates competition and encourages cooperative thriving. Every member has a place in the community and a function that is essential to the fulfillment of others. The community becomes a prosperous ecosystem that is no longer dominated by survival instincts alone. It becomes an extended family that is capable of mutual listening and support.

What I describe is not a state of utopia. It is not an ideal society that is free from all forms of struggle and conflict. Painful arguments and daily crisis will still occur. However, when the birthrights are prioritized in our families, conflict becomes fruitful opportunities for growth. The conflicts become more conscious and all people involved in the conflict get a chance to speak while the others listen. Emotional outbursts can lead to the expression of truth that is actually heard rather than resisted. When someone calls you on your emotional baggage, they help you to identify the block that is preventing you from receiving one or more of these birthrights. The friction of the conflict, when combined with empathy, helps you to unearth your innate gifts and passions. These fruits of the conflict give you a clearer sense of who you are.

Instilling the realization of these birthrights into a family or community is not about perfection. Peace does not mean freedom from all forms of conflict. Peace means freedom from the cyclic sufferings that repeat in each generation of the family. Families will still experience traumatic events such as car crashes and unexpected deaths, but these events won't be characterized by generational physical abuse, such as when one alcoholic passes the affliction onto the next generation. When the birthrights are freely recognized and encouraged among all community members, the fights and feuds move through to a satisfying conclusion. All parties involved will walk away with new awareness. That awareness enhances our ability to forgive each other for mistakes and past hurts.

So often, we attempt to rush forgiveness by willing it in a very mental way. It is often easier and less painful to brush over wounds with a veneer of 'forgiveness' and 'let bygones be bygones' - to spare ourselves the pain of the process and to move on to a state of perceived peace in the family unit.

Receiving these birthrights quenches a deep emotional thirst. When we receive the birthrights, we become in touch with our hearts again. As they nourish us, we reclaim our gut instincts and the passionate fire in our hips. When the thirst is quenched, we can hear the Inner Voice of Truth speaking to us as we navigate our conflicts and choose healthier relationships.

We need not have a perfect society to feel whole. You may have grown up with alcoholic parents. Nothing will change that starting point. But they can get sober and realize their mistakes, and you can get help for your wounding so that you need not hide from your pain in an addiction. The healing process starts off with messiness, but the birthrights help us to bring all of our being to that messiness in a way that transforms it into something clear and meaningful. The messiness challenges us to rise to the occasion with all of who we are, and in doing so, we become the Catalysts that helps other transform from the experience along with us.

The 1st Realization

Humanity currently resides in a state of Survival Mode

Vision for Realization #1

I closed my eyes and returned to the vision of people treading water out at sea. I was alone on the shore. There were thousands of people in the ocean. They didn't know that they were out at sea, because they were born that way. It was normal to them and they didn't know how to change. They couldn't see me on the shore.

Although they were all treading water, not all of them had the same experience. Some smiled and spoke to each other casually. They were dressed nicely and wore joker masks with permanent smiles... They ate well and had parties as they floated on their rafts.

Other swimmers wore vests that made them more buoyant. They just stared off into the distance and repeated the same routine over and over again. They weren't necessarily drowning, but they weren't heading anywhere in particular either. Nothing ever changed.

The swimmers who had it the worse were the ones without rafts or vests. They flailed and coughed up water. Some of them slipped below the surface and didn't return.

One swimmer seemed to notice me on the shore. She stared in my direction. It made me wonder, "could she see me?" When she waved at me and I waved back, I got the confirmation that I needed. Out of the thousands of swimmers out at sea, one of them recognized the one person standing on the shore. In that moment, she realized that there was another way of life that was not about treading water, but about standing on the shore.

From the safety of the sand, I could see that all of the swimmers were just surviving, some better than others, each in their own way. None of them knew what if felt like to stand on the shore.

None of them were thriving.

> *My mission in life is not merely to survive,*
> *but to thrive.* Maya Angelou

Every human being has been in some form of survival mode in their lifetime. The rigorous birthing process, however beautiful it may be, plunges us from the safety of the womb and completely disrupts the comfort we once knew. Even in a healthy birth, the newborn child is emotionally shaken by the sudden change in environment. Our very arrival into the world is a dramatic process.

As we mature into adulthood, any number of challenges can make us feel like we are just getting through the day. Financial struggles, relationship conflicts, a job loss, so many forms of crisis can shake us emotionally and put us in survival mode.

Survival mode serves a purpose. It allows us to prioritize our safety and security in order to focus on the task ahead. With that focus comes a tunnel vision where we pay attention to staying safe or completing a task that is necessary for our continued sense of security. Everything else that does not support this immediate enhancement of our safety or future security becomes less important.

The problem with survival mode arises when it doesn't shut off properly after the crisis or struggle is over. For instance, there are times when we need to undergo surgery. Once the surgery is done and we have physically survived it, we are still left with the need to recover from the emotional experience, including all the fears of risks of the surgery itself. We need someone to be there when we wake up and to hold our hand, to comfort us with hugs and comfort to reassure us of our safety. This reassurance helps us to turn off our survival mode and come back into a fully functional, thriving state again.

But most people don't fully come out of survival mode after a crisis. In fact, when we experience multiple traumatic events, we are more likely to stay in a perpetual state of survival as a precaution against future crises. We stop trusting that we are safe and fear that something is going to get us. This common situation of being in constant survival mode puts us out to sea. Even when we are physically safe, we might be in an emotional state of survival mode because we believe that something could hurt us again.

When we're out to sea, we endure the repeating patterns of suffering. We are born into these patterns, so it is our starting point. The Buddha called this constant state of suffering "Samsara," a Sanskrit word that translates to mean "cyclic existence" in a life that contains suffering.

Samsara has also been referred to as the "sea of suffering,"[3] a reference to how we suffer unconsciously until we become self-aware.

If we are born among swimmers, then we will inherit their way of life, a life that can be deeply entrenched in survival mode. None of us are immune to this state of being. Even those born into wealth will have to deal with divorces, rejection, suicides and addictions. Money may play a role in putting a roof over your head and feeding your family, but excess money does not shield you from having to do the emotional work that brings you back to a trusting state.

We can recognize the sea of suffering that we are born into by first recognizing that our families are in some form of survival mode. By seeing that survival mode is not the normal state of a human being, we begin to raise our awareness to recognize that we need not stay in this state.

When you wake up to the sea of suffering you were born into, you have a choice to turn survival mode off.

In the case of generational healing work, that sea of suffering comes from the collective unhealed pain of your grandparents and parents. They were born into that same condition with their parents and grandparents. When the same painful situations and repetitive problems are passed onto the next generation, it becomes a cyclic form of anguish that is assumed to be "normal."

---

3   Sogyal Rinpoche. (2002) *The Tibetan book of living and dying.* New York, NY. Harper One.

Expressions of Survival Mode

When I worked as a Healer for a homeless outreach program, I was given an opportunity to intimately study survival mode at its most basic levels. Working with people in various situations of homelessness helped me recognize that are different levels of survival mode, that is, different levels of homelessness that all qualified for our aid. Archie was a "couch surfer." He didn't have enough money to pay rent for a place to live, so he rotated living with various friends and family members. He often had a meal with his family when they came home from work and always had a roof over his head to protect him from the natural elements. While he had a roof over his head and at least one meal a day, this didn't mean that he had enough to eat. He struggled to pay his bills and worried about wearing out his welcome with friends and family. He was technically homeless because he didn't have a permanent address and he wasn't always sure where he would be sleeping in the future.

Brenda suffered a more severe form of homelessness. She slept outside on the streets with no roof over her head. She often did not eat every day, even though she worked one or two low paying jobs. She didn't have anyone to stay with, and wasn't able to seek refuge in any of the homeless shelters as she felt they were either too full or too dangerous. Both of these examples illustrate people who are just getting through the day - albeit at different severities of being in survival mode.

While I was working with that homeless outreach service, I was also seeing clients in my private practice as an Intuitive Healer. These clients were from very different life circumstances compared to my clients at the homeless outreach center. They had secure homes, enough food to eat, and higher paying jobs, and some were quite wealthy. Being exposed to these clients at different ends of the spectrum helped me to observe that people, that even those with more privileged life circumstances, can still be in survival mode.

One of my private practice clients was Claire, a millionaire who owned her own company. Although she took a few lavish vacations each year and owned more than one property, she was constantly worrying about her investments and the pressures she felt to provide for her spouse and children. She feared that all that she had built could slip away in a stock market crash or in some real estate deal gone sour. In her most dreadful fantasies, she fell ill, and her family became destitute because they would have to sell it all off to pay for her healthcare. The anxiety was so intense that it kept her up at night, and she rarely got more than a few hours' sleep. She was fatigued all the time, and always running on adrenaline. And although she may have eaten Filet Mignon for dinner that night, she too was in survival mode, because she couldn't relax and trust her life. She was always worried that something could go wrong, that she could lose it all and become homeless.

If you think back to the vision of the all those people out at sea, you could liken Claire to the swimmer who smiles on the raft. She projects an image of being happy, yet deep down inside, she is still emotionally out to sea because she lives in constant anxiety and terror. While this is certainly a more physically comfortable life circumstance than Brenda's, who lives on the streets, it is not a state of *thriving*, and the constant anxiety could lead to physical health problems down the road. It is easy to mistake someone smiling and floating by on the raft as being the same as the person who is thriving on the safety of the shore. It is easy to miss the signs that point to someone being in survival mode (even to the point of being suicidal) when they are cushioned by material comforts.

Drew was a middle-class father who drove a luxury SUV and owned a boat. His wife left him for another man, and she decided to move to another part of the world. He is now a single father raising two kids on his own. He wouldn't describe himself as "rich," but he has a big house and enough money to pay the bills. As he goes through his crisis, he too, is in survival mode. Although he is not homeless on the streets, he lives in a state of painful grief, much like the swimmers who are wearing the vests out at sea. He is financially secure and is able to provide a good education for his children. But his daily anguish made it hard for him to relax and open up emotionally to new people, which led to feelings of loneliness and insecurity about his future.

My four clients: Brenda the homeless woman, Archie the couch surfer, Claire with her millions in the bank, and Drew the divorcee, were all living completely different life circumstances, yet shared one common thread of humanity. They were all existing in survival mode. Their levels of survival mode were completely different; however, they all had varying unmet needs, which meant that each, in their own way, was just getting through the day.

If at any time, any of them became actively suicidal because of their emotional anguish, they would be in the deepest form of survival mode. Even if Claire, cushioned by her wealth, were to reach that desperate stage, she would, in that moment, be in a deeper form of survival mode than Brenda, who may just have scrounged a meal from the trash. In that moment of desperation, the millionaire is the one who is closer to dying than all the other clients. Social status and large financial incomes do not get us out of survival mode on their own. Survival mode comes down to unmet needs.

Needs

Abraham Maslow was a first-generation Jewish American Psychologist. His parents escaped Russia during the Czarist persecution during the end of the 19th century. [4] He was born and raised in Brooklyn, where his family still endured anti-Semitic abuse. He even shared stories where he was physically attacked, having stones thrown at him, for being Jewish. These early experiences helped him formulate his theory that came to be called Maslow's Hierarchy of Needs.

Maslow made an earnest attempt to prioritize our needs as human beings, depicted here in a pyramid. [5]

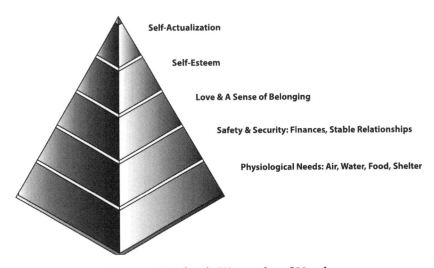

Figure 4. Maslow's Hierarchy of Needs

---

4   Boeree, C. (2006). "Abraham Maslow". Webspace.ship.edu. Retrieved 2012-10-21.

5   Maslow, A. H. (1943) A theory of human motivation. Originally published: Psychological Review, 50(4), 370-396.

Figure 4 shows that the most primal needs of our bodies are our most urgent needs at the bottom of the pyramid. Our motivation for meeting these primal needs will be strongest until they are met. After all, what good is a hug if you are physically dying of thirst? The thirst for water is the more urgent need, and the hug can wait until later. As we travel towards the top of the pyramid, we see needs for financial security next, which means paying the bills so that you can continue to afford clothes on your back and a roof over your head. These are your needs for sustained security, which are not as urgent as our immediate needs for food and shelter, but are the next important in terms of priority. Next, we need a sense of belonging and the experience of feeling consistently loved. This is followed by building a strong sense of self-esteem, where we truly accept ourselves, loving who we are and feeling confidence in our abilities.

Self-actualization means that you have achieved enough self-sufficiency to pursue our goals and dreams. This doesn't mean that you are completely financially and emotionally independent, rather we have a healthy balance in our relationships and with the flow of our money. You are self-actualized when you are fulfilling a sense of purpose in a way that is balanced with the needs further down on the pyramid. In short, you are thriving and your community benefits greatly from your presence.

This pyramid illustrates that someone who is hungry will be focused satisfying their hunger more so than fulfilling their sense of purpose in life. So, Brenda will be more motivated to secure a meal than attempting to sort through the greater sense of purpose in life. One way to think about survival mode is that having unmet *physical needs* puts us in a deeper state of survival than having unmet *emotional needs*. In the same way that there are levels to our needs, there are corresponding levels of survival modes associated with those unmet needs. When we feel the unfulfilled longings that make us want to change our careers, we will be in a milder sense of survival mode than if we are experiencing emotional abuse in a relationship or when we endure food insecurity. The deeper the unmet need, like a scarcity of water due to drought, the deeper the state of survival mode we will enter.

While physical survival needs may be more urgent, this in no way means that emotional forms of survival mode, like being in a state of grief after losing a parent or spouse, are any less important. All needs are important, and meeting them is necessary for coming out of survival mode. But is it necessary to prioritize someone having a physical heart attack over someone who is grieving from a broken heart.

Stepping out of Survival Mode

Before we can step out of survival mode, we first need to recognize when we are in it. How do we know when we have slipped into that state of mind?

It's easiest to recognize survival mode when we have just entered into a crisis. Our daily routine is disrupted. We may initially feel shock, which eventually wears off, and then opens up to a whole bouquet of emotions. All luxuries, recreation, and many daily responsibilities are pushed to the side so that the focus can be on problem-solving and crisis management. When crisis first hits, we do not feel like ourselves and the normal comforts of our life no longer work in the same way. We may no longer derive the same pleasure from unwinding to our favorite music, or going for a stroll on the beach, for example.

But as the initial stress of a crisis gradually fades, we can get numb. If we chose not to grieve a loss, or if we are so emotionally overwhelmed that we throw ourselves completely into work as a means to avoid dealing with the pain, our survival mode becomes harder to detect. We get used to it. If those around us are also in survival mode, there is no one that contrasts from our state of mind to help us recognize our own mental state.

Many forms of meditation are designed to help us separate from the emotional and mental roller coasters of our thoughts. By observing our mental state with some detachment, we are able to witness the survival mode. A mind that is in survival mode will be overactive. In this state, there is almost no break in the thoughts flying through the brain. We attempt to solve the same problems over and over again, sometimes triple checking the results to make sure the solution will bring us safety.

What makes survival mode so much different to a calm state of mind is the rapid pace of the thoughts. We feel agitated. Sometimes we look for more distractions to stimulate our busy brains, because there is a way that the adrenaline rush can feel temporarily invigorating. We can become adrenaline junkies and workaholics, attempting to maximize our rapid intellects instead of addressing the underlying, emotional reasons that we still feel unsafe, even though there is no imminent harm. Or sometimes, survival mode comes from a state of dread about what is happening, or will happen, to someone you love. As one woman who had recently learned that her mother was diagnosed with dementia put it, "work keeps me sane," because keeping busy helped her to avoid feeling the emotional distress of seeing her mother's reduced mental state.

One way to step out of survival mode is to go from a *thinking* state of mind to a *feeling* state. In other words, we stop paying so much attention to our busy thoughts and we start feeling our bodies. We have the power to redirect our attention from our thoughts in our head to the feelings in our chests.

Exercise: Deep Body Listening

This exercise comes from a student of mine, Dina Bernat-Kunin LCSW, who helped me develop the group approach to Bloodline Healing. This exercise can be repeated as a way of stepping out of survival mode at any time. It is also a great exercise to do repeatedly, before you try any of the processes that appear later in the book, as a way to become *present*. Deep Body Listening is a body dialogue process that supports the realignment of the mind and body. Bringing special attention to the parts of ourselves which need it the most repairs the body's emotional wear and tear. This enables the creation of a healthy connection with each body part and each part's voice within us.

The intention of this work is to recognize how our bodies communicate. We do this in order to access our unacknowledged emotions so that we do not live with the Invisible Burdens. The idea of listening to our body is often thought about as monitoring the aches and pains. Yet, pain is an opportunity and an invitation from our body to hear a deeper story, feel what it is holding onto, and discover the buried texts of our life experiences. Hidden beneath these many layers is the place where we connect to our essence. This is a clearer, freer, and more joyful self that can emerge and be revealed.

We all possess many kinds of voices, each with its own particular needs and unique expression. Bringing attention to our body allows for an opportunity for the body to be listened to and heard. Just sustaining attention in our body is itself a gift. This is the gift of our body not holding onto big, challenging feelings alone. All you have to do is follow your body's lead and trust its wisdom.

- Choose a comfortable place that is free of distraction. Put your phone on silent and turn off electronic devices.

120

- Close your eyes and breathe slow and steady breaths. Inhale through your nose and fill your belly, then exhale through your mouth. Gently open your mouth as if to bite into an apple and allow your breath to exit. Follow your breath all the way down your body. As you do this, bring all of your attention and focus into your body. If your attention pops back into your head, just notice it without judgment, and bring it back to your body by using your breath. Take 4 or 5 of these breaths and begin to feel your body.
- Take a moment to notice whatever you notice. Run your attention from your head and scan down all the way to your feet. Notice sensations, temperatures, colors, emotions, sounds, or smells. This is your way of beginning to let your body know that you are here and paying attention.
- Now, ask your body out loud three times:

Where do you need my attention the most right now?

- Pause briefly between each asking and just listen and feel. Allow your attention to go wherever it goes. Do not judge where it takes you, just follow. You may notice sensations, like buzzing or tingling. You may feel a pain. You may start to be aware of a heaviness or a tightening of some area. You may just simply have a knowing. Let your attention go to this part of your body.
- Once you are there, just let your attention hover over the area. Notice how it feels to stay there and sustain your attention in this place. Is it comforting or difficult? Remember, do not judge, just notice. Take a breath and as you exhale slowly allow your attention to move into your body. Let your attention move at

its own pace and let it stop naturally on its own. Do not push it any deeper.

- This is the place for your deeper listening. Let your body know that you are ready and willing to hear whatever it has to say or communicate to you. Notice and feel everything you can about this place. Does it feel heavy, does it appear dark or light, is there a color, are there any sensations, does it feel open or constricted, and do you feel an emotion? You may even hear its words. Stay here quietly, feel and listen, and breathe. You can spend as much time here as you like. If emotions arise just allow them to move through you by feeling them and breathing steadily.

- When you're done let your body know with your words that you are not alone. Thank your body by expressing your gratitude for holding whatever it has been holding onto for you, that you had not acknowledged and felt before.

- Wrap your arms around yourself and give yourself a hug while you slowly open your eyes. Sit up slowly. Rotate your ankles, bringing your attention to your feet as you stand up. Pat your body down until you feel you are standing securely and balanced.

Your Unmet Needs

When everybody else that we interact with on a daily basis is also in some form of survival mode, it is hard to understand which of our needs have gone unmet because everyone else also has unmet needs. Someone who is thirsty in the desert isn't going to tell you that you could really use some appreciation at work, because all they can think about is quenching their thirst. They can't see past themselves because too many of their own unmet needs have accumulated and made them feel desperate.

Comparing yourself to other people who may have more unmet needs than you do is another version of the Pain Contest. When it comes to facing a future in which we have no alternative but to provide care for others for many years to come, self-care is essential. This could be in the form of an ageing parent with a debilitating disease, a partner who may have suffered from a debilitating injury in an accident, or a child born with some form of physical or mental disability. By neglecting your own needs, you will limit how much you can help others throughout your lifetime. Self-neglect leads us to suffer emotional consequences like depression or physical stress-induced diseases, including emotional eating disorders that could lead to heart disease and diabetes.

Take this quick survey of your needs and check in with how you are doing. Be honest with yourself. You can't fix an imbalance until you recognize it. To each of these statements, assign a number between 1-5; with 1 meaning "Disagree," 2 meaning "Somewhat Disagree," 5 meaning "Sometimes," 4 meaning "Somewhat Agree," and 5 meaning "Agree."

1. I sleep enough most nights of the week.
2. On average, I eat three healthy meals a day.
3. I feel secure that I will have a roof over my head tomorrow.
4. I have at least one solid friend that I can rely on in a crisis.
5. I have enough money going into savings to be on pace to retire at a reasonable age.
6. I feel secure in my financial situation for the next year.
7. I have a solid, loving partner in my life that I feel I can grow old with.
8. Faced with hard times, I have two or more people who I can stay with until things get better.
9. I get several hugs a week.
10. I have a friend, partner or therapist that has seen me cry before.

11. I feel clear about my purpose in the world.
12. The work that I am doing on a weekly basis is fulfilling my sense of purpose.
13. I feel seen for who I am by my closest supporters.
14. I am loved.
15. My closest supporters respect me unconditionally.
16. I love the person who I am today.
17. I have one or more communities where I feel like I belong.
18. I feel satisfied with my sex life.
19. I'm on pace to meet my long-term goals in life.
20. On a daily basis, I consistently take a moment to be mindful of my inner state of being.

This quick survey is just to give you an idea of which of your physical and emotional needs are being met or going unmet. It also gives a sense of your higher needs to love yourself and feel a sense of purpose in the world. Just conducting the survey obliges you to think about all of your needs that are necessary for thriving rather than just a focused few.

Take a moment to tally up your score. If you score was close to 20 points, you are in a deep state of survival mode and have several unmet physical, emotional, and higher needs going unmet. This is a sign that you need to ask for help in the form of support groups, new friends, and a counselor of some kind. If you are close to 100 points, you are currently in a state of thriving that can sustain for years to come. A score of around 60 points means that you are doing ok in your life, but that more support and clarity of your needs is necessary to transition from a highly functional form of survival mode to a state of thriving. Generally, around 80 points or more is where thriving begins to really take root, 90 points is where the thriving becomes sustainable, and 100 points is where you become a shining example of a healthy, wholesome human being to other people.

The 1st Birthright

Recognition

When we become self-aware of our survival mode, and the unmet needs that create that state of being, we claim our first birthright of Recognition. We begin to claim this birthright by recognizing our personal state of being. Are we in a rush? Are we feeling overwhelmed? Are our self-expectations too high? Once we recognize how we are doing, we gather enough presence of mind to see past ourselves and our own needs. We are able to more clearly recognize the state of mind other people.

When a parent is in survival mode, the child will feel invisible, like their needs are not being recognized. When this is the case, the child will learn to meet the needs of their parents in order to get attention. Many clients have shared that they felt that their parents were there in body, but that they were not emotionally available. They may have been physically sitting across from them at the dinner table, yet their minds had wandered to a faraway place, leaving the child feeling alone and emotionally neglected. That is what it feels like to interact with someone who is deeply in survival mode. You are only able to capture their attention when you are giving them something they really need. Otherwise, they will distract themselves with other things.

When we are recognized by someone we love, it's as if we are being bathed in rays of warm sunlight. In that moment, we are seen and our place in that person's life is reaffirmed. That basic Recognition makes us feel wanted and important. This creates a sense of belonging in a relationship or in our families. If you ever doubt your need for Recognition, take note of how you feel when you post a photo on your social media account and lots of people like it - or don't.

As a little kid playing in the park, do you recall how you shouted for attention from your parents or grandparents so that they could see how high you could go on the swing? It's those moments of just being seen that give us the recognition that we need to build up our self-esteem and maintain our long-term well-being. We don't realize how important Recognition is until we don't receive it on a regular basis.

Recognition of when someone is emotionally available to exchange needs is an important part of forming mutually supportive relationships. Rather than pouring a lot of time and energy into a one-sided relationship where you are the giver and the other person is the receiver, you can choose more emotionally available people to co-create mutually beneficial relationships. That simple Recognition comes from stepping out of your own survival mode and recognizing your own unmet needs. That awareness alone will help you see when other people have unmet needs and may not be able to help you at the time you need it.

Survival Mode Traps

Because of the prevalence of survival mode in our societies, it helps to recognize the traps which suck us back into survival mode once we have begun to step out of it. Recognizing the traps will help us stay on the Path of the Catalyst so that we can continue to regain all the birthrights without returning back to square one. Studying the traps will help you to avoid them in the future.

Glorifying Survival Mode

We've learned to glorify survival mode. When the boxer we are rooting for is on the ropes, they take the body blows and we feel the emotional strain along with them. Then, when he rebounds and knocks the other guys out, we are taught to cheer. Why? The fight was completely manufactured between two people who barely know each other. Who really won?

While war is a part of our current human reality, we need not glorify it. Many veterans have shared with me what they thought the experience of war would be like. What they envisioned before going away to war was nothing like the reality they actually experienced. We can honor our veterans for being our protectors without creating a fantasy about the glory of war. Instead, just ask a veteran to share what war was for them. We can share our gratitude for their service without glorifying what they had to do to survive.

We even praise people for working three jobs to make ends meet. Sometimes that is necessary to get through hard times. But at some point, in order to step out of survival mode, we must realize that we are in it in the first place. That means that we must release the glory and face the reality of our lives. Embracing that we are survival mode leads to a path of empowerment, a path where you grow in awareness so that you can do something about the survival mode. To do so, we need to look at our needs.

The Head Trap

Albert Einstein once observed, "We cannot solve our problems with the same thinking we used when we created them." I would expand this to say that the problems we create while we are in survival mode cannot be solved while in survival mode. The hasty, adrenaline charged state of rapidly moving thoughts is not the best state from which to see the bigger picture when we make our decisions. This is why meditative and contemplative processes are so important. We must surrender the haste, release the tunnel vision that helps us focus in stressful situations, and take a deep breath before making decisions.

There is a prevailing belief in many modern societies that our intellect will be able to solve all of our problems. But our deeper instincts and intuitions, the many ways that our Inner Voice of Truth tries to steer us in the right direction, is a valuable part of the decision-making process too. These forms of deeper intelligence do not come from the head, rather they are interpreted there.

The fearful reliance on our heads [minds?] as the sole source of answers is an enthralling and dogmatic autopilot that can crash us right into another cyclic catastrophe. There is wisdom in taking a few deep breaths and tapping into a wider array of inner resources before making your next move. By doing so, the analysis of our intellects becomes an important contributor, and not the heady dictator.

The Emotional Blood Clot

There is a very popular form of support after a death that I call the "blood clot." After the death of a loved one, the remaining family members will come together in a tight bond. They will rarely leave each others' sides. Their bonds become more robust. If they live far away from each other, they will call several times a day. They help each other through the painful grief together.

When the physical body is cut, it naturally scrambles to stop the hemorrhaging by sticking clumps of platelets together and creating a tight seal. Once the seal is plugged, it can get to the task of rebuilding itself in an orderly fashion. When the emotional body of the family is cut, then the remaining members clump together tightly to preserve the remaining body. This is a highly effective way of getting through the most painful parts of grieving. However, it is possible to take this survival mode tactic too far. I often see people still in the blood clot formation a decade or more later. That is when it becomes unhealthy.

I have seen this happen many times when a father of the family dies, leaving behind the mother and a few daughters. They try to fill in for the missing male support in their lives by taking on pieces of the role that the father once fulfilled for the family. This blocks the way for new people, including new males, to come into the picture to help out. The remaining family members essentially take up all the parking spots, blocking new people from helping out. The tight-knit circle becomes too tight and the survival mechanism is held onto for too long.

When the blood clot becomes the new way of family bonding, it prevents the final stages of the grieving process. The bonds attempt to fill the void of not having the deceased person there with them. But without fully acknowledging the space that invites the rebirth, the last tears never fall, and new relationships never have a chance to form.

For the emotional blood clot to further heal, there needs to be an intentional separation that allows the living to move forward. This allows the grieving process to complete and restores the person to a potentially thriving state instead of keeping them in survival mode. Very often, because we are not given guidance on how to navigate these separations, we stay stuck together. We scab up, stuck together, never addressing the deeper scar. We stay extra close so that we never take a step back to see the pending work that we still haven't done.

Grieving is one of the most effective ways to come out of the emotional blood clot. Crying and writing about our loss helps us to discern between the heavy feelings of are our personal emotions, and those that belong to other family members. Sometimes we go deeply into empathy with someone else and we take on their feelings as if they are our own. When we gain clarity on what anguish belongs to us as an individual, we can then begin to separate from the blood clot in a healthy way.

Survival and Racism

Survival mode seeks to keep us safe and to get us out of immediate danger. When we are in survival mode, we have tunnel vision which helps us to focus on imminent danger and potential threats. In the same way that we have checklists for a crisis, such as when a pilot has to land a damaged plane or a fireman has to douse flames in a burning house, we too have a very strict script that we follow to keep us out of harm's way.

Our brains work to categorize potential threats by looking for any distinguishing factors that make another individual different from us. If someone looks like us, talks like us, follows the same faith, belongs to the same country, speaks the same language as us (and even has the same accent as us), we are more likely to trust them. The more familiar a stranger appears, the more likely we are to trust them. When people are different to us in culture, appearance, faith, and language, then we will over-emphasize their threat to us, even when there is no objective evidence that they mean us any harm. But fear heightens our state of survival mode. With more fear comes more emphasis on discriminating who will hurt us, even if no real threat is present.

Our survival scripts come from the stories that our families and communities tell us about other races. Some people in America are still repeating slogans from the Civil War, a war that was largely about free African American Slaves. Those slogans are repeated each generation, so the new generations inherit the racist scripts that become heightened when people are in survival mode.

Racism is a complex subject that deserves its own book; however, it's important to recognize how being in survival mode can enhance racist scripts that we have ingested from our upbringing. It amplifies racism and can even be used to justify it. While it might not be your fault for what you heard growing up, it is everyone's responsibility to recognize these scripts when they arise. You're not a bad person for thinking racist thoughts. The question that invites your integrity is, "Do you believe your racist thoughts to be true?"

Exercise: Look in the Mirror

This exercise was taught to me by a therapist. The intent of the exercise is to witness yourself. So often, we look in the bathroom mirror to change our appearance through shaving and applying make-up. We only look at the surface layer and often try to anticipate which parts of us people will notice. But this is not true recognition because it doesn't see a person past the cosmetic surface. The simple act of seeing yourself is the act of giving yourself the birthright of Recognition.

Follow these steps:

1. Look at yourself in the mirror and observe your body language. Describe what you see: What is your body telling you?

2. Look at your face in the mirror and go beyond observing your hair, teeth, and skin. What does your face tell you? If you see some kind of struggle, acknowledge it by asking yourself, "What's bothering me?"

3. Now look into your eyes. See beyond the color of your iris and let that deeper you show itself. Maintain eye contact with yourself. Describe how that feels.

The **30-Day Challenge**: The whole activity only requires a couple minutes for each step. Challenge yourself to do this exercise each day for a month after your morning hygiene ritual. Write down a sentence or two for each of the above steps every day. Don't read it until the end of the 30-day challenge. At the end of the month, read each entry and see what you notice about your progression of actively recognizing yourself. You may be surprised by the insights you discover. It only takes 30 days to start a new habit. For extra encouragement and satisfaction, do this challenge with a friend, then get together at the end and read your entries to each other after sharing a meal. Having another person also recognize both the struggles and moments of self-recognition will enhance the inner work that you have already done over the past month.

Claiming the Birthright of Recognition

When we can begin to recognize ourselves beyond our suffering and survival mode, something deeper begins to emerge. We recognize how powerful we truly are inside. When we really see that enormous potential inside of us, we can clearly see the first reward of walking the Path of the Catalyst. Recognition is essential for coming out of survival mode and heading towards a life of empowered thriving.

Author Marianne Williamson said it best when she shared a well-known quote in her book *The Return to Love*. **This quote is often mistakenly attributed to the great leader Nelson Mandela, who spoke about similar themes. Williamson said:**

Our deepest fear is not that we are inadequate. Our deepest fear is that we are powerful beyond measure. It is our light, not our darkness, that most frightens us. We ask ourselves, who am I to be brilliant, gorgeous, talented, and fabulous? Actually, who are you not to be? You are a child of God. Your playing small doesn't serve the world. There's nothing enlightened about shrinking so that other people won't feel insecure around you. We are all meant to shine, as children do. We are born to make manifest the glory of God that is within us. It's not just in some of us; it's in everyone. And as we let our own light shine, we unconsciously give other people permission to do the same. As we are liberated from our own fear, our presence automatically liberates others.

The 2nd Realization

We all carry Invisible Burdens, the unfinished stories that we inherit from our families

Vision for Realization # 2

As empowered as I felt while standing on dry land, I couldn't leave the swimmers behind. I felt called to help them. They were in survival mode. They couldn't see me. That constant adrenaline rush made it hard for them to recognize anything outside of their daily routines, even a sincere helping hand. In a sense, they only engaged with people who were familiar to them. They only trusted what they could personally control. Anything off the script of their lives was strange and dangerous.

To them, I was strange.

But locking eyes with that woman, the one swimmer who could see me, to see her wave gave me hope that another person could make it to shore. She waved her hands above her head more vigorously, signaling to me that she wanted help. I dove through the water and pumped my limbs, swimming towards her. I evaded the panicked swimmers along the way, knowing that they could pull me under at any moment.

When I reached her, we treaded water together and looked into each others' eyes. She was scared, but she wanted to know what it would be like to walk along the shore. After reassuring her, I pulled her towards the shore. She tried to swim, but she didn't move. It was as if she was dragging something heavy behind her. A chain emerged, a thick tether to something unseen below the ocean's surface.

After we took a deep breath together, I guided her under the water, following the chain that was wrapped around her waist to discover the origin of the other end. The chain was connected to a heavy rock below her. The rock had many chains, connected to other treading swimmers above us. They were all trapped together.

We resurfaced. "Who are these people?" I asked the middle-aged woman. "They are my family," she replied. The rock below, which kept them chained to their spot in the sea, was the shared burden of the family. It was the collective history of her family's unfinished stories. It was the unexpressed heaviness from family funerals. It was all of the regrets of their ancestors for the dreams they never got a chance to live. It was the shame that their family endured for being different, that shame that was never released. Everyone still carried it.

The chain was attached to the woman's thick, heavy vest. This vest didn't keep her afloat like a life preserver. It kept her weighted down, making it hard for her to swim away even if she did cut the chain loose. I pointed the vest out to her, and she didn't see what I was pointing at. She had worn the vest her whole life. She was so used to carrying it, so used to seeing everyone else in her family wearing theirs, that it was invisible to her. This was her invisible burden, the piece of the unfinished family story that had been given to her to complete.

This invisible burden kept her out at sea. It kept her from experiencing the freedom of coming to land.

"I can't bring you to shore," I admitted. "Even if we broke the chain, your burden is too heavy for us to swim back to the shore." The woman looked at me with sadness in her eyes. Then she looked at her kin. She didn't want to leave her family behind. They were completely unaware of the chains around their bodies. It was normal to them. It's all they had ever known. That invisible burden was a hidden part of their everyday reality. It was familiar. She was sad because she wanted to go to the shore. She wanted to fall on the sand and rest. But she wasn't ready to leave her family.

The Invisible Burden

Our parents, our grandparents, and our great-grandparents all have unfinished stories. These stories are filled with dreams. Some of those dreams came to be. The unmet dreams became sad, unfinished stories that sank to the bottom of the sea. The rock beneath the sea represents the unseen, unconscious stories that a family still carries. When some of these stories are assigned to a specific family member by the elders, those specific stories inform the scripts that they grow up with. Were you named after your grandmother who had dreams of becoming a famous ballerina? Have you heard the innocent comments about how much you resemble her, how good a ballerina you could possibly be? Have you felt the weight of the expectation and seen the look of hopeful pride in your mother's eyes? This is the weight of the unfinished story bearing down on you. You may hate ballet and want to play volleyball instead. Choosing whether or not to take on this family expectation and its invisible burden, therefore becomes a conflict for you, and you may spend many years prancing about resentfully in a tutu if you feel you have no choice.

If your elders grieved about and accepted that they were unable to fulfill their dreams, then they most likely didn't pass them onto you. But so many people do not grieve. Most people reach the end of their lives with regrets that they didn't travel, they didn't marry their true love, that they followed the expectations of other people instead of doing what they really wanted to do in life. They stuff down their grief, deep into their bodies. They bury their unmet dreams deep inside, smothering it with a tar-like disappointment. This is how a burden begins to form.

You, too, have dreams of what you would like to experience in your life. Deep inside, you may feel the longing to be an astronaut, to write a book, to take time out to travel and teach English abroad or to ditch the long hours at your corporate job and start your own business selling organic produce. You may feel that you have so much inside that you wish to share and express through art, music, and song. Whatever that dream may be, it makes your body come alive and your heart open up when you think about it.

Everyone has dreams about their lives, yet so few people see them come true. Most people bury their dreams because they were deeply hurt, the idea was rejected, or circumstances physically prevented them from making that dream come true. Perhaps you had an elder who you felt would support you in your dreams of becoming an artist, but instead scoffed at the idea and shamed you. A war in your home country could have interrupted your education, dashing your dreams of becoming a doctor before you had kids. An early death in the family can shift responsibilities to the younger generations prematurely, which may have put paid to your plans to travel through Europe. The desire for these dreams to come true doesn't go away - they just get buried.

Too often, the unmet dreams, and all the emotions about the dream not coming true, become the problems of the next generation. More senior members of the family may not have had the courage to face their regrets, so they expect the younger generations to live it for them so that they can live vicariously through the children and grandchildren. The baseball player that made it to the minor leagues, but never made it to the major league, will likely expect one of their children to become a big league player. Their unmet dream gets passed onto the next generation as a demand.

Body Blocks

In the vision, I describe the invisible burden, that specific unfinished family story that has been assigned to you, as a vest that hugs around the woman's body. The reason I say that is because often, people will carry these burdens energetically in their physical bodies as tension. It weighs down on them, but they are so used to carrying it, that they don't realize how much pressure and tension it is actually putting on the body. Most practitioners refer to these invisible burdens as blocks.

Body workers, acupuncturists, somatic therapists, and intuitive Healers know that our bodies can hold *blocks* that prevent a healthy flow in our bodies. These blocks interrupt our health and can hinder us from living our lives to the fullest. Each system of healing has its own names for the *blocks*. At the core of these blocks is an unfinished story, some type of traumatic event that was unresolved, so it is held inside until you are strong enough to unpack it. These blocks remain trapped inside the muscles, organs, and nervous system until we begin to open it up.

Invisible Burdens are specific kinds of blocks, in that they are bundles dumped onto the next generation by the elders of your community. These blocks don't originate with you; rather, they pre-date you being born and are passed on to you. This is different to when a teacher scolds you for misbehaving, and her harsh words leave an anxious knot in your stomach.

In this instance, your behavior was directly related to the situation you created. You actually had something to do with the formation of this block. With Generational Dumping, you have no choice. You don't choose who you are named after, nor do you have any control over your family's expectations of you.

Even though the unfinished story that is packaged inside the invisible burden did not originate with you, carrying this burden does become your responsibility. With that package comes a scripted role that you must fulfill in order to be part of the family. To be free of the script, you must release the burden. This is why when people move away from home and assume a new life and a fresh identity, they wind up repeating the same script with other people. They take the burden with them. Until you become *conscious of the burden and release it*, you remained tied to the script. If you were the rescuer of your family, you will continue to be the rescuer of your new relationships, until you face what you are still carrying into the new relationship with you.

As long as you carry the burden, there is a way to be pulled back into the family script.

A Teaching on the Invisible Burden

I was invited to speak on public television by Hawaii State Representative Lyla Berg on her show "Voices for Change." The layout of the ʻOlelo station was simple and clean, decorated with green backdrops with patterns of Hawaiian leaves. A carved koa wood bowl sat on the table with sea salt sprinkled inside it, an offering to the ancestors of this land. The set looked like Public Broadcasting Service at a luau.

"I call it the invisible burden," I said. Lyla's eyes were warm and sharp. She had been asking the tough questions for years. How do we change education to better support our children emotionally and culturally? How do we effectively address homelessness? How do we prevent child abuse? What will motivate politicians to make necessary changes in our society? Now, she was asking me the tough questions.

"So, you're saying that this 'invisible burden' is weighing us down and preventing the big changes that need to happen. But what exactly is the invisible burden?" she asked.

I lift the purple school bag with turtle designs onto my lap. I chose a school bag because the burdens we inherit are often transferred to us early in our lives. One by one, I took out items and placed them on the table:

- A composition notebook labeled "responsibility."
- A baseball inscribed with the words: "Make Dad's dream come true."
- An empty beer bottle labeled "family secret."
- A dark stone labeled "grief."
- A thick metal chain labeled "history."

"So, you're saying these are symbols for the things that we are holding on our backs?" she asked.

"Yes, most people just call it stress. But stress is not random. Stress has a story. You can think of the invisible burden as historic stress that we carry around until it gets addressed," I responded. Picking up the composition notebook, I explained that it is an example of good pressure, such as responsibility for getting good grades. This was the kind of weight that can help a child can grow. It's challenging without being overwhelming.

The baseball represented the unfinished story of a parent. It was the parent's expectation that their child fulfill their unachieved dream. We all know the little league coach who once dreamed of playing in the major leagues. Very often, they will push their child to be the baseball player they always wanted to be. But does the child want to play baseball? Are they here to serve another purpose?

The items seemed to get heavier as I progressed. The empty beer bottle labeled "family secret" was a common example. Very often, we are taught to protect the privacy of the family, even though addictions often lead to domestic violence and emotional damage to children. Holding a secret can weigh upon a person. Healing often begins by sharing the secret with a safe person. Secrets have mass, they drag on us, but by their very nature, they are not known to the outside world.

I turned the dark stone over in my hand labeled grief. "It is possible to hold another person's grief," I said. Take for example a mother whose daughter died after being kidnapped. The mother went into depression, spending all her days in her bedroom, searching for the will to get through the day. When she became pregnant again, she began to brighten up again. The mana (the Hawaiian word for 'life force') that a woman gets when she is with child was reviving her. That energy temporarily pushes through the hefty grief. Her new daughter gave her a reason to live. The mother, not having completed her grieving process, passes that grief on to her new daughter, like muddy breast milk. The mother expected her new daughter to be a replacement for her deceased daughter, the one she couldn't protect. As long as the new daughter took on the deceased daughter's role, the mother could hide from the grief that she didn't have the emotional strength to face.

The new daughter took on her mother's unexpressed grief like a thick, suffocating blanket. This living daughter eventually became an alcoholic as a way of coping with the pain that she carried on behalf of her mother. The mother enabled her daughter's addiction by giving her money, not out of care, but because there was a trade off happening, and the mother didn't want to carry that pain anymore. Eventually, the mother began to face the pain of not being able to save her deceased daughter. That's when the family began to shift. By the mother taking responsibility for her own grief, the living daughter then sought help for her alcohol addiction. It was a chain reaction. Healing in families often begins with one person being very brave and facing the hard truth."

"Interesting," replied Lyla. "And the chain?"

"This is the weight of history. I chose this symbol because it was heavy and has many links, which stretch back many generations. We often carry this weight without even realizing how history is still affecting us today. For instance, many families are still feeling the after-effects of Pearl Harbor. It doesn't go away in one generation. It takes several generations to heal."

"So is there anything else we need to know about the invisible burden?" she asked. I revealed a blue gift box with a white bow on top. The label said "gift."

"Underneath the heaviness of our burdens and struggles, reside our deepest, innate gifts," I said. "These are the special abilities that we inherit, such as the artistic talent that we share with our grandfather or the big-hearted empathy of our mother. Underneath the heaviness, are the gifts we are meant to share with the world. By lifting the heaviness, we allow our mana to flow."

Inherited burdens offer both limitations and benefits. If held onto for too long, burdens can restrict the emergence of our gifts and prevent us from claiming our most authentic and satisfying lives. But while we hold a burden, it teaches us about carrying responsibility. They also give our emerging gifts something to push up against, like inner growth weightlifting. Burdens give us enough challenge to discover what we really want out of life.

Sometimes, we need to decide what we don't want anymore before we discover what we truly do want.

Many people hold onto their burdens for too long, which can stifle inner growth. Burdens give us a temporary sense of control, because they help us bottle up strong emotions that we might find uncomfortable. As long as we participate in the family script by continuing to carry these burdens, we are assured of some place in our families. We are so powerful that we can delay our destiny, we can avoid taking the risks to make our passions become a reality. If we stay attached to the role given to us by our families when we were children, then a part of us never grows up into an independent adult. Clinging to our burdens, however painful or abusive they might be, gives us a way to hide from facing who we are underneath those blocks.

Though burdens are not inherently bad or good, it is important to decide when it's no longer healthy to carry the burden. Determining whether a burden is healthy or unhealthy is how we build self-awareness. We start this process by learning more about the details of the burdens we carry.

Now that we have the concept that we inherit specific unresolved family stories in the form of burdens held in our bodies, let's look at a more concrete example of a client becoming aware of what he inherited.

The Murmurs in Our Blood

Adam the Skeptic- Second Generation Holocaust Survivor

Yet they are in us, those long-departed, as potentialities, as a burden upon our fate, as blood that flows murmuring in us, and as a countenance, that rises from out of the depths of time. —Rainer Maria Rilke[6]

Adam was a second generation survivor who lived in a posh beach community south of Los Angeles proper. Originally from the East Coast, he

6   Rilke, R. M. (1946). *Letters to a young poet*. London, England: Sidgwick & Jackson

146

relocated and founded his own firm that dealt with conflict resolution. He worked as a consultant in conflict resolution with very large organizations such as the United Nations. His maternal grandfather had managed to escape Germany during World War II, when his mother was just a little girl. They fled to Austria. Under increasing pressure from the Germans, they lived in constant fear that they would be reported to the Nazis by their neighbors. Adam's family was lucky enough to be one of the few who were allowed to emigrate to the U.S. from Europe, but not all of his family survived.

His mother expected him to be a big money lawyer when he grew up. She prized justice, and wanted to be sure that a good man like her son was keeping people honest. Witnessing some of her family members die made Adam's mother suspicious of unknown people. But being a lawyer felt too rigid for Adam. He also thought about becoming a Rabbi. His way with words and keen insights would have served him well. But in the end, he chose the field of mediation with a focus on international affairs because it gave him more of a sense of freedom.

Most people looked at Adam as a confident, articulate, and highly successful businessman. This was true. But few people guessed that his mother survived the Holocaust. The terror of being a child survivor stayed with her. Her adulthood helped her learn how to package the fear in a better way, a more efficient and socially acceptable way. Even so, some of that family fear was passed down to Adam through his mother. Underneath his impressive exterior, there was incessant worry that did not make sense for the competent millionaire sitting in front of me.

Adam at first was very skeptical, but I assured him that I had no intention to convert him to my beliefs in ancestors.

"Okay, that's a relief," he said. "I didn't mean to offend you... or your beliefs. I just don't want to be bullshitted," Adam said in a calmer voice.

"Your skepticism is welcomed here. I think a certain amount of skepticism is healthy in this work, because it helps you to sift out what's truly happening and what's your imagination. Think of your inner skeptic as the bouncer to the door of your mind. It's there to make sure no 'bullshit' gets in. Just be careful not to go too far into your skepticism, because that leads to cynicism, which is not helpful."

"Wait, what's the difference between skepticism and cynicism?" Adam asked.

"Skepticism is the screen door that keeps the flies outside, but still lets in the sunlight. Cynicism is a rusty, iron storm door that lets nothing inside, not even sunlight. It's hopelessness in disguise. Having a healthy skepticism with at least an ounce of hope is a workable recipe for healing."

"Got it," Adam said, becoming visibly open in his body language. "The reason I came to see you is because I've been constantly worrying about money. My company is doing well, considering the recession, but I've been gradually downsizing. I have money saved, but I still worry about what will happen if I hit a bump in the road. I just keep thinking that if I could make a certain amount of money, then I will be safe. I want to be financially independent, because then I will be safe."

No matter how much money Adam made, he was still living with the anxiety that he inherited from his mother. He feared the disapproval of his family, of being a failure, or his business somehow failing. Though he had never been to Germany or Austria, he had vivid nightmares where he had to escape planes that dropped bombs all around him. In the dreams, he had to keep moving. He was born into his fears.

After talking about his anxiety, I invited Adam to lay on his back for some hands-on healing work. His eyes were hyper-vigilant and watched every movement. I asked him to breathe a few times and tried to help him sink into a new experience. As I made contact with Adam through that heart-to-heart connection that activates a greater flow, I felt the presence of his maternal grandfather.

"Adam, you are a lot like your maternal grandfather, aren't you?"

"It's funny you should say that. My mother just told me that the other day. I have his charm. He must have used his people skills to get away from the Nazis. He made his neighbors allies so that they wouldn't turn them in."

"What do you think happened to your grandfather when he died?"

"I guess he went somewhere else. Like, a soul. I don't think he's gone forever."

"Do you still have a connection to him? Rather than thinking about it, try feeling your body."

"It's interesting, because I was expecting to feel him outside of me, because of what I just said about him having a soul. But I actually feel like Grandpa is inside my body."

"Good. Breathe into that feeling inside your body. You share the same blood as your grandfather. You have some of his natural gifts of charisma and a silver tongue. He's a part of you. Describe to me that sensation in your blood." I sat beside Adam and placed one hand on his heart and the other hand on his shins. That gentle, warm contact helped him get out of his busy head.

"It feels like heaviness in my stomach and chest. The heaviness is beneath your hand and goes all the way down my body. I also feel anxiousness in my limbs, like I just want to run off the table. I'm very anxious right now," he said.

I backed away and asked him to shake out his limbs. He flailed about; first, like he was stretching before a jog, but with encouragement, he whipped around like an octopus out of water. Upon prompting, I asked him to vocalize what he was feeling. The chattering sounds that came out of his mouth sounded like he was shivering from being too cold.

"Good Adam," I said as I asked him to lie calmly again. My hand touched his heart. "You said that you are feeling your grandfather inside your body."

"Yes. It's so unusual because he died before I was born. I'm surprised that I am having all these feelings as I connect with my Grandpa."

I invited him to allow these feelings of heaviness and anxiousness to seep out of his body like steam so that a cloud formed above him. After a few deep breaths, he shared that he felt like he was getting lighter. As Adam became lighter, I was sinking deeper into a waking trance, a state that expert medicine women and men can move to at will. That's why so much of Iroquois medicine was built around song and dance. It taught me to get out of my head and into that pocket of vibrancy that rests beneath our intellects. In that pocket is where the flow happens, almost like a car clutch that stops the gears from rotating so that you can bring the inner human workings back into alignment. Adam's inner engine was always revving too high, over-sharpening the blade of his mind.

My trance sight revealed a dark caked-in blackness inside his chest and stomach. It was breaking up like tar chips. An electric fog released from his arms. Then the tears came. His chest shuddered and heaved. His voice chopped out sounds of a crumpled cry. Adam's body looked like a reverse rainfall; droplets of emotion rose up to a collection of clouds above him. The cloud took the form of a human body, like a mirror image staring down on him from above. Once the crying subsided, I removed my hands from him, and supported him with my words.

"Feel the thick air above you, Adam. That's the invisible burden that you've carried in your body, connected to your grandfather."

"When I first felt a connection to Grandpa," Adam said, "it felt like he was living inside my body. But now I don't feel that heaviness in the same way. I feel relief."

"Do you know why you were crying?"

"I felt this deep sadness about Grandpa. He was able to get us out of Germany during the Holocaust. I wouldn't even be alive today if it weren't for him. That made me sad because he died of a heart attack shortly after rescuing the family. He never got a chance to fully celebrate that the family was safe. I think my mom was really devastated. Our family finally made it to safety, yet her father was still taken away from her in a different way. I couldn't see this before, but now that the heaviness is lifting, my sadness is becoming clearer to me."

"How are you feeling right now?" I asked.

"Not nervous! That's a big deal for me!" Adam's face looked less strained. He breathed a few times. "I can still feel that heavy air above me."

"That is the burden of survival. It's a hefty mist of the fear and grief that you inherited from your maternal grandpa through your mother. That often happens when women lose their fathers early. They secretly lean on their sons, especially if you remind them of their father. You have his charisma, his way of relating to people. When your mother leaned on you emotionally, you filled some of the void that her father's death left behind. That tight bond also comes with emotional dumping, meaning that whatever she feels, you are also obliged to feel."

"That makes so much sense," Adam admitted. "I have another sensation... it feels like a hand on my shoulder. But you're no longer touching me."

"Let yourself feel that contact with your grandpa in a new way. Feel his soul."

"So that feeling inside wasn't the presence of my grandpa. It was what he left behind when he died early," Adam shared. "This hand I feel on me isn't heavy. It's more comforting... it feels invigorating too."

"With the help of your grandpa, I want you to take a deep breath and blow away that cloud above you. With many huffs, the rooms seemed to lighten as he blew away the gaseous exhaust that hung over him.

"Adam, allow yourself to have a connection with the spirit of your grandfather, even if your mind struggles with what you believe. I'm sorry that your family had to go through all that it has endured. But you can be the one who celebrates your family in the way your grandfather couldn't. This way, your kids don't grow up with an anxious father. They'll grow up learning how to celebrate their family."

Adam's body was holding onto the inherited feelings from the Generational Dumping. Because his mind was so busy focusing on other thoughts, he wasn't able to tap into what he was holding inside his own bloodstream.

Like Adam, we all hold something inside our bodies which intimately connect us to our bloodline family, even when we do not feel a significant emotional bond with them.

The 2nd Birthright

Awareness

Awareness is the ability to perceive ourselves and how we relate to the world around us. When we apply this awareness to generational healing, we turn those perceptive abilities to identifying the burdens that we have inherited. Remember, burdens are the packages of unfinished stories that we receive from our elders. Many of these burdens contain the cyclic patterns that have caused suffering in our family for generations. Alcoholism, and the physical and mental forms of abuse that come with it, rarely happen in only one generation. Sexual abuse, abandonment, and divorce also can happen to multiple generations in a family.

When we are able to recognize survival mode, we create separation between ourselves and the very impulses that would keep us repeating our old scripts. It creates enough space for us to make other choices than what the script tells us to do. When we bring our awareness to our bodies, we begin to recognize that we are carrying burdens that impede the flow of our life. It is the same principle behind watching your own breath in meditation. The mindfulness practice brings us fully into the moment and creates space between our thoughts and the ability to perceive life as it is. Without that precious space, nothing new can enter, and change cannot happen.

Let's get clear on the burdens that you are carrying. To do this, we will need a basic family tree.

Core Practice: Family Tree Scanning

In our workshops, we break into small groups on the first day in order to share our family trees. We do this exercise in the spirit of discovering both the gifts and burdens that we inherit from our family trees. You can think of this activity as a fair accounting of the pluses and minuses that come with being a member of your family.

For the sake of identifying what burdens we may be carrying, set the intention to discover what burdens you are carrying on behalf of your family. Be aware that you might be carrying burdens from one or more branches of your family tree. It is not uncommon for an individual to gravitate to one side of the family more than the other. It depends on your individual story. If you are drawn primarily to one side of your family, it's just an indication that a dominant role that you are playing comes from that part of your lineage. Follow the story without the need to apologize to the other parts of your family for not paying more attention to them. When a marriage or partnership is formed, the family scripts collide together. Certain scripts win and are passed down to the children.

It helps to try this exercise with your program buddy. The act of being witnessed while sharing your family tree is an incredibly powerful experience. Just the act of filling it out begins the process. Many times, you will find yourself talking to people that you haven't talked to in years in order to gather photos and information on family members. Many family secrets get revealed in this process which fills in some crucial blanks. Expect emotions to surface during this process as well as a sense of satisfaction of finding answered to lingering family questions. You can also share this activity with a therapist who will surely already have a solid background in genograms.

Steps:

1. Complete the family tree below. Don't worry if you don't know all the people in your family tree. Try to complete the boxes for your parents and grandparents. Fill in their full names (maiden names for the women if you have them), where they were born and their approximate dates of birth. These pieces of information help to coordinate your family member's story with any wars or historic events that may have been happening simultaneously. If you know your great- grandparents information, then fill that in too. Again, if you only have partial names or you don't have information for a parent or grandparent, you can still do this exercise. Fill in the information based on what you have.

2. Now introduce your family tree. If you are doing this alone, it still helps to speak aloud when you are introducing your family tree. This activity can be enhanced by sharing your family tree with a witness, such as a program buddy, a trustworthy

friend, a partner or therapist. There is no one right way to do this. Trust the process. Just start by introducing either your father or mother, then let the storytelling unfold. Remember, you subconsciously have a sense of the burdens that you are carrying. You just need to give your attention to the family tree for it to surface.

3. When you begin to feel a charge, meaning emotions start flowing when you introduce a family member, stay with that family member. This is a sign that you are close to an unfinished story that is still impacting your life. Trust the process and stay with that family member, even if it surprised you that they are your focus today.

4. Either ask yourself the following questions or have your witness ask you:
    Q: What do you have in common with this family member? (Are they your namesake? Did other family members say you look like them? Do you have similar talents, vocation, or aspirations?)
    Q: What hardships did they experience? Can you relate to these hardships? If so, how?
    Q: What responsibilities or expectations do you carry that are related to this person?

5. As you answer the questions, allow your witness to point out what they see in your facial expressions and your body language. Feel your body and notice if there is any pressure, pain, or other sensation as you talk about the family member. This is the place in your body where you are holding some kind of burden

connected to their unfinished story. This new Awareness has begun the surfacing process of your burden.

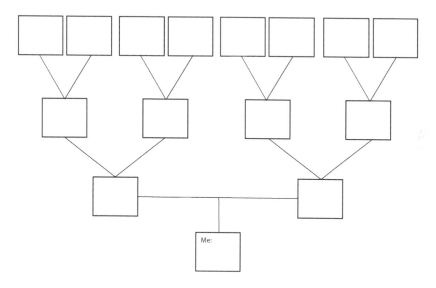

Figure 5. Basic Family Tree Template

Reflect on what you discovered from this exercise. Are you able to feel the location of where you are carrying the burden(s) in your body? Is the story of the burden becoming clearer? Are there family members that you can talk to gain more information about the family story that is emerging?

This exercise can be repeated multiple times as a tool for building awareness. It will be necessary to repeat this exercise for the work we will do directly with the invisible burdens in the next realization. Becoming aware of all the burdens that you are carrying is empowering because then you can do something about it. Each time an unseen story is acknowledged, you have options to complete that story or release responsibility for it, if it no longer feels relevant to who you are today.

It will take time to identify all the burdens, so don't rush the process in some kind of drastic purge. Rushing the process is not advised. The more you know about the family member's story, the more visible the burdens become.

Save this information for another core practice that will be done in Realization #3. Once you have completed the Family Tree Scanning practice, do the next core practice called Basic Body Scan immediately afterwards.

Core Practice: Basic Body Scan

In order to identify where you are holding the tension connected to the burdens that are beginning to emerge in your family tree, do this Basic Body Scan immediately after you have finished the reflection questions in the Family Tree Scanning Practice.

Steps:

1. Rub the top of your scalp with your fingertips. Focus on the sensation of feeling your scalp.
2. Placing your hands at your sides, take five deep inhalations through your nose and breathe out slowly from your mouth in a way that makes a hissing sound (like a leaky car tire).
3. Now ask your body (aloud) to reveal where you are holding the burdens that are beginning to emerge from the family tree.
4. Feel for any sensations that may arise. You may even hear a word pop up in your mind, as if your body has sent you a message from below that has bubbled up in your mind. Pay attention to your body's responses. Where do you feel tension? Do you feel heaviness, cramping, pain, or pressure in any part of your

body? Does any area tingle after you ask your body this question? Write down any sensation, any messages, and any changes that you detect after asking the question. Save this information for the core practice to be done in Realization #3.

Because these practices can bring up strong sensations in your body, it may be helpful to see a body worker, energy worker, or somatic therapist of some kind as you engage in these processes, to further enhance the release that has begun from bringing your Awareness to your burdens.

Realization # 2 Traps

Reentry Pain

Many people experience Reentry Pain when they feel their bodies deeply again. Most people in modern society have spent so much time in the heads that they have lost touch with their bodies. In fact, sometimes, we don't want to feel our bodies because they carry uncomfortable burdens and repressed emotions. This is why most people do not remain grounded. It is easier to avoid feeling the momentary pain or anguish of being in touch with the physical body, which in turn connects us to the emotional body.

Once we are in survival mode, it is easier to just stay there instead of going through the uncomfortable feelings that we haven't faced yet. But the initial discomfort will pass if you breathe and release it.

Pressure and pain are not "bad." They are part of the language of the body and usually occur when we have ignored a story that we are carrying, for too long. At this point, the body is screaming at us to listen to it. Think of the pain as a road flare meant to get our attention. If you have the persistence to stay with the feeling, the pain will break, and a new piece of information or memory will eventually emerge.

The Head Override

The voices of the noisy thoughts in our heads have such a dominant presence in Westernized societies. The thoughts are not always the most enlightened voices that we hear. They are often fueled by excessive worries or anger about the past. But they are not always relevant to what we are going through in the present moment. When you are trying to access the Inner Voice of Truth that resides deeper in the body, it is very easy for a noisier, worrisome thought to grab your attention and pull you away from access to your best instincts. The fast-moving thoughts in our minds are not always right. Very often, they are regurgitations from the scripts written in the past that do not accurately fit what we are going through here in our own lives. The louder head voices can override the deeper wisdom emerging from inside of our bodies.

Within the family scripts, there are phrases designed to stop you from doing the inner work. These phrases were crafted long ago by elders who were trying to hide the abuses they were inflicting on the younger generations. When people are looking at their burdens for their first time, these phrases will emerge to protect the image of the family. We are all conditioned to do so with a variety of messages:

Don't tell the neighbors our business.
Be a good son/daughter and make your family proud.
You have to go to that holiday dinner to show face.
Snitches get stitches.

160

These are all various messages that say, 'be loyal to the family by protecting its secrets.' But how valid are these messages if you and other family members are enduring secret harm? Don't allow these phrases from the family script to derail your progress.

Just because you remember a memory of a loved one hurting you, doesn't necessarily make them a "bad person." That's just another role that you have put on them. Nor are you a "bad person," or disloyal to your family, for acknowledging and expressing when someone has caused you harm. You are allowed to be sad, disappointed, and scared. Feeling angry doesn't make you an "angry person." That's just another label that hooks us back into the script.

It's cleaner to just recognize when a mistake has been made and hurt has been caused. This applies to if you were hurt or caused someone harm. Owning what happened allows it to be expressed and released so that you can move on. If someone has intentionally hurt you, you need not protect them. This just prolongs the catharsis. You are not a *bad person* or any less loyal when you are honest about the impact.

Recognize the phrases and labels from the script that tell you to stop feeling the burdens in your body. No one is helped in the long run by carrying the burdens that no longer fit you.

The 3rd Realization

Unburdening is the process of releasing the painful stories of our ancestors

Vision for Realization #3

She had a choice to make.

We were still out to sea, her and I. She wore a heavy vest, her burden to be the emotional caretaker of the family. That role chained her, tethered her, to that mass of collective family pain that was hidden beneath the surface of the ocean. I was treading water alongside her, waiting to see if she was ready to take that next step of releasing that burden.

She looked back at her kin. Her siblings regarded her as a second mother. Her parents swam around like lost children. Without her, how would they make it on their own? Her deceased grandparents sunk beneath the surface long ago,

163

but still, it felt like they were still there. There were so many dreams that were never experienced and so much grief that was never expressed. If she left her family now, they would be a mess. She could hear the familiar script running in her head, repeating that unspoken rule of her family. "Never leave home."

I pointed to her body, bringing her attention back to the burden that she carried. It looked like a lead vest, heaviest on the shoulders and smoothest over her heart. It was her uniform, the heavy garb of the family rescuer. She looked down at her chest, realizing for the first time that she was wearing the heavy vest. The burdensome vest had subtly grown throughout her life in a way that she could not even detect how heavy it hung on her. She had held it for so long that she had grown numb to its presence. Because she had never taken the vest off, there was no relief, no contrast for her to become aware that she was carrying weighty responsibilities on behalf of her family. She had always just known that it was her job to carry these things in silence.

The vest had a chain attached to it that went all the way to the ocean floor. This chain kept her tethered to the chunk of family grief below the surface where the drowned family members laid to rest. The grief was never expressed. It was rarely talked about. To bring it up in conversation was considered rude and resulted in people pulling away. The grief slept beneath the surface.

Reaching for my bare chest, she realized that I wasn't wearing a vest. Her brows furrowed, her facial expression shifting from confusion to amazement. Everyone in her circle of friends and family wore some kind of heavy vest. It was the first time that she had encountered someone without one. As strange as this experience was for her, she was drawn to it. Something inside of her began to cry out to her, a sensation that started deep inside her torso and began pushing upwards. Something deeper was trying to make its way to her conscious mind, but it needed more time to surface. Her body began to ache as she thought about the burden she was carrying. The more she became aware of the vest, the heavier and more suffocating it seemed to get.

I helped to her to realize that the vest represented the role her family had put on her. She had become the mother to everybody that she knew, even to her own parents. All her obligations, all the family expectations, and all the responsibilities that other people had dumped onto her created the vest. It also held the unexpressed dread and shame of a family that was just surviving through the day. Her family had been through so many early deaths and so much abandonment. Her eyes popped open with the realization that the vest was not hers originally. It was forced on her early on in her life. She was obliged to wear it. When she was a child, she had no choice. But the more aware she became of it, the more opportunity she had to choose a different way of living her life.

"You have a choice to make," I said to her. "Now that you are aware of this burden, are you going to keep it?" Looking back at her kin, her weepy guilt seemed to shift into an intolerable rage. For her whole life, she was expected to be more than a child of the family. She was pressured into growing up too fast, becoming an emotional caretaker to the other members of her family, including her parents. She never got to just be a kid. Instead she was forced to sacrifice the play and exploration of childhood to get her family through hard times. Her resentment surfaced, angry about being a servant to her family. All she wanted to be was a member of the family who felt a sense of belonging just because she was born into the family, not because she took care of everyone else. As her faced burned red, she realized that she was a person who had never truly lived her own life. She lived by the demands of her family, rescuing people who always seemed to have more urgent needs than her own. A burning, like lava crawling up her throat, reached the back of her mouth. Then came the scream, a shrill release of rage as she slapped and splashed the water around her. Her family watched her tantrum, mouths open in shock, as the caretaker of the family shouted her protest at an unfair system.

Then, she looked down at the chunk of rock below the surface and cursed at it. Her whole life had been lived in the shadow of that grief, the collective pain of an eternally sad family just below the surface of the water. She was always aware of it, a heaviness in the background that no one spoke about directly. It wasn't even hers to begin with and her rage made her jerk at the chain that held her to it. As the resentment flowed out of her mouth, the vest began to glow from the heat. Then the vest began to ooze.

An instinct took over and she began to claw at the vest. She pulled it apart like gooey chunks of tar, throwing the chunks into the ocean. Her family continued to stare at her, stunned and disturbed, as their surrogate mother, the emotional rock of their family, finally allowed her emotions to spew forth. She had always put her own needs last, but today, she was going to express herself without reservations. As the pieces of her burden fell below the surface, she felt like she could breathe again. She smiled with relief.

Burdens Tie us to the Script

To leave the painful scripts of our families, we must release the burdens which bind us to the expected behaviors expressed in those scripts. It's not enough to just change our behavior or paste affirmations on our bathroom mirror. We must also release the invisible burden held inside the body to fully separate from the script repeating in our heads.

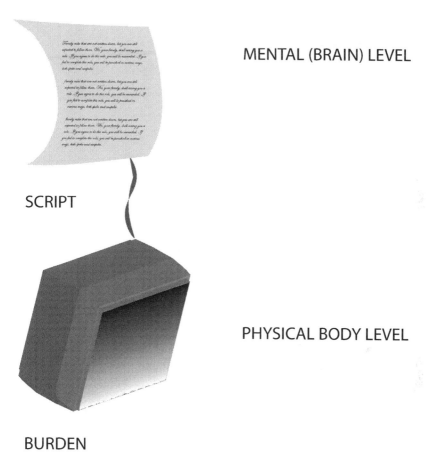

MENTAL (BRAIN) LEVEL

SCRIPT

PHYSICAL BODY LEVEL

BURDEN

Figure 6. Burden with Script Attached

Figure 6 demonstrates how we hold our scripts on the mental level and the burdens are held on the physical level. In practical terms, the script is the series of repetitive thoughts, often with the voices of people that we've heard the scripts from in the past, which repeat over and over in our brain. The burdens are held in the body as physical tension in specific a location(s) where the burden(s) reside.

Scripts are attractive because they give us roles in our families and communities, much the same as actors are assigned different roles in a play. Each of us will have a role in the family which obliges us to fulfill certain tasks as demanded by the script. When we don't follow the script, we lose the benefits of peoples' approvals of our roles and we can be punished in various ways by our family members.

A dutiful mother is a popular role that many play. She is expected to make her children school lunches, drive the children to where they need to go for their activities, and to ensure her family's well-being. If the mother of a family stops doing her job, she breaks the script of family expectations. The family's first reaction would most likely be one of shock. Their next reaction would probably be to make picket signs saying, "Bring back our Mom!"

The mother of the family doesn't need to quit her role completely in order to leave the painful scripts that she inherited. But there is more to being a mother than to be in service to the family. A woman has her own needs and her own dreams in life. Eventually, the scripted family needs will clash with her own needs and dreams. When the scripts become too restrictive, the family will demand that she sacrifice her own needs and desires for the sake of what the other family members need and want. Prolonged neglect of her own needs, because these scripted demands are reinforced with punishments (sometimes subtle and sometimes overt) will lead to internal conflict for her. Subtle punishments can include damaging comments belittling her efforts to return to the workforce and more pronounced punishments can include the guilt trips she is subjected to when things don't run according to plan, in the otherwise orderly home. These punishments can include emotional withdrawals from her which can lead to feelings of loneliness, isolation, guilt and low self-esteem, all of which are emotionally damaging.

I highlight this familiar script, that dynamic where the needs of women come after the needs of boys and men, because it's so prevalent among many cultures. These abusive scripts can be tied to a multitude of burdens that mothers carry. Mothers need not unburden all the responsibilities that they carry in order to weed out the unhealthy scripts. They just need to locate the ones that are emotionally and physically damaging, those scripts that make them feel like they are less valuable of important as a man, as well as those scripts where they are carrying responsibilities on behalf of others in an unhealthy, enabling way.

For instance, it's not a mother's responsibility to ensure that her child is never bored. Nor is she solely responsible for making sure that they are happy. Life is sometimes boring, and we all go through periods of unhappiness. While a good mother might wish excitement and happiness for her children, it is possible to go too far in her self-expectations to give her children everything that they desire. It's not a mother's responsibility to ensure that her children are always engaged with their lives, nor is it her job to make sure that they have everything that they need when they grow up to become adults. Doing so will rob them from learning about the responsibility to self soothe and may hinder their motivation to discover new passions to assuage their boredom. Imagine if a personal trainer did all the weightlifting for you, because they didn't want you to be uncomfortably sore the next day. The workout would be pointless. Don't steal the burdens from other people because they all come with a lesson. Releasing this burden allows the child to grow.

Even the most irresponsible or withdrawn members of our family are still fulfilling roles. For example, take the alcoholic, jobless uncle who passes out drunk on your couch because he has nowhere else to go.

Even he has a family role. If you look back at his childhood, you may see a young boy who took beatings on behalf of your father, because their own was an out of control alcoholic. To the younger generation, he's seen as just a lazy freeloading bum. But what you are seeing is only the aftermath of the abuse, not the full story, because your uncle and father never speak about those times. This is a sign that the family pain that they carry is overwhelming. Your father lets him sleep on the couch, because he remembers how his brother protected him in the past. Your uncle gets drunk to blur the memories of the beatings he took. By knowing this story, you'll be able to recognize that your uncle has actually provided a service to the family. He was a protector of your father in the past. That was his role. By sparing your father the physical abuse he absorbed the family pain on his behalf. He holds the burden of that pain, and all the grief, fear, and hatred that comes along with it. The younger generation didn't see him when he was in his courageous protector role, only in his current state of being downtrodden. Every day is a struggle to contain the pain in a way that it will not be inflicted onto the next generation. He doesn't want to be like his father who spilled his pain onto other family members, so he numbs the pain and tries to be a storage container for it. Each day is a battle to stop the transfer of abuse in the family lineage.

Even the abusive grandfather, the one who abused your uncle, served a role in the unfinished family story. He was the authoritarian who went too far and became the outward expresser of the family pain. Instead of talking about what he went through, he *showed* the family what he went through and inflicted the same harm on them. He too carried this pain on behalf of the family, yet he could not, or would not, contain it. While this might not be a favorable role, he was still serving a part in script of your family. Abusive grandpa made the pain of the past overt by re-enacting what happened to him. This gives context to the family story which helps you to understand why your uncle is always drunk, and why your father takes care of him by letting him sleep on the couch. Your father feels that he owes him a debt of gratitude.

Each of these roles comes with a predictable script that longs to be expressed. It is constantly looking for fresh vehicles who will assume a role in its play. It is the burdens that we carry that bind us in a silent agreement to take on a role. It repeats itself until one script carrier breaks free from that repetitive routine. If we release the burden, then we can leave the script.

Deep down inside, we yearn to be free. We all long to release our burdens by expressing the unfinished story from which they originate so that we can walk our own path. This phenomenon drives so much of what makes us human beings. It is the motivation behind many of our actions and choices. The only thing more powerful than an unexpressed story that is buried inside of you is the act of telling that story.

Gifts and Burdens

Because we have focused so much on the abusive scripts and the most painful burdens first, it may give you the impression that burdens are "bad" or always unhealthy. Chosen responsibilities can also weigh heavily on us. You may take on a very challenging legal career that puts a lot of responsibilities on your shoulders. Holding the weight of those responsibilities can feel burdensome after a while. However, if this career is fulfilling and chosen out of free will, then it is a chosen burden. The main difference between a healthy responsibility and an unhealthy burden is that it is chosen.

But inheriting invisible burdens as a child has another benefit, whether they are chosen or not. With every burden comes an innate gift that resides underneath the burden. Burdens aren't meaningless. The unfinished story of the inherited burden will play a role in awakening a dormant gift underneath the burden.

Each of us is born with innate gifts that will bring us the greatest sense of fulfillment in life if we share them. You can see this when observing children. Two children taught by the same piano teacher and having similar amounts of practice will progress at different rates. One child will go on to perform as a concert pianist and the other will become a stock broker who hardly plays. Why?

Each child has their own talents and strengths. By contributing those gifts to the world, they enhance their family and communities.

We don't inherit every single burden that our family has ever carried. Each person will inherit specific roles based on their strengths. An elder may see something in you, meaning they see an ability that makes you a good candidate for that role. If you feel that the role was dumped upon you against your will, then it is possible that you were being exploited for the gift you carry. In either case, our burdens give us clues as to what gifts may be waiting underneath.

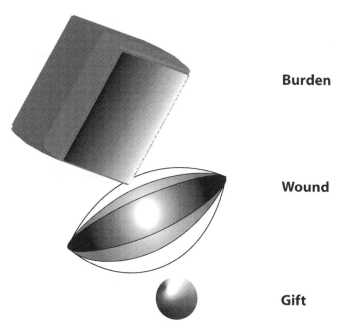

Burden

Wound

Gift

Figure 7. Position of Burdens and Gifts in Relation to a Wound.

As seen in figure 7, the burden sits on top of the wound and the gift resided buried beneath the opening of the wound. The burden and gift have a special relationship with each other in that the burden helps us to discover the gifts that come from being wounded. The burden on top covers the wound, shielding it from being open. Practically speaking, we can stay busy, constantly going from one responsibility to another. By constantly doing task according to the burdens we carry, we never slow down enough to feel our wounds. By hiding in our burdens, we avoid feeling the emotions inside of the wound.

Once a burden is moved, and the emotions flow out of the wound, the gift that is buried inside of the wound can begin to shine through. It often takes the strength and abilities, our gifts, to carry the burdens and complete the unfinished stories that they represent. In this way, burdens can help us grow.

But, eventually there comes a time when the inherited burden has served its purpose. At that moment, our Inner Voice of Truth give us signals that its time for the burden to go. The burden is no longer beneficial and becomes a limitation that keeps you trapped in a script that holds you back from your potential. In order for us to be able to cast away the burdens which no longer belong to us, we must become fully aware of why we carry it. We must be able to see what holds the burden to us, what part of the story keeps us stuck to the script. Once we figure that out, we can release the burden, thus breaking the script, and then claim the innate gift underneath.

The Invisible Burden Dissected

After the airing of the "Voices for Change" television interview that I did in Hawaii, many people wanted to know more about the Invisible Burden. What exactly does this ancestral bundle contain? Most people could relate to the symbolic items in the school bag, but how does the Invisible Burden relate to wounding?

Our wounds are sandwiched between the burden on top and the gift on the bottom. You can think of our burdens as socially acceptable shields that conceal our wounds. They are made up of the responsibilities, family expectations, unexpressed emotions, and heavy beliefs into which we are born.

On an intellectual level, the top layer of the invisible burden contains the acceptable scripts that our families teach us. This includes the family expectations of how we should behave and who we should be when we grow up. Expectations are not just thought forms or scripted responses.

They also come with an emotional push from other family members, like a congealed force that can make us physically uncomfortable. We can feel like we are being "pushed around," even if another person doesn't physically touch us. Though this emotional force is not typically visible, we are able to feel when it happens.

Judgments are another emotional force that we can push upon others. The reason people find judging others so satisfying is that the sharp words and uncomfortable tension creates distance between people. When two people trigger each other, they are rubbing up against each other's wounds on the emotional level. Judging someone is a form of shaming. We put someone else down by throwing some of our own shame on them, which pushes them away and gives temporary relief from having to feel our own emotions. The benefit of judging is that we don't have to feel our own stored emotions. It is a distancing tactic.

The bottom part of the invisible burden sits inside the wounds of our emotional body. The foundation of the burden is our beliefs about ourselves. When I worked with spouses who endured both emotional and physical forms of domestic abuse, I always wondered why they didn't leave the abuser. Even when offered shelter and financial assistance, they often still went back to their partners and endured further beatings. The reason they kept going back is because of a deep-seated belief that they were not worthy of true love and safety. They believed that they were unworthy of proper treatment and that their partner was the best that they could do. These heavy beliefs are at the very heart of the dysfunctional scripts we carry and are the deepest part of the burden.

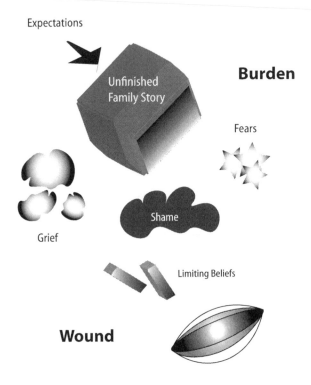

Expectations

Burden

Unfinished
Family Story

Fears

Shame

Grief

Limiting Beliefs

Wound

Figure 8. Anatomy of the Invisible Burden

Let's take a closer look at what makes up the invisible burden as shown in figure 8. The bottom of the burden normally sits inside the opening of a wound. It acts like a cork to the unexpressed emotions that are held inside of the wound. In figure 8, I have separated the burden from the wound so that you can clearly see the components. When the burden is moved, emotions such as shame, fear, grief, and other feelings are released. Think of the unexpressed emotions as the glue that keeps the burden lodged inside the wound.

When we follow the script, the burden will stay lodged inside of the wound until we break the script. It is held in place by the pressure of family expectations to carry the burden according to the role given to us by the script. The core of the burden is the unfinished family story that we inherited from another family member, usually someone older than us. This story becomes your responsibility, as defined by the script.

Underneath the unfinished family stories, and the emotional layers below them, are the limiting beliefs about yourself and your ability to follow your true passions. It is often necessary to do a fair amount of cathartic release before you will be able to name the limiting beliefs clearly. While positive affirmations are a good practice for setting new intentions, without the cathartic release of emotions and the direct communication in our relationships about changing expectations, affirmations are not enough to change limiting beliefs on their own. This is because hampered emotions and the pressure of responsibilities and expectations prevent you from having enough mental-emotional space to make any meaningful change to your beliefs. You cannot just will the change through repetition. A great deal of emotional vulnerability and clear communication must be part of the healing process to successfully change an ingrained belief.

When we change the self-belief that keeps us attached to the burden, the burden finally breaks free, thus releasing the script that is attached to the burden as seen in figure 6. When the burden breaks free, there is often emotional release as well as the physical discharge of bodily pain and tension. This is called a block release.

Burdens in the Wounding Process

Invisible burdens are an essential part of the wounding process. Very often, these packages of expectations and unexpressed emotions are hurled at you during a conflict. The script will often give you a reason as to why you should be holding onto the burden on behalf of someone else. Perhaps your mother is sick, and she just can't face the challenge of raising your little sister, so she gives the responsibility to you to care for her emotional well-being. When you fight her expectation, she verbally assaults you or pulls away from you emotionally until you become submissive to the burden again. There is no end to the family pressures to hold onto the burden and to follow your lines in the script.

Feeling the pain inside of our wounds gives us motivation to address the imposed burdens. When a burden is forced upon us in a violent way, the verbal and sometimes physical impact inflicts an emotional wound that we can feel inside of our bodies. Even in the case of a burden that was gradually passed on in a gentler way, the emotional strain of carrying the worry, grief, and resentment associated with doing a good job in the eyes of your family can lead to physical tension, stress, and physical pain. It's not until we start feeling the pain of the wound that we are even in touch with how deeply we have been impacted by the dumping of a burden.

Burdens have other secret benefits. People who carry the most burdens also tend to be given the most authority or some kind of special pull in the family. A matriarch who carries a lot of responsibility for hosting the annual Christmas lunch will have the final say over who gets invited to her house and who does not. Few people will argue with her over the matter because they fear the cook might go on strike and the holiday will be ruined. Carrying big burdens that came with deep wounds gives people the ability to "pull rank," which means that because others are dependent upon what they are offering, the burden carrier can have things go their way.

The Moment of Passage

The passing of burdens from one generation to the next can be hard to detect. It often happens in covert ways with little conscious conversation about what process is happening. This is why it takes so long for people to even figure out that they are carrying a burden. But one of the easiest times to witness how burdens are passed on is when someone in the family is actively dying.

When family members pass away, in particular elders, they leave behind their unfinished business. The best-case scenario is when the family knows that the passage is going to happen, such as a hospice care situation, and the dying family member can intentionally meet with their kin to share their final wishes. This allows people to say what they need to say before the death, which helps complete a healthy grieving process. It also makes it clear who will hold the roles of provider, matriarch/patriarch, and the tasks that come with those roles. This is also an opportunity to hand down special projects to be finished by other family members, such as books or building a house.

By consciously talking about the impending end of life passage, each family member has the opportunity to become aware of how responsibilities are shifting. Because a great amount of burdens are transferred when an elder passes away, taking inventory of the family responsibilities can be a way to ensure a fair division amongst the family. If we lose track of these responsibilities or neglect to acknowledge when someone is the authority for holding those responsibilities, many extra family fights and sibling rivalries will emerge. It is far more effective if the ranking elder who is passing away is present to discuss the matters in front of the other family members as witnesses. This allows everyone to fully recognize the burden shifts that are occurring and can potentially prevent family fights over inheritance or social power struggles.

My team and I developed an unconventional approach to addressing the aftermath of when burdens are not consciously assigned by a dying elder. It's called an Ancestral Dialogue. This is a process that can be used right after a funeral or even years after the passing of a loved one if something feels like it is still lingering from the death. The goal of the process is simple; identify the burdens and responsibilities that were given to the Catalyst from the deceased family member. Once these burdens are recognized, then the Catalyst is given an opportunity to speak about the impact the burdens have had on them with supporters. In this way they have an opportunity to decide if they wish to carry or release the burdens they uncovered.

Core Practice: The Ancestral Dialogue

When someone passes away, they join our Ancestors. I like to think of our Ancestors not only as those who have lived before us, but also as the collective body of our family stories. They have lived stories which required them to hold certain roles in our families before us. These roles are like having parts in a family play, such as the archetypal roles of mother, father, sister, brother, abuser, protector, artist, innocent child, and mentor. The most unconscious of our family members follow their scripted parts in our family saga without realizing they are even playing a role. You can easily predict what they will be doing that day. Those of our kin who truly care about the role they play, such as being a good parent, take the job seriously. However, they too live according to a script, and if they don't have the courage to speak out against for example, abuse that they know is wrong, then they an example of a family member who is only partially awake.

The Catalysts in the family are the most aware members of the family. They bring the torch of awareness to the family scripts, illuminating which scripts are secretly harming family members. They expose the absurdity of having the same fights, the same repetitive wounding, and the resulting hopelessness that comes from the fear of going off the script. The Catalysts know that they are playing a role and change roles when their Inner Voice of Truth tells them to do so. They are passionately aware and use that awareness to challenge the unhealthy scripts of the family.

The Ancestral Dialogue is an opportunity to talk to your deceased family members about the cyclic abuse that is happening in your family. Yes, you read that correctly. When we facilitate an Ancestral Dialogue in a workshop or session, we ask the participants to speak out loud to the deceased.

This novel idea of having an Ancestral Dialogue first occurred to me when I was working with second and third generation Holocaust Survivors. The families of survivors seemed to be living with the "ghosts" of those family members who didn't make it. By "ghosts," I mean that the memory and lasting impact of what happened to their deceased kin seemed to overshadow everything they did in their daily lives. Whether you believe in spiritual contact with the deceased or not, the residual impact of having a family member perish in the gas chambers is not something that a family forgets. Many children and grandchildren of survivors who lost grandparents, aunts, and uncles in the Holocaust have expressed a similar sense that they felt the presence of these family members, whom they had never met, around them. For some, they felt the stories told to them by their parents around them. For others, it felt like a lingering anxiety about the survival of the family because of what happened to the deceased. Others believed that their deceased kin were walking alongside them in a more spiritual sense. In all cases, the mark of what happened to their family was something that they also carried. Asking them to speak directly to family members who were first to receive that mark produced unexpected emotional breakthroughs.

I knew it was taboo to ask people to speak to the deceased, because there is such a stigma around death in many modern societies. Asking a participant to speak in front of other people was even more taboo than doing it during a phone session. But once participants had a chance to express how silly, nervous, and ashamed they felt about doing so, and after they had a moment to judge the Ancestral Dialogue as being weird, crazy, and scary, I was consistently surprised by how committed each participant was to having that conversation. Something inside of them understood that this was a rare moment to express their truth of what they experienced in a family that was still recovering from what the previous generations had gone through.

While Jewish Holocaust Survivors were the original inspiration for the Ancestral Dialogue, it didn't take long before I offered this core practice to people of all cultural backgrounds and various family tree histories. It's worth repeating that your family doesn't need to be survivors of the Holocaust for you to have an unresolved story lingering in your family tree. This is not a pain contest. All families have an unfinished conversation that can be potentially resolved using an Ancestral Dialogue.

As the workshops became multi-cultural gatherings and I offered this work to clients of all backgrounds in sessions, I could see how simply speaking to your deceased loved ones could bring resolution between the living and the deceased. There's a prevailing belief, among many cultures that I've encountered, that unsettled arguments with people who've died are not able to be to be resolved. It's incredibly frustrating to inherit a painful, partially completed family story, only to be taught that there's nothing you can do about it because your loved one died.

But I didn't invent the concept behind the Ancestral Dialogue. People do this on their own, in private, when no one is watching. They speak to the gravestone, even if they aren't sure that someone is listening. They have a dream where they speak to their late grandma or grandpa that feels cathartic to them. During a meditation, they see their faces. Many people talk to the deceased before they go to bed, including them in their prayers. There are even cultural events like the Day of the Dead in Mexico, or All Souls Day, where the deceased are acknowledged directly. It is not uncommon to want some kind of contact with either the presence or the memory of a deceased family member. What is taboo is talking about it publicly or sharing that intimate moment while other people are witnessing. Once workshop participants and clients move past their initial hesitations towards trying an ancestral dialogue, I'm consistently astounded by how much benefit they get out of these conversations. Engaging in an Ancestral Dialogue speaks to their courage to break the limiting beliefs that are littered within many cultural scripts. These limiting beliefs prevent meaningful resolution from happening after a family member has passed. Whatever your beliefs are about the afterlife, or lack thereof, one thing that everyone can agree upon is that our deceased family members have left behind some kind of legacy that could potentially impact our present day lives.

What makes the Ancestral Dialogue so poignant is that we instinctively gravitate to these defining moments, that experience that forged a certain role that we play in the family script. By honestly speaking to the deceased, we can enlist an untapped source of support. We can also confront an abuser who died before you had a chance to express what happened, for the sake of releasing a burden of rage and grief surrounding the abuse.

Keeping a family secret prevents that catharsis from happening and keeps the client in a role of the secret victim which stifles the healing process.

Ancestral Dialogues ignite the unburdening process. This is because speaking directly to a deceased family member who has a higher generational rank than the abuser can be empowering. This is especially so if an abuse happened after a protector, such as a matriarch or patriarch, passed away. Many abuses would not have happened if the authority figures of the family were doing their job of protecting the younger generations. But if a protector dies, they can no longer directly ensure the well-being of the family. When clients talk to their deceased matriarch or patriarch about how they were abused, the release of that secret pain shakes the burdens of being a secret keeper loose. For many, it was the first time they had spoken about the abuse aloud, which invited the living practitioners and other participants to support them.

A Dialogue Goes Both Ways

A skeptical man once came to one of our introductory workshops. As he described it, "I was dragged here, kicking and screaming by my partner." His partner had attended a previous workshop and hoped that by bringing the skeptical man to the introductory event, he would start doing the inner work on himself. Many people who had been dragged to such events in the past just suffered in silence, so I found his vocal protest about being at the gathering to be very refreshing.

He stared at his watch, waiting for the two hours to finally expire so that he could punch his timecard and run out of the room. But before he left, he was forthcoming enough to articulate why he found the idea behind the Ancestral Dialogue to be uncomfortable. To paraphrase what he said:

I understand the whole concept of talking to the deceased, like when you speak to a grave site. It's similar to when you speak to God when you pray. I'm okay with us talking to them. It's when they start talking back that you need to be taken away in a straight jacket.

I thanked him for being sincere. At least he felt safe enough in our circle to share what he really thought. He had repeated a belief that so many of us are raised to believe. Once someone dies, contact with them also ceases. There are no second chances. If you didn't get what you needed before they passed away, then you missed your chance to get things off your chest. Now, you must live with the grief, the guilt, and all the heartfelt notions that you never got to say, for the rest of your life.

Many people believe that there is an afterlife. Some even believe that there is an intermediate space where the living and deceased can have meaningful contact, such as in their dreams or in a mediumship type experience. A few believe that guardian angels are the spirits of departed loved ones. Those who believe that they are being watched over by a loving, trusted presence feel an immense comfort. For people who hold these beliefs, an Ancestral Dialogue will feel as if they are channeling messages from some intermediate space where the deceased loved one resides.

For those who do not necessarily believe in an afterlife or contact with the other side, the experience of an Ancestral Dialogue may feel like they are tapping into what Carl Jung called the "collective unconscious."[7] More specifically, you can think of each family member sharing a subconscious link. This is why, at times, one family member can sense when another family member is in danger even though they have not received a phone call or text message. Many have shared with me that they still feel this visceral bond with someone who is deceased, even though they never

---

7   https://www.britannica.com/science/collective-unconscious

received a message from them before. It was more of an unspoken knowing. The Ancestral Dialogue may be a way to tap into that unresolved story that still murmurs in the blood somewhere. It gives a dedicated space to focus and invite such information to the surface. While a participant may feel the presence of an ancestor, they might not believe or experience that the discoveries they are making about the family story through the dialogue are direct communications from them. This doesn't make the information any less valid. When a piece of information rings true, it has a certain feeling of truth.

For those who don't believe that we can fill in the blanks in our family tree by some intuitive means, then you can rely on the family stories gathered by elder informants in your family. Just the act of filling out a family tree and opening up boxes of old photographs can spark dialogues about deceased family members. This process can reveal a lot of information that can help you identify the patterns that you are stuck inside.

Ancestral Dialogues are an opportunity to vent about what has always bothered you about how your family behaves. This is where the Ancestral Dialogue can be cathartic theater, allowing the Catalyst to express how upset they have been about the fighting, the colluding, and the abuses that have hurt them and their family. The simple act of expressing emotions in a non-judgmental space makes room inside internally. The strong emotions pass like storm clouds and leave a clear sky afterwards. Once the emotions have passed, the mind is clear to consider how other family members may have felt, which awakens empathy. The catharsis creates room for you to reflect and lay out all the puzzle pieces on the table in front of you. You might not receive some new piece of insight from an outside source; yet, having the space to lay everything out may give you a new perspective that tells you why your family behaves the way it does.

In all cases, the Ancestral Dialogue is only as real as your willingness to be completely honest about your hurts and burdens. Speaking aloud about what you have experienced is a universal part of the healing process, regardless of the modality. If you are speaking the truth, the healing process will be genuine, regardless of what beliefs you carry.

Core Practice: The Ancestor Table

The Ancestor Table creates a neutral point of reference which helps participants to focus their Ancestral Dialogue. When we face the menagerie of unresolved stories of our family tree, it is imperative to focus on one family member and one specific unresolved family story at a time. One of the advantages of the Ancestor Table is that it is possible to put a photo of the deceased family member on the table to help the participant to pinpoint what they want to say. When a photo wasn't available, some people spoke to an empty chair by the Ancestor Tables as seen in chair work in Gestalt Therapy.[8] As the emotions around the unfinished story are expressed, the table becomes the place to orientate the conversation.

Ancestral Dialogues don't conform to any one religious or spiritual practice. They are amorphous on purpose, allowing them to adapt to the specific needs of the speaker. Because all cultures have ancestors, the Ancestor Table does not belong to any one tradition. When people adorn the table with photos and keepsakes of their kin, it personalizes the experience in a shared way with the other participants. The table invites sharing in a way that is beyond competition, outside of religious rules, and free from cultural hierarchy. Think of this as a cross-cultural

---

8   https://www.counseling.org/docs/david-kaplan's-files/wagner-moore.pdf

sharing where no one culture is dominant. This is a special circumstance where everyone is allowed to share in a respectful way.

In the 1990's, a German psychotherapist Bert Hellinger developed a therapeutic approach to healing generational wounds called Family Constellations. The Good Therapy organization described the development of Family Constellations as drawing "from a number of other modalities, including Gestalt therapy, psychoanalysis, Virginia Satir's family sculpting, psychodynamic therapy, hypnotherapy, systemic family therapy, and Zulu beliefs."[9] In this approach, the participant chooses other people from a group of supporters to stand in as family members in a extemporaneous arrangement where a scenario is acted out. This brings clarity of family dynamics as well as the opportunity for emotional catharsis, among other benefits.

One of the most common questions I am asked is, how is the Bloodline Healing approach different than Family Constellations? Bloodline Healing differs in its execution in that other workshop participants do not "stand in" as the deceased "grandma" or "daddy" roles. Instead, the Ancestor Table is often used as the main point of reference. The reason the "stand in" method isn't used is to ensure that participants develop their own interpretations of what was happening in their family trees rather than going on another participant's improvisational read of the unfinished story. This is not a criticism of the innovative approaches shared in Family Constellations; rather, it is an alternative style choice that puts more of the onus for interpretation onto the participant who initiated the Ancestral Dialogue. Since we are handling sensitive situations involving the deceased, it is essential to have this boundary to ensure the utmost respect for a very intimate act involving a matter that has many cultural

---

9   *Family Constellations.* Good Therapy Organization. 5/9/16. https://www.goodtherapy.org/learn-about-therapy/types/family-constellations

taboos. Another point of difference between Bloodline Healing and Family Constellations is that the focus is placed on the deceased rather than people who are still alive, because it is a way of seeing the bigger picture of the inherited stories that were re-lived by multiple generations. Feedback from workshop participants who had experienced both forms of work has been that the different points of emphasis complement each other well, and I encourage people to also explore Family Constellations work.

To paint a picture of what an Ancestor Table could look like, I'd like to share one of my favorite Ancestor Tables that happened at an intensive workshop we held at the Brandeis-Bardin retreat center in Southern California. The workshop space was a large annex-style classroom. We decided to convert a baby grand piano that was also already in the classroom into the Ancestor Table. Aviva Bernat was assisting as a facilitator and she placed a tablecloth that she had gotten from a previous Hawaii retreat on top of the piano. I placed a glass bowl of water with Hawaiian sea salt on top to represent the cleansing nature of the ocean. Dina Bernat-Kunin, Jessica Gelson, and Anna Molitor placed tea light candles and directed the participants to bring up photos of their deceased loved ones to the Ancestor table. By the end of table set-up, we had a beautiful assortment of precious keepsakes, sepia-hued photographs, flowers, candles, and a vessel of Hawaiian seawater.

Every Ancestor Table is unique to the workshop participant or client making it. The most important guideline is to make your table personally meaningful.

Exercise: Making Your Own Ancestors Table at Home

Before you attempt your own Ancestral Dialogue in the privacy of your home, create your own Ancestor Table to be the focal point for this work. Begin by setting a clear intention for your table before you begin constructing it. Here is an example of a clear intention.

I am creating a clear space to explore the legacy of my ancestors.

Intentions are very important because they set the tone for the work that will happen next. They help create a clear environment for you to see the truth about the burdens you have inherited and the gifts that have been passed onto you from your lineage. Feel free to make your own intention, but be sure to say them in the positive. Having negative statements in your intention creates a reactionary response. Instead of speaking a reactive statement: *My intention is to stop being depressed and anxious,* try a more empowering statement: *My intention is to express my feelings and reclaim my inner peace.* You can speak more than one intention if you feel it is necessary to say more than one sentence. If you find that you have several intentions, take a moment to make a list, then edit the list down to the most important statements before beginning creating the table.

If you are creating an Ancestor Table with your program buddy, you can choose to share the same table, or create separate tables in the same room. If you share a table, it is ok to change things around as each person takes turns having an Ancestral Dialogue.

There are no set rules to creating your Ancestor Table; however, here are some guidelines to help you get started after you speak your intention.

- Place some type of cloth or covering on top of a raised surface of any height that feels most comfortable to you. It is also ok to put a mat on the ground or set a chair in front of it. Make the space your own.

- Add photos and keepsakes that feel relevant to the ancestors who have been on your mind. Trust your gut instincts when selecting these articles, because you may be surprised by which ancestors may reveal themselves in the work. Everybody has their A-list relatives who they want to talk to, but they might not be the ancestors you need to talk to because the A-list ancestors might not be part of the burdens you are carrying. Don't worry about including every person in your lineage on the first attempt because you will quickly discover that the Ancestor Table is an evolving project that shifts its focus based on the time of the year, holidays, the milestones in your life, and most importantly, which burdens you are working on. The Ancestor Table is not a static shrine, it is an ongoing process.

- Beautify the table with flowers, fruits, incenses, colors, symbols and whatever else feels right to you. Follow your instincts.
- Since you are in the safety and privacy of your home, it is also acceptable to place an urn with cremated ashes on the table if it feels right to you to do so. Again, there is no obligation that you include this if it doesn't feel right in your gut.
- Most importantly, remember that there is no wrong way to do this. It is just about what feels right to you.

Prioritizing Burdens

In Realization #2, we began to become aware that there are Invisible Burdens in our family tree. In core practice Family Tree Scanning, we began to identify which family stories you may be carrying. We also did a Basic Body Scan to see where in your body the tension from these emotional burdens may be physically located.

From the Family Tree Scanning practice, you may have more than one family member in your family tree that had a charge to it. From the Basic Body Scan, you may have had more than one area of your body speak up. This is a sign that you have more than one invisible burden to examine. To successfully clarify an invisible burden, we need to focus on one at a time. If you only had one name and one area of your body come up during the last two core practices, then proceed to the next section.

In the case that you have more than one family member and more than one area of your body giving you sensations, we need to identify which burden you will address first. Follow these steps:

1. Choose one of the names that were revealed from the family Tree Scanning. Say it aloud. Now ask yourself if this is the most important burden to address now. Feel your gut for a response. In general, gut feelings such as tingling, an openness, or warmth are affirmative responses. Negative responses tend to be sensations that are collapsing, constricting, dull, or numb. Write down your family member's name and whether you had more of a "yes" response or "no" response from your gut.

2. Repeat the same procedure with the next family member name that came up and write down the gut response next to their name.

3. After all the names and responses have been logged in, prioritize which burdens you will address first, second, third, etc.... If you still find it difficult to prioritize which burden will go first, then just randomly assign a number 1, 2, 3... to each ancestor name that came up, knowing that you will address all of them one at a time. At least you now have a working list for the following core practice.

The 3rd Birthright

Choice

See your sons and your daughters. They are your future. Look farther, and see your sons' and your daughters' children and their childrens' children even unto the Seventh generation. That's the way we were taught. Think about it: you yourself are a Seventh Generation! - Chief Leon Shenandoah, Tadahdaho (Head Chief) of the Six Nations Iroquois Confederacy

Abigail's Choice - Third Generation Holocaust Survivor

The more I helped my clients cleanse the heavy blood in their veins, the more I could see the unacknowledged generational power grip that older generations had on their offspring. The older generations had found very effective ways to train and position younger family members to suit their personal needs in ways that were not always beneficial to the family as a whole. It often created a situation that was either subtly or overtly harmful to younger family members who had to suffer in secret. To maintain control, the older generations used intimidation tactics in the form of verbal threats, withdrawing support financially and emotionally, or even physical abuse to ensure that the young generations continued to hold onto responsibilities that were not their own.

Breaking free from these unhealthy patterns often involves some type of separation. Sometimes, this separation comes in a clear form, like someone moving out of a house. Other times, a relationship shift happens where the frequency of communication fades without explanation. These relationship shifts often are part of an unspoken rite of passage, where the burden carrier relinquishes their role in the family script. This directly shifts friendships, family relationships, and even romantic partnerships.

A great example of an unexpected rites of passage happened with a client named Abigail. She had just finished an extremely taxing PhD program in Psychology and had gotten married in the same year that she graduated. Shortly after that, she had a baby girl named Aliza.

Abigail was a third generation Holocaust survivor on her mother's side of the family. Still recovering from her strenuous PhD program, and still adapting to the rigors of being pregnant for nearly nine months, Abigail understandably felt physically fatigued and emotionally worn thin. Even so, her demanding mother, a second generation Holocaust survivor, expected Abigail to be just as emotionally available and generous with her attention as she had been before becoming a mother. Her mother felt threatened by the impending arrival of a newborn infant, a competitor to her getting her own emotional needs met from her already drained daughter.

Abigail and her mother were emotionally joined together her entire life. It often confused Abigail. She didn't feel like she was her own person when mother was around because she had a way of invading Abigail's personal space and dominating her attention. On one hand, Abigail truly loved her mother and wanted to be a good daughter. But she was still coming into the realization that she had been recruited early on in her childhood to carry emotional burdens on behalf of her mother. This burden-sharing made them appear as if they were attached at the hip.

As much as Abigail felt comfort in the closeness with her mother, she also wished to have her own voice and life outside of her mother's needs. When baby Aliza was finally born, the conflict between her and her mother came to a head. The overwhelming event of birth brought Abigail to her breaking point, as the emotional needs of her mother clashed directly with her crying newborn daughter.

Abigail booked a session with me because the fights with her mother started in the hospital as she was going into a slow, prolonged labor. As much as Abigail wanted to focus on the life altering experience of giving birth to her first child, her mother's emotional pulling was competing with the demands of giving birth. Her mother wasn't supporting Abigail. She was protesting the loss of attention.

Abigail recognized that the demands of her mother were unreasonable given the circumstances. This was her Catalyst Event, those extreme moments in our lives that push us beyond our limits and make it clear that something has to change. It's the optimal moment to make a break from an unhealthy script.

According to her family's script, Abigail had been both the "harmonizer of the family" and her "mother's emotional caretaker." This role demanded that she give up her own emotional needs in service of her mother and the rest of the family. This script had also spilled over into her relationship with many of her friends and community members. The script around these roles was further reinforced with the belief that her mother had suffered more than she had, so Abigail owed her mother this service.

But as Abigail hit her exhaustion point, and the contractions of her womb grew more intense at the hospital, she could no longer hold back her fire. She became resentful, even snippy, at her mother and other family members who badgered her for more attention during the birthing process, paying no heed to the obvious situation fact that Abigail needed to care for herself and her newborn baby. As Abigail's outpouring of support to her family dried up, her mother became aggressive and domineering. She was competing with her soon-to-be born granddaughter and pulling rank as the senior family member who had endured the most pain because she was closest to the Holocaust.

Even after the healthy birth of Aliza, Abigail felt torn. She needed her mother's help to raise her baby. Abigail needed her mom to be a grandmother and truly wanted to enjoy the process of being a new mother. But as her outpouring of support to others shifted to her newborn baby, Aliza, the family members began to pull away in protest. They went on strike, pulling away emotionally and refusing to converse with Abigail until she started offering them empathy and attention again. But she didn't have the energy to do what she had done in the past, because she still had to take care of her new baby.

"Rationally, I can see that there is a big cost of me leaving the role of being the harmonizer to my family," said Abigail. "But in my heart, I know that I can't do it anymore. It's not humanly possible to be a mother to Aliza and keep up this role in my family."

When I asked Abigail to voice the fear that kept her in this limbo, she expressed how she feared losing her mother if she didn't play by her rules. "I lose my voice around my mother," Abigail confided. "Part of me is scared of her... of what would happen if I stood my ground. But my heart tells me that this situation is unfair. I compromise myself too much. It's like she scrambles me somehow, even when she is being attentive. It's like I can't find what I need in her presence. My whole existence is subservient to her needs. That is not the best thing for me or my daughter."

I described to Abigail that her situation was as if her mother was energetically suckling from one of her breasts and her baby is drinking from the other one. You can't nurse both of them and be healthy.

It's that heartbreaking choice that many new mothers had to face when they were put in this generational tug of war. Do they go on trying to take care of the other generations, or do they honestly choose to prioritize the younger generation? Most try to do both, which inevitably harms the younger generations who cannot fend for themselves. The parent in the middle generation suffers as well as they age prematurely from the stress and neglect that they experience.

In the scramble for positioning in the family, her mother never fully acknowledged Abigail's promotion to motherhood. Not only did she need more support, but she also needed the newfound authority of becoming a mother to be acknowledged.

Abigail felt a powerful connection emerge with her maternal grandmother.

Along with the presence of her grandmother, she could also feel a few other great-aunts from past generations gathering around her, as they engulfed her in celebration at becoming a mother. The occasion unfolded on its own, as our session quickly became an honoring ceremony where Abigail could feel the support from her deceased kin that she was not able to receive from her mother. I sang her an Honor song to mark the occasion of her new motherhood. Support flooded to her from the connection she felt from her grandmother. She was encircled in a sphere of gentle respect.

During her time of struggle with her mother, this event would remind Abigail that she could still feel respect and support.

In order to create the space for her motherhood to expand and bloom, I helped Abigail realize that she needed to make herself distinct from all the anxiety that she took on from her mother. She knew where the anxiety came from. "My nine-year-old grandmother always carried a butcher knife with her on the New York City subway," Abigail said. "She was afraid that the Nazis might come back again. My mother took on a lot of that anxiety." So did Abigail.

"When my grandmother lost everyone, my mother was chosen to replace all of them. It had been an enormous pressure on her. And I was chosen to be her sidekick, the faithful partner who would support her in that gigantic task. It was my job to be the favored child and to figure out how to meet that unsolvable demand. That's why I became a psychologist, so that I could somehow figure out how to cure the pressure on my mom. I'm worried about what will happen to my daughter, Aliza. She's the first grandchild, and I don't want her to be chosen to replace those who died. It's unfair."

I asked Abigail to make a wish in the witness for her daughter, with her kin in spirit as witnesses.

"I wish for my daughter to be free from taking care of the older generations. I want her to have a balanced connection between her family and herself," Abigail's tone gained more confidence, as each sentence became more adamant, almost defiant. "Aliza needs to be protected from all the octopuses with tentacles that will suck the energy from her. I wish for Aliza what I also wish for myself."

Making that wish awoke a buried fire about the unfairness that the younger generation had to endure. I asked her to let the scream go by screaming into a pillow.

"I WANT TO BE FREE! I WANT TO BE FREE!" The wailing made the veins in her forehead pop out. The space around her flashed red and orange. It pushed back the stream of fear that was always flowing to her from her mother. When it was done, jittery fear was no longer in her personal space.

"It feels really good to yell like that," she said. She had claimed her personal space for her motherhood. By doing so, she chose to own the authority of her new phase of life. Her wish meant that she would prioritize the next generation rather than continue to feed the older generations in an unhealthy way.

Two rites of passage happened for Abigail. The first rite of passage was obvious. She had become a first-time mother. The second rite of passage could be easily missed. Abigail was stepping out of the scripted roles of "the family harmonizer" and her "mother's caretaker." It wasn't until she felt her mother's emotional badgering and punishing withdrawal at the same time as her labor pains that she realized that she had been enduring a form of abuse. But stepping out of that abusive dynamic, she ensured that Aliza wouldn't experience the same abuse from her when she felt overwhelmed.

Once we have built up enough Awareness to realize that we are carrying a burden, the option to let it go becomes possible. Without the awareness of the previous two steps, we wouldn't even know that another path even exists. The Awareness from our previous work on the last step creates space for Choice. It gives us options. Abigail's case showed that once she realized the unrealistic expectation that her mother be emotionally cared for, before her newborn child, that she could no longer do both. When she became aware that she could not hold both responsibilities, she had to make a real-world choice. She had to make a decision that could drastically change the way she related to her mother and impact their presence in each others' lives.

Our inherited family stories can be so pervasive that we may believe that our whole lives belong to our family. We grow up with many expectations of how we are supposed to live, and very often, these expectations were formed before we were even born and before our families had a chance to witness us as unique beings. These expectations are the teeth of the script that bite into us and holds on no matter how hard we shake. Awareness helps you to recognize how the burden and its script is stuck to us. The more Awareness we gain, the more we can own our most authentic lives.

Unburdening gives us an opportunity to exercise our free will. The first choice to make is whether or not to keep holding onto the burden now that you can see where if came from and how it is impacting your current life. To unburden a family story that no longer feels right to carry is exercising your birthright of Choice.

Carl Jung saw the process of individualizing from our families, along with facing the conflicts that inspire us to walk our own path, as a necessary part of our growth. He summed up the benefits of this process by saying, "Besides achieving physical and mental health, people who have advanced towards individuation, they tend to become harmonious, mature, responsible, they promote freedom and justice and have a good understanding about the workings of human nature and the universe." [10]

The very process of choosing to live our own life makes separation from our family a necessary rite of passage. Whether you get married and move out of your childhood home, or you go away to a university, eventually, we leave the everyday routine of our familiar life. Those who never leave home will have a greater struggle to even realize that they are living by a predictable script. It's not until they see a different way of life that the option to separate even comes into their awareness.

---

10   Jung, C.G. *Psychological Types*. Collected Works, vol. 6, par. 757.

Necessary separation from the family, and the inherited script, begins with separating from the burden that is tied to the script. By unburdening, we begin the separation process and make room for the discovery of how we feel in our own space. Think of this as the energetic shift to the blueprints of your relationships that will eventually translate into meaningful conversations and new boundaries in your friendship and family relationships.

Once a burden has been released, there is a rush of relief. This relief is the experience of reclaiming your personal space. Your body discharges the tension that came from the pressure and expectations tied into the burden. Your mind begins to relax when you realize that a change has already begun in a problematic relationship and you become clear on what conversations need to happen next. Your lungs fill up easily, as if they are celebrating the new-found spaciousness in your psyche. Unburdening is not just a mental exercise; it is a whole-body experience. Once an unburdening has happened, there is even more space available to make choices about what you would like to do in your life.

Elements of a Complete Unburdening

The Ancestral Dialogue begins the unburdening process, but this powerful form of cathartic conversation alone might not be enough to bring a complete resolution to an unfinished story. It often takes additional elements to process a surfacing burden.

As I witnessed many of the dialogues early in the work, there were many benefits realized just by going through the act of speaking to the lineage. Some participants' processes were very fluid. Once they were given a dedicated space to share, all the unfinished business was addressed very organically. By the end of the dialogue, they felt clear on what they had just let go of and how they were going to make tangible changes in their current relationships.

But for others, telling the story wasn't enough. Even when they experienced a deep emotional release, they were often left with a question after the dialogue: "Now what?" Though they felt better that they had gotten so much off their chests, they still weren't aware of how this burden fully impacted them. Nor did they have a clear sense of how to make actionable change in their relationships in order to create more freedom in their lives.

Because the invisible burden has many layers, it is sometimes necessary to address each layer of the burden in the event that an Ancestral Dialogue does not organically expunge all the script, pain, and patterns that have been trapped inside of us for many years.

To help, lets highlight the elements necessary for a complete unburdening process.

Speaking the Unspoken: Once you discover that you are part of an unfinished conversation, the act of telling your side of the story becomes an empowering event. Very often, the things that you need to say are not included in the family script. The act of speaking what you need to say breaks the script, creating space for your emotions to flow. Sharing this experience with a trusted supporter, a therapist, or group of people enhances this experience, because being heard for what you endured and being recognized for the heaviness you have carried on behalf of loved ones is very validating. It makes the invisible burden become tangible. You can feel the burden while your supporters are able to see it. Rather than just being numb to what has been endured, the validation helps you to see that the burden is a real thing that you have lived with for many years.

Sharing secrets in a safe environment breaks the scripts. Confiding about a secret harm makes the burden surface so that it can be worked with in an empowering way. The Ancestral Dialogue invites hidden harms to be expressed, which jump starts the healing process and creates momentum for the rest of the unburdening process to occur.

Self-Recognition: Being heard by others creates an uninterrupted space for you to recognize what you have been through. To witness yourself, firsthand, for what you have accomplished and what you have endured in order to be part of your family is part of healing. Your supporters model for you how witnessing is done. When this support is given, they show you how it feels to be validated so that you can replicate that experience for yourself firsthand. You essentially learn how to treat yourself in a healthier and respectful way.

Catharsis: As this conversation continues, and the emotions begin to flow, a deeper release happens in our hearts, in the deepest parts of our mind, and even from inside our physical bodies. Catharsis is the process of releasing the emotional glue that keeps the burden stuck inside. Without the emotional content of the story, only so much of the burden can move. It is human to want to cry, to scream, and to express ourselves through our bodies from a deep place inside of us. But societal pressures and social norms too often hinder our opportunity to let it happen. This why creating an Ancestor Table and making the time to have an Ancestral Dialogue is so precious. Let yourself feel however you feel. Emotions clean us out in ways that our brains will not immediately understand, nor do we need to know what the rationale behind our feelings are right away. Trust the process of catharsis long enough for the feelings to run their course. Your conscious mind will eventually piece things together in a way that answers the question, "Why am I crying?" Give the process enough time to happen without shutting it off in a controlling way.

Identifying the Responsibilities Held on Behalf of Others: When you grow up shouldering responsibilities for your elders, it may seem like a normal part of the routine. In many cultures, the oldest child must help raise the younger siblings, or sometimes, take full responsibility for raising the children, regardless of what age they may be. It has also become very common for young parents to allow the grandparents to do the heavy lifting of raising a child. Responsibility shifting is so prevalent in every culture that we easily lose track of who was supposed to do what.

These shifts often happen in moments of crisis, like when a parent or grandparent dies. Everyone tries to scramble together to fill the void of the missing family member, then get so caught up in their lives that they forget to divide the responsibilities evenly after the crisis period has passed. This results in a jumble of responsibilities that never get sorted out. Eventually, carrying other responsibilities on behalf of others for prolonged periods of time eventually leads to unhealthy forms of enabling in relationships. It also leads to burnout from being overwhelmed by too many expectations. Meanwhile, other people may carry too few responsibilities and go through great efforts to avoid taking on those responsibilities again.

Just because the dumping of responsibilities may be culturally acceptable to the way you were raised does not mean that it is good for you as an individual. As a child, you have no choice. But in adulthood, we do have a choice. We, as adults, become the experts of our own well-being. If carrying too may responsibilities feels unhealthy, then it's a sign that one or more of them needs to be unburdened.

As we sort through the responsibilities that we have, it is important to ask ourselves, "Is this responsibility healthy?" Paying your bills on time, providing for your children, working hard at your job and earning a degree are all beneficial responsibilities that can feel burdensome at times. These healthy responsibilities are not a problem. Identifying the unhealthy dynamic of carrying responsibilities on behalf of others, such as paying the bills of an alcoholic who is not getting help, actually enhances your ability to fulfill the beneficial and necessary responsibilities that are part of a fulfilling life.

In crisis torn families, a very common example of unhealthy responsibility shifting is when a child becomes accountable for their parent's well-being. The excuses for this hidden form of abuse are endless. "My father had a rough life. My mother is ill. My sibling is too immature to handle his duties. My family doesn't speak a certain language. He or she is an alcoholic." Even hearing these common phrases may elicit an emotional response. Be with the emotion that comes up as it is certainly a clue to a responsibility that may be worth examining.

The responsibility of caring for your parents' well-being, long before they are elderly and bedridden, is a very prevalent scenario. I had a client that grew up on a farm. Even though she was only 11 years old, she would often need to babysit her drunk father at the barn after work. Before he would pass out, she helped him into the old pick-up truck and drove him home on the other side of their fields. She didn't have a driver's license, nor should an 11-year-old need to drive their drunk parent home. But she feared leaving him out in the elements when he was drunk, so she took on the responsibility of getting him safely back to the house. It was so normal for her to do this as part of her weekly routine that she didn't realize that this was inappropriate. As an adult, she could look back and realize that this was not the normal life for a young adolescent, but even at the age of 50 years old, she was only beginning to understand that she was still holding onto a responsibility on his behalf. This pattern was still in the works in all her relationships with men. She pushed herself to go above and beyond in order to take care of them to the point of enabling them to dump their responsibilities onto her.

Before a Catalyst comes to the point of embracing that they are carrying a responsibility that belongs to someone else, they often need to stop defending the person that is dumping on them. It is truly remarkable how frequently the person who is being hurt, drained, or strained because a loved one has dumped a burden onto them will defend the dumper. Not only does the burden carrier endure secret harm from years of shouldering the load, but they have also been trained, often through manipulation, to stay at their post even when the duty is bringing them harm.

Carrying a responsibility on behalf of other people for prolonged periods of time is detrimental. If carrying this responsibility for a loved one absorbs all your extra time and energy on top of your own personal duties, it can lead to stress related diseases, insomnia, and burn out. Taking care of your parents full time while they are still young enough to care for themselves will absorb any energy that you might put into a satisfying personal relationship where mutual care can be exchanged. If you possess a deep gift/talent that you wish to passionately share with the world, being liable for other people's well-being who are not your children will interrupt your passion. Time will slip by without you ever having the fulfillment and satisfaction of expressing it. Imagine if Chuck Berry decided to be an accountant? The world would have been robbed of Rock & Roll.

But these detriments are often not enough to persuade Catalysts to look at what responsibilities they need to release. This happens because in the beginning attempts at unburdening, the Catalyst does not yet have enough self-value to summon their courage and end abusive dynamics. However, there is a hidden pocket of motivation that seems to consistently propel people to take stock of the responsibilities they are carrying. This motivation activates when they realize that they are doing what was done to them by the older generations, to their own children, nieces and nephews.

Dumping responsibility is a more subtle form of abuse when compared to emotional harassment, physical beatings and sexual abuse. But all forms of abuse have responsibility dumping at the core of the cyclic problem. If a person who has endured any of the aforementioned forms of abuse is so tied up in caring for their abusers first, they will inadvertently neglect their children and themselves. This happens because they are so fearful, ashamed, and trained not to break the script that they will feed the irresponsible loved ones first, feed the scraps to their children, and then eat the emotional crumbs left over for themselves (if any). The priorities of who gets care and how much become completely skewed, creating a situation where the Catalyst makes the hard discovery that they are part of the problem. They are an enabler who gives too much energy, time, and attention to the dumpers, which creates a pattern of neglect for their children, grandchildren, and themselves.

Prolonged responsibility shifting is so dangerous because its damage compounds slowly over time and it never leaves a bruise.

Changing Your Beliefs about Yourself: We all grow up forming beliefs about ourselves based on our experiences. These beliefs can be empowering or defeating, depending on how we fill in the blanks for ourselves after we have been through an experience. Here are a few examples.

"I'm pretty because everyone in high school wants to date me."

"I am unlovable because my father left us."

"I will never have a successful relationship because everyone in my family is divorced."

"I am too tall because all the men that I am friends with are shorter than me."

"I'm a bad sister because I couldn't save my brother from his drug addiction."

"Because of my race, I will never amount to anything."

"I am capable because I am employee of the month."

We inherit many of our self-beliefs from our families and communities. Because your elders were not able to accomplish or change something in their lives, they will assume that you will fail as well. So, they tell you a belief and you take it in. "The world is unsafe, so you should keep your head down and never stand out or else you will become a target of ridicule."

We can also create self-beliefs ourselves based on what we endure firsthand. These beliefs can get added to the script and can even reinforce the script. A young boy who believes that he is unlovable because his father ran off with another woman may have never been told directly that he was unlovable. He may simply look at his neighbors playing with their fathers and feel the void of not having a father figure. He may fill in the blank for himself, that something is wrong with him for not having a father even if his mother tells him every day how much she loves him. Because there is no father present to speak with about this belief, he is not there to challenge the negative belief his son holds. If the father passes away, the Ancestral Dialogue becomes the place where that self-belief can be expressed and re-examined.

Beliefs that we absorb when we are children can stay buried deeply inside of us until we are put into life situations that makes us re-examine our beliefs. Just because we believe something about ourselves doesn't make it true. In the case of limiting beliefs, we will hold ourselves back from fulfilling our dreams until we change those beliefs.

Our self-beliefs are often behind why we take on certain responsibilities. A very common self-belief is that to be worthwhile, we must be useful to others. In the case of the client who was 11 years old and had to drive her drunk father home, she believed that she wasn't worthy of his love because he was always caught up in his own pain and never gave her the guidance, protection, and attention that she needed. She believed that she was unworthy of his full attention and unconditional love.

Even though she got very little from her relationship with her dad, she decided that having very limited contact with her father was better than no contact at all. Every once in a while, they would share a laugh, or he would offer a surprise nugget of recognition for what she was doing for him in between the very long stretches of neglect. This exchange made her feel needed, and her belief became, "If I take care of my father physically and emotionally, then maybe I will get some recognition." That belief made her take on the responsibility for her father's well-being.

After she left home and stopped taking care of her father, she took her self-belief with her. Believing that she was unworthy of love carried over to her romantic relationships later in life, and so she agreed to take over the emotional well-being of her romantic partners as she had done in the past. Because she never changed her self-belief, she continued to live by the scripted responsibilities that were familiar to her.

Until we see ourselves outside of our self-beliefs, we hold onto the responsibilities on behalf of other people. Without shifting the beliefs tied to the unhealthy burden carrying, we settle for emotional crumbs instead of manifesting healthier relationship that truly nourish us.

Breaking Unhealthy Agreements: To complete the unburdening process, we must dissolve the unhealthy agreements in our relationships. At some point, there is an agreement made to fulfill certain roles on behalf of other people. A conscious version of making an agreement would be formally adopting a niece or nephew as your own child because their parents died.

The aunt and uncle essentially become the mother and father. In general, any agreement that is spoken about aloud is a conscious agreement.

But many of the roles we play on behalf of other people initiate without any explanation or guidance provided. An example of an unconscious version of making an agreement is an eldest daughter becoming the next matriarch of the family when their mother dies unexpectedly. The family is distraught and in survival mode because the deceased mother used to take care of everybody, and now she is gone without warning. The daughter isn't told what to do, because the family members are all beside themselves with grief. After the funeral, there is no initiation ceremony, no matriarch manual given, nor are any special instructions prepared for the burgeoning matriarch. She just does the best that she can, and eventually, the rest of the family moves on with their lives without fully seeing all that she does.

It is possible for one person to be conscious of the agreement being made, while the rest of the family is oblivious as to what formal roles have been assumed. In fact, many of the family squabbles that happen after a funeral occur because one person agrees to consciously take on a role, most commonly matriarch or patriarch, yet other people, who do not recognize this shift, will still fight to have the role. The people who start the fight are the most unconscious of the bunch, seeking some kind of compensation or recognition even though they have not taken on the responsibilities of the role. They essentially try to cash in on the hard work done by someone else in an attempt to unconsciously grab benefits without agreeing to fulfill the responsibilities of a role. The conscious person in this scenario is the Catalyst.

We often form trade-offs in our relationships, which means that we carry responsibility for another person's well-being in exchange for them doing something for us. These are not clean agreements, rather they are a *quid pro quo* contract, meaning "I'll do something for you, but only if you do something for me in exchange." In the unburdening process, these types of agreements are the top priority when it comes to dissolving unhealthy agreements because they are not founded on unconditional love and trust. They are built on conditional terms, which often shortchange the more conscious person and become draining and straining over time.

It is also possible for a once healthy or beneficial relationship agreement to run its course. As we change, so do our relationships. We may not need what an old relationship had provided us with anymore. There may be genuine love and respect between you and the other person, but you may need to make space for the next step in your life or for the next partner/ friend to offer you fresh gifts.

To truly release an agreement that no longer fits into our life, we need to disrupt the mental scripts that were taught to us. This can feel like we are "being rude" or breaking social customs. But when we understand that that a certain agreement is limiting, unfair, or even harmful, the bigger infraction comes from us doing nothing to change it. For instance, when an abused spouse recognizes their partner's behavior as abuse, that awareness comes with the realization that they must make some tough choices to be safe if their spouse is not getting help.

As part of the Ancestral Dialogue, we ask people to formally speak aloud the responsibilities that they are handing back to someone (living or deceased). If they wish, they can ask an ancestor to watch over a living person who you are dissolving an agreement with as a way of turning over control for their well-being. Or they can hand it directly back to the ancestor. We also ask the Catalyst to speak their limits aloud, such as: "Dad, I will no longer be your emotional caretaker. I will no longer give you the attention that my mother denied you. I am moving on so that I can make space for my own partner in life." These limit statements can be written down and even hung on the wall as a reminder not to fall back into the script.

Exercise: Using the Ancestral Dialogue to Unburden

Now that we have enough background on the Unburdening Process, it's time to do your Ancestral Dialogue at the Ancestor Table. Stand in front of your Ancestor Table with your family tree. If you are physically debilitated, sit in a position where you feel fully engaged with the ground beneath you. Before you begin the Ancestral Dialogue, stomp your feet on the ground a few times, bend your knees, and feel a connection with the ground beneath your feet. Then, follow these steps:

1. Choose one Ancestor to speak to directly.
2. Say their name aloud and speak to them directly (in the first person). For example: *Grandma Mary, I need to talk with you.* Share about why you chose to talk with them today and reference what struggle they had in their life that feels relevant to what you are going through.
3. Ask yourself, "What do I need from this ancestor"? You might need a shoulder to cry on, meaning that you need someone to hear your pain. You may need to tell them about a secret abuse that you endured. You may even need to confront them about something they did or didn't do that impacted your life. When you get clear on what you need, make a request of them. For example, *Grandma Mary, I need to tell you about how your Don, my father, abused me when you weren't home.*
4. Allow your emotions to flow. Feel your connection to the ground and breathe.

5.   Now repeat a Basic Body Scan and ask your body where you are holding the burden around this unfinished story that you share with the ancestor. "Body, where is the burden?"

6.   As you feel the burden, ask yourself "What responsibility am I holding on behalf of another person?"

7.   Once you identify the responsibility, ask yourself, "Am I ready to release this responsibility?"

8.   If the answer is yes, ask your body to release the burden. Be prepared for your body to react to your request. You may feel a sudden change in body temperature, you may start coughing or dry heaving, or you may feel a moment of discomfort as the burden begins to shift.

9.   Ask your ancestor, guides or higher power to help remove the burden if this is in line with your beliefs.

10. When the cathartic emotional release and the main physical reactions from your body have run their course, once again, feel your feet on the ground and breathe.

11. Ask yourself, "Is there anything else I need to say to my ancestor?" If there is, express it.

12. Close the Ancestral Dialogue by saying so aloud. For example, say, *I am done with this dialogue.* Then specify if you ask for any support from your higher power, guides, or ancestors. If you wish to be alone or have boundaries, speak them at this time. For example, say, *Grandma, I would like you at my bedside tonight to watch over me.* Or, say *I prefer to be alone tonight; please respect this boundary.*

13. Journal about your experience. Writing about this unburdening experience makes it feel real to your brain. You may also realize that you have more emotions to express after the work that

you just did. Additional insights about what your family has been through and how it is impacting your life can also come through in the writing.

Necessary Separation

After the unburdening has happened, it is time to recognize how this release of a family story will impact your current relationships. Separation can be scary at first. Everyone assumes that a separation means a permanent goodbye. But most often, separating from a relationship means establishing new boundaries so that there can be enough breathing room to expand into who you are becoming.

In order to fully realize who we are, we need to experience ourselves outside of our scripts. This often means that some form of separation from the family is necessary to really see what we are made of inside.

These necessary separations take all different forms. A high school graduate may choose to go away to school instead of staying at home. A son or daughter may take a job in another country. Others marry and move to another place to get away from the house they grew up in. One of my favorite intentional separations was when a client left graduate school and took a job that required living on a cruise liner. Each one of these separations has a socially acceptable cover story, yet the motivation comes from underneath our script. It is our inner fire, that life-changing vital force which leads us to do something "different."

In some instances, the wounding is so severe that the early awakening Catalyst will leave the family without explanation. Some even run away, risking homelessness because they feel safer on the streets than in their own houses. Whatever the logical reason, it is a normal rite of passage to separate from our families and discover who we are.

Action Plan

After writing down your reflections, it's time to apply the new insights gained from the Ancestral Dialogue into real, actionable changes in your life. This means once a pattern has been revealed in your Ancestral Dialogue, it's important to look at which current relationships have the same pattern at work. So, if you had a cathartic release while speaking with your deceased paternal grandfather and your father about how they both abandoned the family when the children were young, ask yourself who in your life reminds you of them. Perhaps you are on and off with a romantic partner who leaves you when the going gets tough. Is this a pattern you wish to perpetuate? Can you see how you might be waiting for that partner to come back and finally realize how valuable you are in their life? Are you waiting for them to stay for good?

Once you have identified how an old family story is reoccurring in your current life, you can write down steps in an action plan. Here is an example based on the example of male abandonment:

Sample: My Action Plan

1. Write a letter to my partner that I never send to express all the things I was too scared to say to him/her directly. This letter is for my eyes only, so I can be completely uncensored since they will never read it.

2. Because I feel powerless when (s)he comes and goes as he pleases, I am going to take my power back and set boundaries with them. I will call them up this weekend and share that I have changed. I'll tell them my new boundaries: "Don't come by my house unannounced anymore. Don't text me late at night." This will give me the space to decide whether or not I want to end things permanently with them.

3.   Talk with my friends to see if they know of anyone else that I can date. I want to see who else is out there.

Exercise: Make an Action Plan

Now it's your turn to create an Action Plan. Review your journal and look for the insights that you found most helpful. Based on those insights from your Ancestral Dialogue, write down responses to each of the following:

1.   What repeating patterns did you discover from your family lineage?
2.   Pick one pattern and make a list of the people in your life who fit this same pattern in one way or another. Trust the names and faces that pop up, even if it takes a few moments to realize how they fit the pattern.
3.   Write down what tangible changes will make you feel empowered in each relationship.
4.   Set a timeline for when you will have these conversations or make other tangible changes with your current relationships.

Third Realization Traps

Because separating from a burden begins a shift in how we relate to others associated with that burden, some type of necessary separation usually follows. This brings up fear. When the fear first arises, it can be overwhelming. It's difficult to make sense of it all. Your brain doesn't work the same way. Your thoughts may be erratic, making it hard to discern what exactly you are scared will happen.

Fear is the biggest trap to unburdening. For all the strain and pain that you may feel when carrying a burden, at least it's predictable. Many people opt to endure the heaviness instead of facing the initial flood of emotion that arises when we start moving burdens around.

But fear passes. It is a powerful energy that is a part of the healing process. Fear brings a heightened awareness to our vulnerabilities, which brings us one step closer to our wounds. In this way, fear serves a purpose. Think of unburdening as lifting a heavy manhole cover. As the cover is pulled off, there can be a rush of off gas coming from the hole. That off gas is the fear. The gas alerts you that something is happening beneath the surface and that you must be careful moving forward. The hole itself the wound. When we go to the next Realization, we will talk more about going into our wounds. But before we even get there, we must face the rush of fear until it subsides.

At first, we can't discern the fear that arises. But it helps to think of the fears that come up as being a group of individual fears that we can address one at a time. These fears can be summed up as:

1. Fear of Responsibility
2. Fear of Being Alone
3. Fear of the Unknown

Fear of Responsibility

Necessary Separation gives us the room to claim our gifts. Some leave to be an artist or to learn other languages. But the fear of taking responsibility for those gifts is a struggle for most. Not only must they take space to feel their own individual lives, they also need to shelve the family script of what more senior members of the family expected them to become. This is especially poignant when someone is born into a long line of lawyers, doctors, politicians, or the military. Often people in this situation are told what they are going to be when they grow up, rather than asked.

Taking responsibility for our own well-being, including making a living is another form of fear we can face. In the family script, there can be trade-offs where someone supplies money or housing in exchange for you behaving a certain way. The fear of having to make a living for yourself is very prevalent and keeps people enmeshed in the family expectations.

Fear of Being Alone

As Catalysts swim ashore, they must face their fears of being alone in the world. Chances are, they already felt alone in their families if they are carrying burdens that no one else wants to shoulder. But breaking away from the major family scripts entirely can make you feel even more solitary, because the pleasant moments in between unhealthy scripts can also be disrupted if family members react to your new-found independence. This is why it is so essential to have validation and support when a necessary separation is taking place.

At least in the family script, we have a pre-carved-out identity that gives momentary comfort, even if that comfort comes with the illusion that you are not enduring abuse. To maintain an unhealthy script requires our collusion that the script is normal and healthy when it is actually damaging us physically or emotionally. But when we hear our Inner Voice of Truth, we know when change needs to happen.

In order to find empowerment, we will initially face our fear of being alone. We can't expect support from people who are deeply entrenched in the very script that we are leaving. They are out to sea, and if they aren't ready to swim with us to shore, we can't make them do so nor can we force them to see our point of view. Their survival mode will not allow a break in their tunnel vision and they will continue to believe that they are right in staying loyal to unhealthy scripts. Because more people in any given family will be living according to the script rather than without it, they will have more validation than you will have, even if what they are defending is morally wrong. If you spend time with your loneliness, you will discover that your fear is not about being *by* yourself, but rather it is the hesitation to be *with* yourself, for facing who we truly are underneath the scripts and claiming responsibility for that transformation into our outer world.

One benefit of the community that has formed around the workshops and online training programs is that people get to walk a cohesive path of shared liberation with other Catalysts. The idea that you will be completely alone in your transformational journey is not true on a practical level.

Fear of the Unknown

Perhaps the greatest force that hinders self-realization is fear of the unknown. It is our deep-seated mistrust of life that makes us hesitate in taking the next steps in our growth. We want to know that someone has our back. If we have a car accident, we want to be able to call people and have them take care of us. For all the abuses and flaws that can happen in a family, this is one of the things that families can provide. While some families may overburden or harm its members, they may still rise to the occasion when a crisis happens. In that moment of crisis, everyone is in survival mode together. There is a comfort that comes in that togetherness. However, as the crisis fades, you begin to see who stays in the perpetual state of survival mode, even after the danger has passed, and who goes on with their lives in a healthy way.

Survival mode remains active all the time when we fundamentally do not trust our lives. The state of trusting life feels like your Essence is a star in a reserved space in the sky. You are right where you need to be, and life is unfolding naturally around you.

Prolonged Victimhood

The biggest trap to the process of unburdening is over-identifying with a victim-based role. I think of victimhood has a necessary transitional role that has an expiration date. When someone was just attacked and is filling out the paperwork at the police office, it is completely appropriate to be the victim. At this moment, you deserve the care and attention necessary to heal and seek justice. Very often, if that attention has not been given and justice has not been served, the role of victim is held onto for years later, as if to serve as evidence that an injustice has happened. Once this trap has solidified, it becomes a habit that is tough to release. In fact, we often find ways to use our past victimhood in our relationships to try and get what we need emotionally rather than trusting that if we ask for something, we will receive it.

If someone who was just victimized by a crime was given empathy, validation, and the offending party was held accountable, then there would be no reason to hold onto the victim role. But too often these wounds are inflicted and they fester for years, even decades after the offense. We long to have our pain known and for those who hurt us to realize what they have done. So, we build our lives around that hole inside and the lingering victim role becomes part of our personality and influences how we interact in relationships.

It is also possible to enable someone stuck in a victim role to remain in a position of manipulative power by validating their story. In the case of Abigail's mother, she was carrying a lot of genuine pain that she shared with her parents who survived the Holocaust. But rather than expressing that pain in a vulnerable way, she was using the urgency of her needs in domineering ways that were actually deeply impacting to her daughter. While most people would normally just back away and allow her mother to behave this way under normal circumstance given what her family had been through, the victim role doesn't hold up when they see her badgering her pregnant daughter while she is in labor. Her mother was holding onto the victim role, as if she were an abandoned orphan who was about to lose attention to the new sibling. Yet this is absurd given the fact that she was in fact the grandmother who could be mentoring her daughter through a beautiful, and arduous, rite of passage.

The Ancestral Dialogue reveals the core wounds which put us into some kind of victim-based role. It gives us our day in court and our chance to receive the empathy and support that we never got when we were first hurt so that we don't carry the victimhood into unrelated areas of our life. The role that we play in that story gives us a place in our family, even if it's not the place we wanted in life. From that moment forth we become the silent victim or the screaming rebel (both roles are born from being victimized.) Every moment that the abuse has not been addressed leaves a fingerprint on us. Then everything that we look at has the smudges of fingerprints over it, like looking through a window touched by greasy fingers. The Ancestral Dialogue points out the smudges and helps the Catalyst to wipe the window clean so that they can see and be seen.

The 4th Realization

Wounds are pathways to Empathy and Compassion

Vision for Realization #4

The vest had reached the floor of the ocean. Her chest was bare, and her heart felt open. It was the first time she had been free of the burden, that emotional weight that she had carried since childhood. She was breaking free of her co-dependency on her family, realizing that she no longer needed to take care of fully-grown adults, as she had done when they were all younger. As she looked down at her chest, the place where that burden had lived for so many years, she noticed a wound. It was shaped like a jagged slash down her chest. Tracing the edges of her wound with her fingers, she could feel her heart more intimately. It was filled with a mixture of pain and grief. As she noticed the feelings, they moved out of the wound like smoke from a chimney. She cried, the emotional release bringing her relief.

As her former numbness gave way to a stream of emotions, many memories from the past began to surface. As a child, when she asked her parents for what she needed, they scolded her for being too "needy." When she tried to rebel against the burdens being dumped on her, they punished her and called her "ungrateful." Instead of being loved, she he was punished and called "selfish" until she finally agreed to be the emotional caretaker of her parents and siblings.

This rough treatment forced her to grow up too fast. They conditioned her to devalue her own needs, to go numb, and to be "tough." Eventually, as a ten-year-old, she took on the vest and served her family. When she assumed the role, she was praised for being a "good girl," a loyal servant. To fulfill that role, she had to bury her needs, tears, and eventually the deep rage deep it led to inside her chest. Now that the vest no longer trapped her emotions inside of her chest, they started rising to the surface. She could feel that deeply buried resentment and grief about how she had suffered in silence for so many years.

As he clasped her hands over the open wound in her heart, she cried. This slash in chest was the wound of betrayal. In denying her what she needed most, and ridiculing her for being "selfish," her parents had broken her heart. In her moment of self-empathy, she was able to finally start acknowledging the deep pain of having to betray herself, in return for being a member of the family.

But more than just the pain was surfacing. So, too, were the memories and frustrated dreams. She had wanted to become a dancer. She longed to be on stage, to tell stories using her graceful limbs. In elementary school, she would daydream about her family coming to her dance recitals to cheer her on. She dreamed of joining a ballet company, traveling the world and performing professionally. But her family couldn't see her true gift, nor did they have the mental space to even listen to her dreams. They were all swimmers, trapped in survival mode, just getting through the day. To them, dancing was a frivolous luxury.

As she tore off the vest, she unburdened herself of the role of being her family's caretaker. Now the emotions could flow. Now she could remember what she truly wanted to experience out of life. She was cleansing her wounded heart. She was making room for something inside of her to emerge, to shine forth into the world. From her heart, a fire was emerging. No longer could she ignore her anger about the sacrifices that she had made. The catharsis was necessary to clear the pathway to what needed to come out of her.

Turning back to look at her family, she could still feel the chain in her gut that bound the family together. But she could feel the space between her and her kin growing. The burden of being the caretaker had lifted. The emotions were flowing, and her heart was getting lighter with each release. She wasn't sure how to relate to her family, especially as her yearning to swim to the shore became stronger.

By feeling her emotions, she was waking up to her truth, to what she must do for herself to feel free. But she wasn't yet ready to leave her family. They shared a bond, a heavy bond that was attached to the collective family pain that resided below the surface. She didn't just cry for herself, she cried for them too. Her unfettered heart opened so wide that she could witness their burden. She could feel empathy for the struggle of the family she loved so much. Even for those who hurt had her the most. She could feel how hard it was for them to make it through each day, and how unaware they were of just treading water as they looked at her in bewilderment as she tore off that vest.

Another courageous step had been taken. She was reclaiming her heart, and with it she reclaimed her capacity for empathy. By feeling the wound in her heart, it had become a pathway to an emerging light that had been buried inside of her for many years.

Wounds as Pathways

The wound is the place where the light enters you. ~Rumi

The "light" that Rumi referred to can be interpreted as a new awareness entering into our consciousness. By feeling the pain inside a wound, we discover the untapped strengths inside of us. When we focus our attention on our wounds, they become doorways to new learning. Wounds serve a purpose. They reveal what we truly need in our lives and they challenge us to rise to the occasion in a way that can be empowering.

But if the light of new awareness can enter us through our wounds, as Rumi taught us, then the light of our essence can also shine out of our wounds to the outside world. In other words, our unique identity can radiate outwards to the world through open wounds. Once the wounds are cleaned out through cathartic release of our feelings, there is an opportunity to shine and show something deeper that can be witnessed by people in our lives. Addressing painful abuse can make us dig deep and discover a hidden strength that rises to the challenge of an abusive situation.

When we feel our wounds, we clear a passageway that can be likened to both an inhalation and an exhalation of heartfelt awareness. The inhalation through the wound is called Empathy, which is the ability to experience your own feelings as well as what other people are feeling. The exhalation out of the wound, that warm response to feeling Empathy for another person, is called Compassion.

Empathy and Compassion are the inhale
and exhale of unconditional Love.

Empathy is more than a thoughtful gesture or intellectual acknowledgement of a difficult situation. To illustrate: your best friend

survives a brutal car crash and is expected to make a full recovery. You're about to visit him in the hospital for the first time. Giving him a store-
-bought "Get Well" card with a printed poem inside it is an act of *sympathy*. This gift expresses concern and requires the thoughtful consideration in your brain that acknowledges that your friend went through something difficult. But the act of giving him the card doesn't go deeply into the heart level, especially if the words inside the card are not your own. In contrast, an act of Empathy would be hugging your friend in the hospital bed while he cries in your arms and tells you how scary the experience was for him. It's not just consideration or imagining how hard it was to endure a life-threatening event. It's opening your heart, holding the space for him to cry, and feeling his pain with him. *Empathy* is deeper.

After you receive the intense emotions from him in the hospital bed, it makes you feel grateful that he is still alive. You feel warmth in your heart that moves from your chest to his. Not only can you imagine how hard it was for him in your *head*, you can feel how hard it was for him in your *heart*, and you share warm Compassion to them. Compassion is the loving response to Empathy.

When we tend to our wounds, they become the pathway for exchanging unconditional Love. Empathy is the inhalation that helps you realize the depth of somebody's experience. Compassion is the universal warmth that affirms that someone cares about you, that you deserve a loving response and that you don't need to change who you are to feel that embrace.

Wounds help us to learn how to love and be loved – and this includes self-love.

What is a Wound?

The word "wound" in English comes from a Germanic source that means "a hurt, injury, cut, bruise." As a verb, it means "to strive, to fight, to suffer."[11] Physical wounds are easy to see. A gash in someone's arm is a visible wound. But emotional wounds which come from striving and fighting can leave residual suffering that is often invisible if the story behind that suffering is not shared.

Through the eyes of an Intuitive Healer, those clouds of hurt that we spoke about earlier are the emotional body's reaction to wounds. Our minds and our bodies are linked emotionally, so when we witness or experience a situation that is distressing, the body will react and create clouds of hurt. A wound is that point of impact into the emotional mind-body that is inflicted by a conflict or catastrophe.

If clouds of hurt are the emotional body's reaction to the impact of a wound, then we can trace back the clouds of hurt to their point of origin and arrive at the location of the wound. Very often, that wound will look like a physical bruise, dent, or rip in the emotional body. Symbolic structures, like a sharp object representing betrayal, or a keepsake piece of jewelry symbolizing the loss of a favorite grandmother are often left behind and can give a clue as to how the wound was inflicted.

The wound is the opening where the unfinished stories that we absorb from the outside world reside in our inner world. Many of these stories come from the people who played a direct role in our upbringing. Yet others were absorbed from social interactions or incidents: from school yard fights and bullying to larger societal crises like religious persecution, discrimination and conflicts and wars. Wounds are the living records

---

11   Skeat, Walter W. (2013) *An Etymological Dictionary of the English Language*. Mineola, NY: Dover Publications.

inside our mind-body that tell the story of what we have been exposed to, endured and ultimately absorbed. Think of them as the curriculum of life lessons that can potentially awaken hidden strengths and talents if we give them the attention they need in order to heal.

Hungry Hearts

We all have a hunger in our hearts to be known and loved on a deep level. It is within our human natures to yearn to touch another person deeply, to truly love and know them. Very often it is this need that motivates us to start the process of facing our wounds, and this can often come with overwhelming emotions.

Unless your heart experiences both Empathy and Compassion on a regular basis, your heart will feel starved of love and attention. Most of the world resides in some form of survival mode, which takes the focus of our conscious awareness away from our hearts and into our heads. To feel our hearts, requires that we slow down enough to *feel*. This often means that our emerging wounds will bring us pain that needs to be experienced.

Feeling our wounds is the heart's instinctive way of clearing itself out so that this underlying hunger can be met. The pathway that allows Empathy and Compassion to flow will otherwise be blocked by the emotional blocks that we uncover underneath the burden. As the hunger has room to bubble up, it tells us what we truly need, one of many crucial lessons that our wounds teach us.

If you allow yourself to get close to the hunger, you will encounter its layers. The initial layers often reveal themselves as sadness and envy, like when an emotionally disconnected person watches a couple that is in love dance together. This scene will remind them of the connection and care that they're not experiencing. But staying with those waves of emotions will bring underlying sensations to the forefront. Even people who feel stuck in a loveless partnerships or marriage can feel as they see friends who are in happier relationships.

Once the emotions have washed through your wound, there is a deeper, clearer form of longing in your heart. It's a deep need to connect heart to heart with other people, regardless of whether you are in a relationship with them or not. We need an exchange of love to thrive, that warmth that moves from one person to another when quality attention is given. This longing for quality attention is the motivation behind many of our daily actions, from the clothes we wear to our posts on social media.

As seen in figure 9, longing is the healing force that pulls us through our wounds. On the other side of our wounds, we discover our Inner Fire that burns away the past and reminds us of our passions. This Fire leads to our Gifts, the special talents and abilities that give us purpose. By making life decisions based on our passions and purpose, we become more trusting of our Inner Voice of Truth which has been guiding us to our wounds, passions, and purpose, all along.

That longing to get what we need brings us through the old pain of past disappointments and puts us in contact with a deeper sense of Love. Following our longing brings us to our truest expressions of ourselves. We long to know who we are, to love ourselves for who we are, and to love and be loved in that truth. Longing brings us to that inner space where self-love and love of others happens.

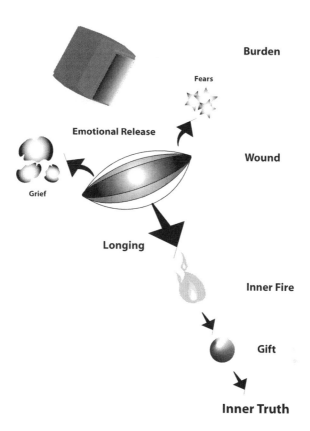

Figure 9. The Movement of Longing
from a Burden to our Inner Truth

Empathy: Receiving the Wound

When an empathic connection is made between two people, they are essentially receiving each others' wounds. When this happens, we hold each others' wounds and we feel them together, providing support that reassures you that you are not alone in your pain. Empathy is a form of emotional holding that brings acceptance to what has happened to you, including to how you were harmed in the past.

231

Now recall the body maps featured in the previously mentioned study "Bodily Maps of Emotions" that resembled the clouds of hurt.[12] These body maps give us a basic visual of what wounds look like in the body. These clouds of hurt are reminiscent of Doppler radars that show storm clouds on a weather map. The clouds show the location and movement of emotions. Think of the wounds themselves as the canyons below the emotional clouds, those splits in the skin of the earth that were torn by the scrapping of glaciers. Likewise, on the body maps, the emotional clouds are covering the deeper wounds, those splits in the emotional body underneath the clouds of hurt.

By sharing an empathic bond with another person, you invite the wound to open up, allowing those clouds to flow from the wound. As the emotions are expressed, the clouds eventually dissipate, like mist evaporating from a canyon. Inside the clarified opening of the wound lie the fiery passions and innate gifts waiting to emerge. Empathy is the force that draws out the pain so that our buried treasures can surface.

The cure for pain is the pain. ~Rumi

The Wounding Process

Wounds help us to reach our essence, the deepest point of origin in our being from where our most authentic identity emanates. A wound begins with a tear in our emotional body from either a conflict or catastrophe. This perforation creates an opening to the essence of our true identity, making the wound like a tunnel into the place where our Inner Voice of Truth originates.

---

12   Bodily Maps of Emotions. 2014. 111(2): 646-651.

The space underneath the opening in the wound fills up with emotions connected to the unfinished story that created the wound. These emotions are made up of those hard feelings sent to us from the person or situation that is hurting us, as well as our own emotional reactions to being wounded.

The emotional pain can be so uncomfortable that at the time it is usually inconceivable to consider that anything good can come of it. In order to cope with the pain, we use the mechanisms at our disposal, which could be choosing to feel the pain and expressing the hurt we feel or to package it up by covering the wound. We cover up the wound by pretending that we aren't hurt, using a mask to hide the cut in our emotional body. At this moment, an emotional burden is formed by a mix of the emotions we empathically took in from our inflictor and our own reactions to the wounding.

This bundle of emotions doesn't come with instructions on how to process the experience in a healthy way. Unless you are able to hear your Inner Voice of Truth clearly, moving through the healing process of a wound can be a process of trial and error. Instead of instructions on how to heal what has happened, we get the familiar script on how we are expected to behave, including how you carry the wound and what you are allowed to express about your experience. These scripts are tied into the family expectations and are enforced by the family members who are in power.

For example, a suspicious daughter follows her father to discover that he is cheating with another woman. The discovery breaks her heart. She fleas the scene without him knowing because she feels ashamed at what she has just seen. Now she hears multiple voices in her head. Some of those voices express their own pain. Some express empathy for her mother who doesn't know what is happening. Then there are the voices that come up from the family script that tell her to protect the secrets of her family, to keep her mouth shut and to mind her business. In this overwhelming moment, when the anger, sadness, and fear about what might happen to her family as so strong, the script can speak to her very loudly. She might not be able to hear her conscience yet.

In the absence of clear guidance on how to address an emotional wound, our best asset is our curiosity about the stories we carry inside our wounds. By looking through the opening to the script, in additions to the clouds of hurt that emerge from the wound, we might also catch a glimpse of something shiny on the other end of the opening. These are our Innate Gifts, our unclaimed talents and abilities that our wounds make discoverable.

When a singer pours her heart out in a song, the truth of her expression touches the listeners. The singer has a gift for making notes and keeping a melody. When the truth of her experience pours through her vocal gifts, a truly inspiring experience is created. To be able to express the pain and triumph, the love and the loss contained in that song, she would have needed to have those experiences through past wounding, to truly share the song with feeling and authenticity. The beauty of the singer's gift moves through the song based on her life experience.

Healing the Wound

When a wound is inflicted, it is highly unlikely that we have the means to attend to it immediately. Almost always, we need to cover it up and hold the emotions inside until we can find a safe place to unpack it. It may take a long time to find that safe place to address the wound, so to protect ourselves we bring our conscious attention away from hurt, often denying that it even happened. This denial allows us to resume our daily routines to some degree, but it also puts us in a state of survival mode.

Once we come out of survival mode, we have an opportunity to rediscover the wound from which we chose to emotionally detach. This invisible burden can manifest itself physically and be felt as pressure, pain, or tension. Because the burden sits on top of the wound and can even sit inside of the wound, it helps us to locate where the wound is inside our bodies. The burden will contain the negative judgments and external expectations connected to our responsibilities to family, community and work. It contains all the reasons why the wound should not be touched and so it acts as a shield that keeps the wound from being reopened.

This shield is temporarily beneficial by 'keeping things under wraps' so that we can function. But in the long-term, the shield delays the healing process because the burden does not get separated from the wound enough to allow the release of the emotions.

This separation between the wound and the burden can be *temporary* for the sake of cleaning out the wounds, or *permanent* if it feels like the responsibilities and expectations held in the burden no longer fit your life.

Temporary unburdening: Ray's father ran off when he was just seven years old, leaving his mom to fend for herself and the rest of the family. His father's irresponsibility left Ray with a sense of abandonment and the determination to be a super responsible father to his own children. By taking some time out from his role as a father and leaving his children in the care of a trusted babysitter for a weekend, Ray was able to take the time for some introspection. This temporary reprieve gave him the space to address his wounds before again carrying the responsibility of being a father to his children and all the family expectations that come along with that role.

Permanent unburdening: Kim, the middle sibling in her family, had never felt recognized by her parents. Her youngest brother demanded constant attention from her parents as they did damage control because of his anti-social behavior. Her parents would be called into school regularly and would receive regular visits from the police because of petty vandalism he would get involved in. As a teenager, he developed a serious drug habit. Kim faded into the background and followed the family script. She covered up for her brother and did not discuss the family issues outside of the family. As an adult, she decided to stop playing that role in the script and refused to enable her addict brother financially or emotionally as she could see how carrying that burden enabled him to remain in his addiction. She released all responsibility for his wellbeing. The burden no longer fitted her life.

Once we are in a safe environment and the burden has been separated from the opening of the wound, the next step of the healing process begins with carefully re-opening the wound so that it can release the emotions that are held inside. The process of unburdening and opening up the wound for cathartic release allows you to hear the script that delayed the healing process to this point. As discussed earlier, when you break the script and allow yourself to *feel*, it's like a director of a movie yelling "Cut!" You put down the expected role and you come out of character. When you are done with the expected scene, you can take the costume off, wash off the make-up, and then come back to the person you are, outside of the role. You are no longer repeating lines or acting in a certain way to please others. You simply feel how you feel. You give yourself permission to just be yourself.

Catharsis creates space inside of the wound. As the expression of emotions cleans out the wound, the opening of the wound becomes the unobstructed space of potential. When enough pain has moved out of the wound, the wound becomes a pathway to our Inner Fire, which is the source of our passion, as well as our Innate Gifts, which are the gifts and talents that give us a sense of purpose. By opening the wounds and discovering our passions and purpose, we move towards connecting with our Inner Voice of Truth, the most authentic source of our identities.

Wounding in Action

Albert is swinging his baseball bat in the back yard to practice his swing. He recently joined a baseball team and his new teammates picked on him for being the new kid. They laughed at him for constantly striking out and not being able to hit the ball. The experience left him feeling ashamed, especially since his family had newly immigrated to the United States, and he only recently started playing baseball. To Albert, playing baseball is not just about fun. It is about being more American, and fitting in. As the newcomer, he wants acceptance, and to win the respect of his peers.

He asks his father to help him learn how to swing the bat properly so that he will be able to hit the ball. But his father hasn't played baseball before. Albert's father feels the pressure to teach his son something that he doesn't know how to do. The pressure of his son's expectation makes him feel insecure, especially since he never knew his own father and had no model as to how to connect with his son. As a fatherless child, he feels shame and fear as he faces the expectation of helping his son fit in. Rather than showing vulnerability to his son and confessing that he doesn't know how to play baseball, he lashes out.

"Albert, you should know how to do this already. Be tough!" he says. He storms off into the house and slams the door behind him, seemingly irritated by his son's request.

What just happened here? Let's put on our intuitive goggles and visualize what happened in the emotional bodies of the father and son during this interaction. Albert had red around his head, because he is mad that his teammates made fun of him for not being able to hit the ball. His teammates all grew up playing baseball together, but Albert was new to the game. In Albert's chest, there is also red, and the rest of his body is covered in a black smoke because he feels ashamed of not being able to play baseball.

Albert needs support. He asks his father, expecting him to be the safe man that will help him through his difficult adjustment to a new language, a new school, and his attempts to make new friends. Albert and his father are connected by a tube of support between their bellies. The tube can be visualized as an emotional anchor, with the parent being a steady support for their child. Albert pulls on the cord with his expectation that his father will be able to save him from future embarrassment by showing him how to develop a powerful swing.

Albert's father, at his son's request for help, begins to feel pressure as Albert tugs on their support tube. Fear arises, like scattered yellow and black bees from his stomach, as his son triggers some old fears about being abandoned by his father. Albert's father never knew his own father and never had a male figure to show him how to take care of a son. He was figuring it out for himself and learned not to ask for help from others, for fear of rejection. The father learned to be tough and self-reliant, believing that by not needing anyone, he would never have to feel rejected again.

After the fear, Albert's father has dark clouds of shame come up and a fiery red glow emerges in his chest. He learned to be ashamed of having needs, because being needy was judged as being weak. His father didn't want to feel all these insecurities, so his motivation switched from helping his son, to finding the quickest escape from the situation in order to avoid the emerging emotions. Instead of trying to help his son, he chose to send a judgment to Albert with his words. "You should already know how to do this. Be tough!"

As these words leave the father's mouth, a sharp arrow-like object shoots into Albert's heart. The arrow sinks into his heart and Albert's chest lights up in frantic waves of yellow, signifying the shock from his father's verbal attack. The area around the arrow turns a deep burgundy and violet, as if a bruise is forming in his emotional body. His father was shaming him for not learning how to be capable at baseball sooner, while also implying that Albert is too soft and needs to toughen up. In a misguided way, his father was "toughening up" Albert, and in so doing, also abandoning him. When his father turned away and walked to the house, the tube of support yanked free from Albert's stomach. His father was just trying to get away from the tense conversation so that he didn't have to feel his *own* shame and fear in that moment. The belly area of Albert's emotional body tore open and began leaking clear clouds of energy. In this moment, Albert felt an intense nausea, like his guts were pouring out of him. It made him feel drained and weak.

The arrow-like cloud that came from the judgmental words of his father pierced his heart. This was a form of betrayal, because Albert was asking for help and his father chose to shame him instead. When the cord of support was ripped away by the father's abrupt escape from the conversation, Albert was emotionally abandoned. This was signified by the tearing away of the cord of support between them. Unconsciously, his father was saying "Albert, don't ask me for this kind of help again. I can't give it to you, and I don't want to feel the emotions that your expectations are triggering."

The breaking down of this wounding moment between father and son is only a snapshot of the repeated multi-generational process. Although

Albert's father did not know his own father, there were still times when as a young boy, he asked other men for help. The judgment passed down to Albert was not new. Many men in his family had heard the message, "be tough, don't be soft," and the wounding was unwittingly passed down to the younger generations. It was meant to tell men to stand on their own two feet and to kill off that need for help from others, in a false effort to become impervious to judgment and rejection.

When a wound of this nature is inflicted, it not only changes a relationship between father and son in that moment, but it often shifts how the son sees all his relationships, including his relationship with his future son. Albert had a genuine need for support as he adjusted to a new life in a new country. He asked his father for help, but instead received a wound. If this wounding is left untreated, it leads to forming limiting beliefs, such as "having a need is bad." That belief can be passed onto the next generation, which will prevent them from being confident members of their families and communities.

Time alone doesn't heal all wounds. When we follow unhealthy scripts, we prevent the wounds from necessarily re-opening so that the shards of judgments and emotional puss can be cleaned out of the wound. Wounds require adequate time to be addressed, as well as the careful attention and guidance in order to fully heal. The time spent ignoring your wounds has no impact on the healing process, no matter how many decades they are denied. Unless we acknowledge the presence our wounds in a meaningful way, they will not heal on their own.

Empowering Surrender

Many cultures view people emotional vulnerability as a weakness. Public displays of emotion are judged and shamed. Part of the reason that unconscious people react by shaming the person who is displaying emotion (the Catalyst) is because emotional expression interrupts the expected script that the family and local community lives by. Being off script makes them feel exposed and unsure of themselves. Without the normal pleasantries and routines, fear arises. As a way of stopping the fear from coming up, stopping the Catalyst from triggering the emotions has been built into many cultural scripts as a way of sustaining the status quo. A common example is the person who cries first at a funeral. Some people will react strongly to the crying and will either discourage the emotional expression or simply leave the room so that their emotions don't also get triggered. Those who are ready to grieve will feel an unspoken permission to also emote because the Catalyst has given them an unspoken permission to express how they feel. They break the script of the normal routine and go with the flow of their emotions.

This shaming is so prevalent across numerous cultures that it's difficult to see how surrendering to your feelings can be an empowering act. However difficult it may be to find emotionally safe places to explore a sense of surrender, there are great benefits to doing so. Cleaning out the wound makes room for us to claim the rewards inside the wound. Surrender begins with allowing your emotions to flow without being censored or needing to explain why you are upset.

Empowering surrender happens when you allow your heartbreak to happen. Instead of burying and denying your emotions deep inside a wound, instead of fighting to control how you feel, letting your wound release the hurt can have a positive effect. While the initial pain of the wound may be overwhelming, these feelings do not last indefinitely. You are feeling them as they are being let go, and eventually, when they have been fully acknowledged, they leave your body. In the same way a broken bone heals back stronger if given the right care and attention, our hearts can grow back more aware and resilient as a result of recovering from a betrayal.

Passing through the wound means that we stay honest with ourselves about how we feel, even when we are expected to behave in a certain way. Be real with yourself and share your story with your most trusted supporters. By doing so, you not only surrender to how you feel, but you begin to surrender to how you, as a unique individual, have been shaped by these hardships.

Wounds Are Specific

As the waves of emotions flow from a wound, our mind becomes temporarily overwhelmed, making it difficult to track the details of the surfacing memory. This is the point in the healing process when people say, "I don't even know why I am crying." Intellectually, it is true that they don't consciously know they are feeling intense emotions. But just because we can't articulate *why* we are having emotions doesn't mean that the wounds are random. Emotions take time to surface from our unconscious awareness before we understand what memory we had been holding inside.

Wounds are astoundingly specific. Before Maya Angelou found her voice as an author in her first book, *I Know Why the Caged Bird Sings,* she spent many childhood years in silence after being wounded by her family members. She was judged by her family in emotionally damaging ways. But her withdrawal into silence, after being wounded, helped her to recognize her own independent voice outside the emotionally harmful script of her family's voices. Her gifts of writing and keen perceptive abilities were developed as a form of expression to address the inner pain she was feeling. Without the wounding, she might not have had the same motivation to seek solace and the resulting expressions that came from it. In her writing, she expressed both the pain and insight that her family could not hear. The wounds she inherited played a direct part in discovering her voice as an author. The writing process was a part of her healing process, opening up wounds, expressing her challenges creatively, and ultimately claiming her gifts which have touched millions of people.

In the previous example of Albert who was verbally wounded by his father when he asked him to teach him about baseball, the father's response was very specific. The father didn't indiscriminately shame Albert by saying something like, "you will never amount to anything," or, "you're not American, so you'll never be good at baseball." The father said, "You should know how to do this already. Be tough!" While the response is not what Albert expected, the wounding by his father was a direct challenge. However painful it may have felt to Albert to receive a challenge instead of empathy and support, Albert still had a choice in how he was going to approach the wound. He could choose to be heartbroken and to collapse into defeat. Or, instead of giving up, Albert could summon his willpower and meet the challenge of his father by becoming an expert in baseball.

Ancestral Dialogue: Breathing Through the Wounds

Releasing burdens can greatly enhance your ability to feel your body. With the newfound relief and space after the unburdening, we can feel the location of the wounds in our body more completely. Our body awareness becomes more acute, so finding the wounds, hiding underneath the burdens, becomes easier.

- Begin this exercise by vigorously patting down your body with your palms. As you slap the body, it becomes more alive. This helps you to think less and feel more.

- After a minute or so of the vigorous pat down, take five deep, conscious breaths by inhaling through your nose and feeling the air leave your body through your lips.

- Invite a safe and supportive ancestor to make a heart connection with you. Their job will be to hold you emotionally with empathy. In the event that this directive is outside of your beliefs, recall the memory of a deceased family member who loved you or a safe friend (living or deceased) who makes your heart feel warm. You can also do this as a partner exercise with a program buddy or therapist by asking them to connect empathically to you.

- Now resume breathing normally while you feel your body. What sensations do you notice? Where do you feel tingling? Where do you feel pressure or pain? Where do you feel movement?

- Pick an area of your body to focus on with the intention of finding a wound. It may be an area that you have recently felt during the unburdening, or it might be another area that needs your attention.

- Once you have settled on one area of the body that feels like it might be a wound, allow a vision of the wound to appear. In your mind, it may look like a split or scar of some kind. It might look like an opening. It can even appear as a dark spot, like a bruise on that area of your body. There is no standard or "right" image or symbol. Just trust what arises.

- Allowing your breath to continue normally, feel the air around you being pulled in through the wound and into your body with every inhale. Feel the exhale coming out of the wound when you breathe out.

- Continue to breathe through the wound for several minutes. With each breath, you are getting more in touch with the

feelings in the wound. Each inhale and exhale cleans out the wound, helping to clear a path for your innate gifts to surface.
- Observe whatever physical sensations, emotions, images, or memories pop up, allowing the wound to tell its story to you, making it conscious.
- When you feel like the wound has given you the experience it was offering today, journal about the experience.
- As you read over what you have written, see if you can feel some empathy for yourself and for what you have been through.

Doing this exercise build up your capacity for self-empathy. Exploring the story that you are carrying gives you more awareness about who you are now as a result of the past.

As you do this, you may experience physical sensations that are very powerful or unexpected. Keep in mind that your physical body is very connected to your deeper emotions. It is possible for the physical movement of emotions to manifest physically. One such common example is when someone feels like they are going to vomit because of strong emotional news that has nothing to do with what they've just eaten. If you feel like you are having dry heaves or a coughing fit, just breathe and allow your body to have its reactions. The reactions will subside given time. The body is wise, and it knows how to release emotional experiences if you create the space for it to do so. At the end of the cathartic release, you will feel relief and spaciousness.

Wounds Inspire Empathy

It helps us to relate to those who have endured similar pain when we've been hurt. When we learn that others have been through a similar ordeal, we're able to extend a sense of Empathy towards them. In that moment, we can feel what the other person is going through. The breathing in of their experience into our hearts is Empathy. It is the inhalation of the exchange of Love.

In this way, shared pain can forge a bridge between two strangers. I have witnessed how people from completely different backgrounds are moved to hug each other after only a day or two of meeting at my workshops. Because they share common ground through what they have survived and endured, they're able to empathize with each other. All it takes to forge this new bridge is to be vulnerable enough to share what you have been going through.

Empathy becomes a gift in that it allows a deeper connection between people than the scripted routines of day-to-day interactions. Empathy allows us to open up and be vulnerable, allowing meaningful exchanges of common experiences. When being truly vulnerable, we are not reading from a polite script, rather we take a risk and express our authentic feelings, ideas, dreams, and desires.

To open our hearts to another person is to take a risk, because by sharing something meaningful about ourselves, we can either receive supportive empathy from the listener or can leave ourselves open to being judged or criticized. We are essentially letting down our defenses, our disguises, and breaking protocol of what we are supposed to talk about with new people. We are facing our fears of being judged, rejected, or shunned for revealing what we have been through. Practicing empathy in safe environments, such as with trusted friends, support groups, and with counselors, can help us to expand our hearts and make new connections with like-hearted people.

The most immediate reward we receive from practicing empathy is the sudden realization that we are no longer alone in our pain. When that empathic bridge is formed, we are not suffering in silence, rather we are releasing pain in unison with other sentient beings. A loving field forms around people who share openly from their hearts. Within that field, empathy draws out the dormant emotions that have been held inside for a long time. Empathy clears the path for the warmth of compassion to extend from one heart to another.

Wound-Based Identity

Wounds are the openings to a deeper sense of identity that is connected to our Inner Voice of Truth. Wounds are not the actual source of our identity. When people hesitate to care for their wounds, they can get stuck in a wound-based identity. This is an image of who they *think* that they are rather than an earnest revelation of the loveable being they are on the other side of their wounds.

We can attach our identity to any pain that we've endured. A woman who has been body-shamed for being overweight can see herself as the "big girl" in a group of friends. She can even make daily life decisions, such as what to wear that day, based on that self-image, and may not even stop to notice how she truly feels about herself when she looks in the mirror. Instead of seeing herself as a loveable person, she self-inflicts the shame, judgments, and ridicule she's been subjected to. This wound-based identity will often eclipse her talents, kindness, and character that would otherwise inform her identity if she hadn't been emotionally wounded.

To transcend wound-based identities, we need to look beyond our wounds to discover our passion and sense of purpose on the other side of the wound's opening. Specifically, we transcend wound-based identities by discovering our Inner Fire as the source of our Passion, and our Innate Gifts as the source of our Purpose. It is the passionate expressions of our special talents that can help us heal the wounds. Expressing yourself not only helps you cope with suffering; it also helps you to experience a more authentic part of yourself. For instance, singing about your hurt makes you feel better. The more you self-soothe in this way, the more you discover that you actually have a strong and engaging voice. You feel passion surge through your body when you sing, making you feel alive and empowered. It makes you want to explore this part of yourself more fully. Rather than being the child that was abandoned, you become the singer who moves people to feel their hearts.

Innate gifts are a cleaner way to discover our identities rather than getting stuck in an image of ourselves based on what we've endured. Think of gifts as the light at the other side of the tunnel that is the wound. Gifts are not the ultimate definer of our identities, but they are important stepping stones to our deepest truth. We are meant to discover our gifts as we clean out the wounds of the past. They are the rewards, the wisdom connected to who we are inside. Gifts bring us in touch with our purpose, which helps give meaning to why we had to endure the pain of the past.

Group Empathy: Helen's Keening

A workshop participant, Helen, demonstrated the sheer power of group empathy in her Ancestral Dialogue. Group empathy is when the experience of one member of the group is being open-heartedly received by numerous people at the same time. Helen was a lively woman in her late 50s, a strong Irish American woman who came from a lineage of tough matriarchs. Several members of her family had died young, and her family was emotionally overwhelmed by the accumulated burden of unexpressed grief. Her mother and maternal grandmother had both died early. Shortly after losing them, her husband died. There were also cousins, aunts, and uncles who had passed away, leaving her feeling very alone in the world. There was hardly anyone left in the family, except for one young daughter. As she shared the layers of devastation with the group, her story reminded me of Frank McCourt's memoir *Angela's Ashes*.

Not only was she carrying the grief of losing the people whom she had personally known, she was also carrying an enormous package of unexpressed sorrow that her mother and maternal grandmother experienced. Both of the previous matriarchs had lost children and their husbands. It made them sorrowful. Their grief from these deaths either pre-dated Helen's birth or happened when she was only a child, so she grew up in a household filled with unexpressed sorrow. She absorbed it like a sponge. Neither Helen's mother, nor her grandmother, ever cried about loss in front of her. They were taught to be staunch Irish women who showed their spine in the face of adversity, never their tears. They learned this way from the countless matriarchs who had done the same, unwittingly handing down their sadness to the next generation of women. They silently shared the pain as part of their unspoken bond. By not crying in front of their daughters, they never got to show the younger women how to release the pain. Helen absorbed that grief, like thick dark clouds that became packed ash in her chest and throat.

Helen was surrounded with highly empathic staff members and participants, including a big-hearted facilitator, Dina. As we faced the ancestor table, Helen made a wish that she and her daughter be healthy and at peace. Then she shared the long list of people who had died in her family. The group gathered closer and people shared how they could collectively feel the pain that Helen had absorbed. She had been an empathic sponge for so many other women, particularly the matriarchs. Now, it was her turn to release.

Dina placed her hand on Helen's chest and began to wail what she sensed in Helen's heart. Dina's shuddering cry splashed over the rest of the group. To me, it looked as if bluish-purple waves washed over people's heads and then sank into their chests. Tears sprung forth in the eyes of many participants and they too began to grieve. We could feel the sheer mass of the unexpressed sorrow. When I looked at Helen, it looked as if there was a jagged meteorite-shaped burden on her shoulders. It was the combined responsibilities that were left behind by numerous deaths along with the unspoken hurt that was never buried when the bodies were laid to rest. Helen's heart looked like a red crater surrounded by a body filled with dark tar. As I scanned what she carried, it was clearly more than one person could bear alone. The grief appeared to have bottlenecked because there was only one matriarch left to hold it. The tears shed by Dina and the participants siphoned off some of the burden. The grief that Helen carried touched the grief inside of them, creating a bridge of relating. By opening that group empathy, the participants were helping Helen by relating to her, but also helping themselves by giving themselves permission to acknowledge their own pain of losing loved ones and the struggle of carrying their burdens alone.

That's how grieving works. When one piece of grief moves, all of the stored memories that relate to loss move with it. That's the beauty of group empathy. Everyone gets to benefit. The tears of the participants eroded away Helen's tough Irish exterior, like ocean waves lapping against a statue made of black volcanic rock. *Lap, lap, lap* until, eventually, the floodgates opened, and Helen's face exploded into wet sobs. She slammed her hands on the pillows in front of her, angrily shouting at her deceased mother and grandmother. "How come you never cried when Daddy died!? How come none of you ever cried at any of the funerals!" Helen screamed. "It made me feel so weird about being sad. How could you be like that?!" She was breaking the script by letting her feelings pour forth. Painful pockets of repressed grief rolled up her spine, causing momentary flashes of pain in her head. Her heart beamed orange in the center and red at the edges, like a neon curdling custard pie. The rage flowed and popped her head like a hot popcorn kernel.

When the fire cooled, Helen cried gently. Many of the women in the group hugged her, forming a compassionate cocoon. In that embrace, she also felt the nurturing apology of her mother and grandmother in spirit.

"Mom and Grandma, I can feel you with me," she said. Expressing the anger had helped her to crack that hard shell. She felt the cool streams of support from the former matriarchs seep into her body. It felt soothing, helping her to forgive the way they were, the way they had taught her to be. It helped to calm the inflamed ache in her head and neck.

"Be sure to pass this on to your daughter. Show her how this is done," I said to Helen. "It's okay to cry in front of her about the loss of your husband. That's how the script is fully broken, when the next generation grows up differently and doesn't have to face what you had to endure."

When the group empathy had subsided, Helen turned to the group to share a story.

"I went to Africa in 1986 to help build a hospital for children as part of a charity effort. While we were there, a young African woman was holding her infant. The infant was breathing its last few breaths of life. Everybody knew that the baby was dying. All the other women of the town gathered around her in a circle and hugged the distraught mother. The young mother cried out in pain, and the women surrounding her began to cry as well in a collective grieving. They held the baby until it passed away. In that moment, I realized how much trouble we are in. We Americans are fractured. I know that because we wouldn't do what those

African women did. It was so human. Now almost 30 years later, I finally get to experience what that felt like. Thank you."

After her process, I shared with Helen that her group process reminded me a lot of the ancient Irish practice of Keening. To mourn the loss of a family member, the pre-Christian practice vocalized the pain together in groups.[13] This ensured that the family did not hold the pain, and it was also a way of honoring how much they missed the deceased. She had instinctually tapped into an ancient practice of her ancestry.

Exercise: Keening to Your Ancestors

This exercise can be greatly enhanced by doing it together with other people to create a sense of group empathy. It can also be done alone in front of the ancestor table.

- Choose a safe Ancestor
  - Tell the story of what you are still grieving to them
  - Put your hand on the part of your body that is holding onto the tensions, stress, or pain as you speak about the story.
  - Make the sound of the anguish that you are holding inside of your wound with the intention of sharing that pain with your ancestors. You are not actively hurting or burdening anyone by sharing your pain. You're simply releasing the pain with the empathic support of your lineage.
  - Whether you believe that someone is listening or not, remember that you are listening to yourself while keening. The catharsis will help clean out the wound and help the deeper layers of the wound to become clear.

---

13   Keller, M.S. (2013). Expressing, Communication, Sharing, and Representing Grief and Sorrow with Organized Sound

The 4th Birthright

Compassion, The Exhale of Love

When the Dalai Lama visited Hawaii in 2012, he used the traditional Hawaiian greeting called the honi when he greeted the local students. The honi is when two people touch noses and breathe in each other's breath. That breath is referred to as *ha* which means the "breath of life," Each person is both inhaling and exhaling the life force from each other. [14] Every greeting also includes the word *aloha*, which can be translated as to direct (alo) your breath of life (ha) towards the person you are greeting. By engaging in the Hawaiian honi, the Dalai Lama was partaking in a

---

14   Pukui, Haertig, Lee (1972) Nānā I Ke Kumu Look to the
      Source Vol. 1; Honolulu, HI; Hui Hānai

physical expression of taking in another person's breath and sharing his own breath in the greeting.

The act of sharing Empathy and Compassion, the inhale and exhale of love, when we are exchanging intimate stories connected to our wounds is a deeper form of this same exchange. After we receive the emotional state of another person through Empathy, the inhale, we are touched by their story. Our heart reacts to this story in a kind way that helps us to relate to their struggles and their will to grow. We put ourselves in their shoes and feel what they are going through. When the inhale of Empathy is complete, our heart's natural response is Compassion.

The warmth that emanates back to the person whom we've just empathically received is Compassion, the exhale of Love. It completes the heart connection between both people, allowing each member to exchange breath, both the inhale and exhale of each other's experience. With the vulnerability of heart sharing, we exchange meaningful energy that furthers our true understanding of each other. Wounds, and the emotional stories held inside of them, can inspire meaningful connection by inspiring Compassion.

In order to prepare our hearts for making a Compassionate connection with others, it helps to release whatever heavy emotions may be held inside your chest. Grieving is the act of catching up with your heart, giving it a chance to express how it still feels about the unresolved past. Paying attention to your heart by giving it self-empathy makes space for warmth to be created.

Grieving: The Art of Recovering your Heart

If each human being was allowed to fully experience their feelings precisely at the moment when they were hurt or frightened, grieving would be a less mysterious process because all the emotions we felt in that moment would immediately be expressed. There would be no mistaking how we felt in that moment, because the emotional response would happen without delay.

Instead of immediately feeling and expressing our feelings during a crisis, what often happens is that we switch into some form of survival mode so that we can escape from potential harm or somehow manage the situation. Because most people are not skilled at stepping out of survival mode when the danger has passed, the feelings such as fear, sadness, and anger get stored up inside the heart.

What makes grief confusing is that the stored-up feelings are not directly related to your current reality. While feelings of the past can be brought up by similar circumstances, the stored-up feelings come from events that had already happened a long time ago. The head's intellect is linear and wants to match events and emotions up chronologically. The heart has its own way of processing the past and doesn't necessary distinguish between a heartbreak that happened when you were a teenager and the break-up you experienced this afternoon. To the heart, the pain is all mixed together. When an opening to feel that pain comes, the heart wants to open up and pour it all out without sorting out the origin of the pain. The heart just wants to cry and shout to expunge the past. If the focus of our conscious awareness is in our intellect during this time of emotional release, the catharsis of the heart won't necessarily make rational sense, at least not right away. It's often after the heart has released its emotional blockages that our brain is able to debrief the experience and sort out what feelings came from which memory of past conflict.

The function of grieving is to reconcile the past. It's a way to bring your heart into the present moment. Grieving is our internal process that allows us to catch up with what has happened to us, which makes space for us to exchange empathy and compassion with other people.

Grieving is a form of self-love, because you are dedicating your caring attention to the wellbeing of your own heart. By feeling your emotions, you are courageously valuing how you feel. Why else would you endure feeling uncomfortable physical sensations and emotional releases unless you cared about your heart's capacity to give and receive love?

Unexpressed Grief

Grief is a combination of many emotions. But the two "movers" in the grieving process are anger and sadness. Expressing the outrage for betrayals and losses moves our Inner Fire through our wounds. Crying and releasing sadness unloads the heaviness that is packed inside our wounds. The anger helps us claim our right to be upset. Sadness helps us feel past loss, allowing us to appreciate how much that person meant to us and making room for new heart connections to form.

Unexpressed grief can be detrimental to your physical heath. People actively going through bereavement can have physical symptoms such as indigestion, chest pain, dizziness, and headaches. To avoid feeling the grief, higher amounts of alcohol and painkillers may be consumed eventually leading to possible detrimental health problems associated with excessive use. People in bereavement can get infections more often, have higher blood pressure, and are more likely to have physical ailments than those who didn't lose a close loved one. [15] Spouses who lose a partner have higher mortality rates. Grief can have a profound impact on our physical and emotional well-being.

It's possible to grieve the loss of a relationship with someone who is still alive, such as in the case of a break-up, divorce, or the loss of contact

15   Stroebe, M. PhD, Schut, H. PhD, Stroebe, W. PhD. "Health Outcomes in Bereavement" *The Lancet.* Vol 370 Issue 9603 (2007) Pgs 1960-1973. Print.

with a family member or friend. When we lose a job, we lose access to the work community and a sense of purpose that comes with that roles. These losses are easier to understand than inherited grief that predates your birth.

When we look at the generational impact of harboring grief, there is covert damage to the younger generations, because a parent with unexpressed grief will be less emotionally available. There is less room in their heart to empathically connect with their children, and the warm response of compassion is not generated on a consistent basis. It's as if part of their heart becomes quarantined by holding onto the frozen emotions from the past. When filled with a lot of unresolved grief, the heart is a painful place to feel, so less of the heart is available to supply nurturing, celebration, support, and validation to their children. In my work, I have met many second and third generation Holocaust survivors who are secretly waiting for their mothers and fathers to cherish them in an overt way. The love is there in the hearts of the parents, but the highway to the heart has a roadblock of dead bodies. This doesn't mean that their parents don't love them; rather, it means that the heart's capacity to empathically understand what their children are going through, and offer warm reassurance in response, is compromised by their unexpressed grief. It's not just families of Holocaust survivors that go through this quiet anguish. Any family that lost a key family member or caretaker can have blocks in their heart.

Unexpressed grief can also compromise a parent or elder's ability to protect the younger generations of the family from harm. For example, a parent who survived sexual abuse but has not yet done their inner work to process the past emotions are likely to have blind spots about recognizing potential predators. When their Inner Voice of Truth says not to trust that babysitter or family friend around your children, this will trigger the unexpressed grief in the abused parent, making them feel overwhelmed.

Instead of listing to the instinct, they shut down emotionally and hand their child over to someone who could potentially abuse them in the same way.

When we halt the grieving process the grief gets dumped on the next generation, as we saw with Helen's story. The elders model for the younger generation how to hold onto their emotions rather than showing them how to grieve and release the hurtful past.

Exercise: Tending to Your Heart:

If I had to choose one meditative exercise to do for the rest of my life, it would be Tending to Your Heart. Being in touch with our hearts immediately brings us out of survival mode and back in touch with whatever feelings we have been storing up inside. By feeling that crucial emotional center of your heart, it has a chance to reenergize and to open wider. When our heart is open, we can receive crucial nourishment from our relationships as well as offer our own support most fully.

1. Begin by rubbing your scalp, using your fingertips to firmly massage the top and back of your head to help switch out of thinking mode and into a more sensually aware state.
2. Now put your hands on your chest and gently rub your heart.
3. As you do this, take a few deep breaths and sigh, "Ahhhhh" a couple times.
4. Keep your hands still on your chest and feel for the warmth underneath your hands.
5. Ask yourself, 'How does my heart feel?'
6. Allow whatever feelings are pending to rise up, whether that is a sense of joy, a physical sensation, or some type of emotional pain. Don't force it. Give the heart time to thaw.

7. As you become more aware of your heart, express those emotions in whatever way feels natural. Crying is perfectly acceptable. Even the sensations of numbness, emptiness, or hardness are valid feelings.

8. If you discover some type of pain, ask your heart 'Who hurt me?'

9. You may see a face, you may get a name, you may sense that numerous people have hurt you in a similar way. Take the time to let the story unfold, like a movie in your head.

10. After you have acknowledged the hurt, ask yourself 'Did I have a part in this hurt?'

11. Allow your heart to answer candidly. It may do so in words, or it may be an affirmative feeling such as an expansion in your heart for a 'yes' and a contraction for a 'no.' Practice learning the language of your heart.

12. If you discover that you had a part in the wounding, such as neglecting to protect yourself or if you find that you are judging yourself harshly for not doing more, apologize to your heart for what it has endured. A sincere apology is a form of self-empathy that can be very healing to a hurt heart.

13. If you discover that you had no part in the hurt, simply express to your heart that 'I'm sorry that you are going through this.' You may even notice that you haven't visited your heart in this way for a while. Acknowledging that you haven't made space or time to be with your heart can build self-trust and re-energize your heart.

14. To close, take several deep breaths and notice any changes in the sensations of your chest. Speak out loud that you value your heart and thank it for allowing you to feel love and receive positive experiences in your life. Repeat this exercise as often as you can.

Healthy Inheritance

Healthy inheritance of responsibilities and unfinished tasks from the older generations is possible. To be healthy, the responsibilities and family expectations need to be intentionally transferred and clearly communicated. The younger generation needs the space to ask questions and receive instructions or advice on how best to complete the task being bequeathed. Ideally, this could happen when someone is in hospice care. However, we don't know when the moment of our passing will happen. Taking time to discuss these important matters, openly and honestly during everyday life, can be one of the most precious gifts you give the younger generations of your family.

The missing ingredient in healthy inheritance is Choice. Generational dumping assumes that the next generation will take care of things when the older generation dies. The unacknowledged dumping leaves very little room for discussion, negotiation, and the clean transfer of duties. It almost never happens with guidance on how to assume roles or the support in shouldering the new weight.

In the events of untimely deaths, the family has no time to prepare for what happens next and rarely has the collective skills to handle the grieving process on their own. Asking for help is a choice, a courageous request that ensures that the older generations are held while they grieve.

Last rites are meant to serve as the transition ceremony before a person dies. But in modern times, many of those rites focus on fulfilling religious obligations and do not make enough time to speak about specific familial responsibilities being passed on. These wishes are usually read by a lawyer from the last will and testament after the person has already passed away, leaving no room for questions or clarification. The last will and testaments rarely cover all of the necessary transitions outside of property exchange and financial inheritance. If we could reform hospice care to have a purposeful sit down with family members passing the torch from that person to other specific members, generational dumping could at least become visible. This will enable people to see the benefits and need for a therapist to provide emotional support during the transition. Many have died unexpectedly in tragic events and never received their last rites. The Ancestral Dialogue becomes a highly effective tool for completing the grieving process in these cases.

The Family You Never Had

In the same way that our family gives us scripted roles that help define the image of ourselves we strive to live up to, we also have an image of how our family should be. This image is formed from your beliefs about how parents and grandparents should treat the younger generations and how you expect your family to provide for you. The reality of how your family actually operates and the image that you expect will not always line up.

Deep inside our hearts, we all have the need to be seen, to be heard, to be understood, and to be loved. Because the inherited burdens fill the spaces in our hearts to really receive and give to each other, these needs may only be partially met or entirely unmet, depending on the self-awareness of the family member.

I have encountered a few rare families where there are multiple people doing their inner work and are able to witness each other. They make an effort to connect in a heartfelt way. If you are fortunate enough to have other people in your family who are becoming self-aware, treasure them.

When you walk the path of the Catalyst (even if your family members don't follow your example), you will find other Catalysts who are also doing the work. When people living off the scripts find each other, they have an opportunity to rewrite how they form relationships with each other. This gives the opportunity to create a new extended family with people who are both from your bloodline and from other bloodlines.

The Unscripted Relationship

When we don't fully know who we are, we defer to the script of how other people see us and expect us to behave. The problem with relying on others to define us is that they will see us based on what they need us to be rather than who is emerging from inside of us. But who we are is not beholden to the scripts we are handed, nor do we need to form relationships according to family and cultural expectations outlined in the scripts we inherit.

Our closest confidants are those who are most likely to see the authentic you. Forming an authentic friendship or partnership means you see who the other person truly is beyond your needs and expectations of them. This doesn't mean that the relationship will be free of expectations, demands, and conflicts. That's a natural part of growth. But it does mean that you choose a partner based on the person you see in front of you and that you continue to witness, and be witnessed, off the script throughout the relationship.

The unscripted relationship means that there is no "responsible one" in the relationship and no single person who "wears the pants" in a relationship. There will be power struggles, however, an effort to balance the collective responsibilities with access to decision-making powers are done in a conscious way. You figure it out together without doing things the way your parents or grandparents did it.

Each individual will have their strengths in the partnership. One person may be more naturally nurturing than the other (regardless of their gender), the other may be more analytically inclined or financially savvy. But the power and responsibility in the relationship is shared when you look at all domains, from the bedroom, to the kitchen, from the office to the backyard.

The most important tenet of the unscripted relationship is that you are allowed to be all of who you are in connection to each other. You are both directors of your own lives and are writing a shared story as you walk through life together. The beauty of such a partnership is that you face the unknown while holding hands, each being and receiving a dedicated witness to your evolution. Leaving the limited scripts of your upbringing makes so much more room for the exchange of validation, empathy and compassion. This free exchange of love and support fosters mutual respect in a genuine partnership.

Dependents and Co-dependents

In our goal of forming healthy, inter-dependent relationships, it becomes important to recognize when we have slipped back into old scripts. An easy way to recognize this slip is to identify when we are acting from either a dependent or co-dependent response.

According to Mental Health America, "Co-dependency is a learned behavior that can be passed down from one generation to another. It is an emotional and behavioral condition that affects an individual's ability to have a healthy, mutually satisfying relationship. It is also known as "relationship addiction" because people with codependency often form or maintain relationships that are one-sided, emotionally destructive and/or abusive."[16] Co-dependents can also be referred to as co-addicts

---

16   "Co-Dependecy" http://www.mentalhealthamerica.net/
     co-dependency Mental Health America. 2018

because they enable their partners to escape self-accountability through their reactions.

Dependents in addiction programs are more commonly referred to as addicts, meaning people who escape their pain and self-responsibility through any form of addictive escape. This can be a substance such as alcohol, drugs, or food, or can be an escapist act such as excessive sex and gambling. For the sake of recognizing when we have slipped into a scripted role, we will define *dependent* as when we are reliant on a relationship without taking full responsibility for our actions or contributions to the relationship. In other words, we escape from pain and accountability through our escapes and leave the co-dependent person to shoulder the responsibility in the relationship.

It is common for many relationships to be characterized by some kind of trade-off. One person in the relationship can be dependent on the other for their well-being and even their livelihood, while their partner needs to be needed by the dependent. These tradeoffs exist in the script as relationship expectations.

How a Dependent Heals

A dependent heals by facing their fear of abandonment and learning to take responsibility for their life. Each dependent has a deep fear of being alone, of being separated from the person who will take care of their needs. When the co-dependent caregivers in their life no longer enable them, the dependent must take responsibility for their actions and mistakes. They must take care of themselves, which means letting go of, and doing the inner work to deal with whatever they have endured earlier in their lives.

When dependents learn to be self-reliant and learn to trust in their capabilities to manage their own lives, they also learn to value themselves.

The more confidence they gain in their contributions to others, the greater the sense of autonomy they will have. This will make them less likely to look at people based on what they can get from them and more likely to see past their own needs.

Perhaps the greatest indicator of growth is when a dependent admits to making a mistake and attempts to make amends for the harm they have caused. A sincere apology happens when they don't make the admission of wrongdoing as a way to get more attention for how they need to change or how badly they messed up. Genuine amends happen when empathy is offered by the dependent to the co-dependent, meaning, they actually feel what harm they have caused other people. They stop talking and they start listening with their heart. In this moment, the attention fully shifts from the dependent and is given to the co-dependent.

Very often, when the co-dependent puts their foot down and demands that a dependent change, there will be some kind of theatrical performance that appears to be a turning point in the dependent's life. The co-dependent will try and force the dependent to change how they behave, but this is just more of the trap of their co-dependency at work.

A dependent changes when a Catalyst Event disrupts their script so completely, that they are forced to look at their lives from a different perspective. In addiction circles, this is often referred to as rock bottom. This event cannot necessarily be manufactured by the caretakers in their life, nor forced upon them by the demands of others. This doesn't mean that interventions and necessary separations aren't a part of what leads up to these Catalyst Events. These efforts are often made from a sincere place and can help, however it's important to realize that once you have done what you can, the rest is up to the dependent to make the change. Co-dependents cannot use their influence over dependents to force them to get responsible, to get respectful, or to get sober. But they can leave the scripted relationship in a conscious way, leaving it up to the dependent to get help.

How a Co-Dependent Heals

A co-dependent heals when they learn to value their own needs as much as they value the needs of others. Co-dependents also have a deep fear of being alone, so they look for people who need them. Even if the co-dependent is not getting what they need from the relationship, they feel secure in the knowledge that the needy partner, who they are enabling, will never leave them. The dependent fills the void for the co-dependent, and the dependent in turn usually surrenders a lot of control over their own life. Many co-dependents like to have the control because it gives them sway over the relationship.

While the co-dependent is able to maintain control over the relationship in the beginning, this lasts for only as long as they are able to consistently satisfy the needs of the dependent. This control over the relationship is an illusion. Because co-dependents often struggle to trust life, they prefer to have influence over their dependent partners because the temporary obedience makes co-dependents feel that they can "do something about their lives." They can't control external factors such as the weather or a crisis at work, but they can go home and exchange a trade-off with their dependent in exchange for control over the household.

A co-dependent breaks free of their trap when they finally value their own needs. When they value their needs enough to take a stand in their relationships, they step out of the expected roles in their script and start getting honest with themselves. A sign of healing for a co-dependent is when they manifest relationships in which they are seen for who they are, rather than what needs they meet for the other person. Manifesting a healthy relationship where the co-dependent's needs are an equal priority with their partner is the best indicator of progress.

Even though they have different ways of coping with life, co-dependents and dependents have two important conditions in common. They both mistrust the forces of Life that are beyond their control, and they both fear facing unknown experiences alone. This is why so many relationships follow the co-dependent and dependent scripts. This arrangement is effective for survival-based circumstances. Even when people have enough food, money, and work to make a sustainable living, they can still be in an emotionally-based survival mode based on an overactive fear of all the bad things that could happen to them. Co-dependent/dependent relationships are orderly and predictable, including the explosive fights that often characterize them, which can bring familiarity in times of uncertainty. But these scripted roles ultimately limit growth and true self-discovery.

When facing life decisions, most people make decisions that are safety based. They will say, "better safe than sorry." The Catalyst follows a different mantra: "Better thriving than surviving."

Traps to Realization #8

False Loyalty

Whole families are often in a state of perpetual survival mode. Even if they do manage to keep the lights on in their house, they still struggle to make meaningful lives and keep their families together. One of the glues of the family is a clinging bond that I call False Loyalty.

Think back to the swimmers in the ocean. Each family has at least one person who wakes up and realizes that there is an easier way to live. They try to convince their family to come with them. But change is scary, and families have ways of hammering down the raised nails in the floorboards, meaning the person who stands out in the family will be aggressively put back into their place. To be part of the family, you must pledge your allegiance to it, regardless of what abuse you must endure. Those who try to swim away from their family to the safety of the shore must first survive the separation. Guilt trips, shaming, blame, and threats are the tools used to maintain a false sense of loyalty. Anyone who elects to stop participating in a family trapped in cyclic abuse will experience one or all of these techniques for preventing separation. In the moment that a Catalyst expresses a desire to leave, the family becomes like a trapped animal fending for its own survival. The idea of one family member departing is like losing a limb from the familiar body. The head bites, the other limbs grab on, and the body, as a whole, recoils.

Those who successfully leave are often shamed and branded as traitors. The survivors' guilt interrupts the celebration of taking this important step in life. In some instances, their emotional or physical security is challenged for betraying the family.

Many have trouble recognizing if loyalty is genuine. There is an easy way to tell. Genuine loyalty is a two-way street. It is mutual. It means that a person stands by their kin in hard times, telling the truth to each other and not speaking badly about each other when they are not around. False Loyalty is a one-way street. It benefits and protects selected family members, often at the cost of others, including children. Loyalty must be reciprocal to be complete and sustainable.

False Loyalty is when an individual member of the family must be loyal to the greater family, even when the family is actively betraying or abandoning that individual. When a family fails to protect its members, the trust system breaks down, yet the scripted expectations of how each member behaves often remains the same. To the outer world, appearances are kept up to protect the secret betrayals and abuse. Yet the secret keepers are often the abused parties. So, when an abused family member tries to break free, he or she is often treated like the offender rather than the victim.

Fear of Being Alone

So many of our worries about being judged and rejected are rooted in the fear of being alone. It can even contribute to our survival fears if we believe that we need somebody else to take care of us. This fear can be so overwhelming that it will prevent necessary separations from happening. But feeling fears are part of the healing process.

Fear is the force that herds all of our emotions into tight, manageable packages. Worries about showing emotions in public, including the hesitation to cry at a funeral, reinforce this storage of feelings, and prevent us from reconciling the past. These packages of personal experiences accumulate and become part of the burdens that we have inherited.

There comes a time in grieving where we must face our loneliness directly. While empathy from others and guidance from teachers and elders can help us along the way, the magic ingredient to facing loneliness is courage. Our courage grows as we see that we can survive waves of panic that leave our chest. It expands as we realize that our fear of being a complete outcast, or of not being able to "make it" in life without other people doing something on our behalf, are not accurate predictions of our future. This doesn't mean that you should isolate yourself and reject the helping hands of your supporters. It means that there is a piece of the work that must be done internally, because if you fear being alone, you must face that fear in order to pass through it. What other way can you face being alone?

As the waves of fear pass through you, and you let go of the panic and worry about your safety and lovability, you will notice a voice in your heart. It's a freshly cleared space that makes room for self-love and receiving care from others.

People often start new relationships without facing their alone-ness. Those packages of unfinished memories and unexpressed emotions are labeled with the names of people and events from the past. They sit there unopened, blocking full access to the heart. Though the energy of Eros that happens between new partners feels good, eventually this energy fades naturally, and the heavy boxes stop the flow of love and care between the partners. Both partners are then left with the choice to either work through their past stuff on their own and together, or to part without fully taking inventory of the opening inner work.

If you experience a cycle of Eros followed by the termination of a relationship numerous times, it may be an indicator that devoting some time to catch up with your heart is a good idea. This part of the healing process is not about how long you have spent alone. You can distract yourself for years without even feeling what your heart has been through. It's not about how many years ago someone has died, or how many years it has been since your divorce. It is about the effort and depth you put into knowing your heart firsthand, for yourself. It means you no longer wait for someone else to give you empathy or compassion before you feel your heart. You do it because your heart is worth it and because it needs to be done to be whole.

That space that is cleared in your heart will be pristine. It is the space of potential for self-love to emerge and to invite others to adore and cherish who you are. Your heart is worth the effort it takes to experience this phenomenon for yourself.

Desperate Grab for the Past

Now the wound has been cleansed. Empathy has helped you to acknowledge the pain you once held, and catharsis has released those feelings. What is left before you is a wide open wound. This cleansed wound can now be seen as a pathway to the light on the other side of it. It is time to walk through the wound and claim the gifts.

Because change is so scary and unfamiliar, there will be moments where we cling on to the past. In these fits, we long for the familiar, and however painful and unhealthy it may be, it is all that we know.

When we begin to shift from a wound-based identity to an identity that focuses on our gifts, the craving for the past will grow stronger. There is more inner space than we are used to, as we dump out all the burdens and feelings that once crowded that wound. Now, it is a gaping opening before us, opening us up to rediscover who we are right here and right now. We often don't know what's on the other side, yet a deep curiosity about what treasure and discoveries could emerge keeps us moving towards the opening.

Be more curious than afraid in front of the open pathway.

As we pass through the pathway, we leave behind our attachment to the feelings about our past. The blanket of victimhood loosens its hold, the roles attached to the pain are surrendered, and we begin to have an experience of the gifts that bring meaning to our ordeals. But before we gain confidence in the gifts that leads us to the truth of which we are, we must first endure the void in our identity. Doing the work itself, without any outside trigger like a death or loss of some kind, can feel like we are having an identity crisis. Our identity has nothing to grab onto while it passes through that threshold of the wound. This is when we may contract, recoiling away from the pathway, and we cling to some habit or relationship from the past, seeking a moment of comfort. But as we tangle with elements of our past, we recognize that they no longer comfort us in the same way anymore.

An old relationship moves on, and we feel rejected and scared, because a safety net has been peeled away. We try to get our old job back but find that we are more bored and stifled there than the first time we left it. We can even relapse into an addiction, this time not to escape a pain-filled wound, rather to avoid our fear of the "nothingness" inside the wound. But that void is not "nothingness."

It's freshly cleared space of potential.
It's a clearing of land that is perfect
for building a new house.
It's the space to dance with a new partner
who truly sees who you now.
It's the room to breathe, expand and
develop new dreams for your life.

Rather than fight with the desperate grip for the past, name it. By acknowledging that this reversion to what you used to know is an escape from the unknown, you strengthen your self-honesty. The pangs to escape who you are becoming will settle if you face them.

Too Much Empathy

When we find ourselves in the role of the Good Samaritan, the Bodhisattva, the do-gooder who is making the world a better place, it is hard to recognize when we have fallen into a script. When you are fighting the good fight and working to help others, your gaze is focused on the results of your efforts as well as identifying others who are in need. But when all your empathy s focused on others, you can lose track of the necessary self-empathy that balances out your self-care with the care of others. By neglecting our own hearts, we over emphasize what others are going through and get caught in the trap of too much empathy towards others.

Because the world always seems to need more empathy, it can be hard to tell when we have hit our personal limits because we can simultaneously see the needs of others. It's not noble to ignore the energy levels of your heart, no more than it is wise for an ambulance driver to neglect to check the fuel gauge of the vehicle before racing to the rescue. By de-prioritizing your own needs, you inadvertently devalue your needs. A stalled ambulance with an empty fuel tank is not going to help anyone.

One of my clients captured this trap in words so eloquently. She was an Indian American woman in her 30's, whose parents immigrated to the United States. She often spoke of the strong cultural expectations placed upon her as the oldest child of her family, especially being the first in her family to be born in the U.S. As she was doing some deep work to break free of the script of her family, she shared the following: "Who am I to be happy without my family? Who am I to separate from them while they are suffering? What right do I have to be in this world, have a place in this world, without them?"

While empathy is an important power of your heart to recover, it needs to be balanced with consideration for yourself. Overly identifying with what you feel your family is going through can hold you to sticky guilt trips that pull you back into a scripted servitude to your family. See your family members as people who can embrace their personal empowerment when they are ready to do so. Waiting for them doesn't mean you are a better family member. By embracing your own path, you show them the way to personal liberation.

273

Blazing a Trail

There is a light at the end of every tunnel and there are gifts on the other side of each wound. To make it all the way through the wound and claim those gifts, we must summon our Inner Fire as a healing force. The Inner Fire clears the pathway through the wound so that we can see the gifts of the experience more clearly. It propels us to the other side of the wound so that we can claim the reward and take another step towards fully healing the wound.

Grieving not only reawakens our sense of compassion, but it also re-invigorates our courage to experience our latent gifts in a new way. These are the talents and abilities that give meaning to the wounding and a sense of purpose to our lives. The more we embrace these gifts, the more the struggle that comes with cleaning our wounds seems worth all the effort.

Grieving puts us in touch with our anger, which can be further transformed to help us reach our Innate Gifts. To get to the reward, we can summon the cleansing power of our Inner Fire to finish cleaning out our wounds.

The 5th Realization

We all have an Inner Fire that ignites our Passion

Vision for Realization #5

The choppy ocean slapped her face. Her cheeks were flush with hot blood. Her resentment towards her family for not seeing her and not recognizing all that she had done for them was only the first expression of her Inner Fire. As she felt the growing fire inside of her, her desire to be free also grew.

The more she dreamed of dancing on the shore, the stronger her frustrations about not living that life became. But her Inner Fire was not all about anger and resentment. When she envisioned herself dancing on the shore, a passionate heat took over and rolled from her belly to her heart. Excitement surged through her body as the heat radiated through her skin. She needed to be free. She needed to swim to the shore.

Looking back at her loved ones, she could feel how much she truly loved them. But she also realized that they needed her more than she needed them. They wouldn't grow if she continued to enable them to hide from their responsibilities. No longer would she hold their burdens. The idea of being alone on the sand made her feel guilty for leaving them. Realizing that they wouldn't swim with her made her sad.

"What would they do without me?" she asked herself.

"They will do what they are doing now," I replied. "They'll survive."

"What will I do?" she asked.

"You can live your life according to your dreams."

"But that means that I must leave them behind. They won't listen to me. They won't follow," she said.

"They might not follow you immediately. But you leaving the ocean will prove to them that there is another way to live."

Hard tears fell. She was torn by guilt for wanting to leave them and the fire inside of her that told her to make her dream come true. She couldn't wait to live her own life anymore. She wouldn't wait for them to understand why she would swim to the shore. As she screamed her frustration, the resentment burned so hot that it seemed to dissolve the guilt stuck in her guts. As the guilt melted away, she could finally breathe again. She raged at them for not seeing her, for not considering what she needed, for being so selfish. Her angry hands found the chain buried deep in her guts. It was the tether that kept her engrossed in the past grief and fears of her family buried beneath the surface of the water. It had always been there, secretly binding her. Her hands ripped the chains free from her belly. Then she dropped the chain and they sank to the bottom of the ocean. Her family members stared in disbelief.

We swam together, back to the shore. Her arms pumped through the water, fueled by the liberating fire that consumed her whole body. It was exciting and scary, overwhelming and invigorating. Her family screamed in protest, calling her a traitor and a fair-weather daughter – the one who only shows up for the family when things are going well. They didn't understand the courageous step she was taking. They only knew that she was leaving them.

When we hit land, she gripped the sand, lifting her hands to her face. She was on the land. It had finally come true.

She rose up and twirled in a circle, releasing the sand in playful release. For the first time in her life, she danced on that sand, just as she had dreamed. She danced with fervor, her Inner Fire transforming from resentment and outrage to an invigorating passion. Her creative expression cleansed her. It was how she celebrated her life celebration of her life. For the first time, she truly felt alive!

Reclaiming Your Fire

Our Inner Fire is always present. This fire is our vitality. We can feel it when we are invigorated, passionate, angry, and when we have sex. When we feel threatened, it's that valiant energy that comes forth to protect us. If you are still living and breathing, you certainly have an Inner Fire.

When our Inner Fire is stifled, we lose motivation or feel depressed. When we neglect to express our fire, we can feel listless, lost, and agitated without having a "good reason" to feel that way. These are all signs that we have lost a direct connection to our Inner Fire and have temporarily lost track of what led up to it being smothered or ignored.

When we are in survival mode, our Inner Fire becomes focused, dedicated towards protecting us at all costs. When we feel threatened, we yell at someone to back them away from us. When we are worried about money, we channel our fire into working long hours. Most people in survival mode won't feel relief, except when they express their fire sexually, allowing the fire to play. But when our Inner Fire is not allowed to flow for long periods of time, we not only feel unhappy and physically unhealthy, we also feel like we are not manifesting our full potential, which leads to lingering feelings of being unfulfilled.

Writers, artists and musicians are notorious for having "writer's block," which means that their ability to create has been impeded. The words are not finding their way to the memoir or lyric sheet. The paint brush never truly flows on the canvas. These creative blocks almost always involve some kind of block to our Inner Fire. The fear of people not liking your work or falling behind on a deadline that will affect your finances can pinch off our connection to our creative fires. Coming back into contact with your Inner Fire is essential to being productive and fulfilled.

Our Fire is such an incredibly powerful force for change, that when unleashed with skill, any obstacle can be overcome. Any piece of art can be completed. Any goal can be achieved. So why do so many people have a poor relationship with their Inner Fire?

Most people have placed their Inner Fire into servitude to other people. In their relationships, they give their power away. Essentially, they donate their vitality to outsiders: a political cause, to family expectations, or to completing a work project. Even those who rebel against the system of living a conventional life can splash their Fire around in a stream of chronic partying, yet never really connecting to their Inner Fire to explore the other aspects of it. The underlying reason that so many have not arrived into their fully empowered state is that they do not claim ownership over their Inner Fire.

In order to really get to know your fire, it's crucial to experience it in its natural state. To do this we have to disengage our Inner Fire from all the expectations that we place on it. This requires recognizing when our

Inner Fire is in servitude to other people. In other words, we need to let our Inner Fire *just be* so that we can have an unadulterated experience of it.

A flowing Inner Fire that is aligned with
your Inner Voice of Truth becomes a
powerful agent for transformation.
By freeing up your Fire, you personally
change for the better.
By revealing your Fire to the outer
world, you become seen.
By expressing your Fire through your gifts and
by speaking passionately about what you believe
in, you become a Catalyst who is able to help others
on their journeys to personal transformation.
When they are ready, they too may become
Catalysts and inspire others to awaken as well.

Generational Family Shaming

"We should not be ashamed of anger. It's a very good and a very powerful thing that motivates us. But what we need to be ashamed of is the way we abuse it." —Mahatma Gandhi[17]

The act of shaming has been built into families, communities, and even religions. It's so pervasive that it is socially acceptable. There is a long history of shaming people for the color of their skin, their gender,

17 *The Gift of Anger: And Other Lessons from My Grandfather Mahatma Gandhi by Arun Gandhi April 25, 2017 Publisher: Gallery/Jeter Publishing*

sexual orientation, language spoken, and religion. In modern day society discrimination and shaming of this kind can be identified as hate crimes in more progressive nations, but many countries around the world do not consistently hold the "shamers" accountable.

Shaming exists in one form or another in every family. Some elders hand down negative beliefs about how far the younger generations will get in life because of their sex, age, background, or even their school grades. Putting shame on a misbehaving child as a disciplinary action is also very common. "Shame on you," they say to the misbehaving child. This corrective action doesn't just tell the child that their actions are unacceptable, it also communicates that something about the child is very wrong. Shaming as a mode of disciplinary action is much like pouring hot tar onto a freshly bleeding cut. It will stop the bleeding, but getting the tar off after the blood has clotted is no simple matter. Likewise, putting shame on a child may temporarily stop the acting out, but other behaviors reacting to the shame later on can be expected as the Inner Fire rises in a rebellious fashion. The rebellion in this case is the maturing child trying to peel away the shame that is not a part of who they are at their core.

Shaming can also be a form of distorted venting on behalf of elders. If the elders of a family aren't getting help through counseling or friendships, they will be bottling up their own feelings of shame and fiery rebellion. There is no place for those feelings to go. So, when they are overwhelmed with financial matters or a bad day at work, the bottled-up shame and misguided Fire will spill to the surface. They will take it out on the kids and grandkids.

When parents inflict painful words on the younger generations, they will mistakenly feel justified in their outburst. They may even feel a moment of release akin to hitting a punching bag or having a cathartic therapy session. They will have "won" that exchange by having the last word.

As an adult, they will finally be the one to have their enraged moment that they could never have as a subordinate child. But rarely do the elders realize that in these hurtful moments of shaming, they are not winning anything. Rather, they are inflicting lasting harm onto their children in the same way that it had been inflicted upon them. This deeply unconscious form of Generational Dumping is not corrective action. It is an ineffective way of getting rid of the shame and only offers a moment of relief before feelings of remorse begin to surface. If the remorse is immediately suppressed, it will add more inner pressure that will facilitate another bout of inflicting shame and blame onto the younger generations.

In an effort to clean our Inner Fire, it's helpful to separate the shameful phrases from the heartfelt guidance in the script that we inherit from our families. The negative beliefs that are inflicted on children as part of shaming, are not the words or teachings of our most respected ancestors. Disparaging a family member in the same way as it has been done for generations is not wisdom. Re-inflicting the mistakes depicted in ancient stories, however long ago they were written, is not wisdom.

The passage of power from one generation to another is not always beneficial to the family as a whole. It can be done out of tradition without any consideration to the unspoken shame a family carries. For instance, a good patriarchal grandfather who has dutifully cared for the family can pass the torch as head of the family to a child molester because he is the first-born son and tradition dictates that he is next in line. Likewise, a solid matriarch can pass the torch to a gossiper who selfishly divides the family into sides, creating feuds that can take many generations to heal. Just because it's tradition doesn't mean it's right, nor does it mean that your ancestors (with the best intentions for your family) would have wanted it that way. Blindly following the words of our ancestors without considering the deeper impact of empowering abusers who impose veiled forms of shameful abuse causes more damage to the family. This means that more shame is generated and passed onto unsuspecting children who can't figure out why the adults keep hurting each other. Children don't know enough of the family history to make sense of the greater story. So, they inherit that emotional load on top of their bright Fire that was once so easy to see during their childhood.

Blaming

We're conditioned to have a good "attitude" and maintain a steady mood, but our Inner Fire often does not follow these social cues. We may find ourselves in a situation where someone says something seemingly harmless, yet it may trigger an unexpectedly agitated emotional response in us. Our sexual urges can even be stirred at socially awkward times. This is the Inner Fire pushing to the surface. At these moments our Inner Fire can feel overwhelming and disruptive to the scripts of our daily routines and assuming the responsibility for listening to and caring for our Inner Fire can feel like an enormous challenge. Our Fire can rise up in a way that is surprising to our rational mind.

Once the Inner Fire is released from its repression, it doesn't follow a set script. It burns away the parts of the script that don't fit who we are becoming. It's possible that when the Fire pushes us out of our comfort zones and beyond our limits, that we will resist it. Once the Fire has surfaced, it is very difficult to repress it again. So, we push it away so that we don't need to "deal with it" anymore. The pushing of our Inner Fire onto another person is called *blame*.

Blame is when we surrender personal responsibility for our fiery feelings, like anger and resentment, and place the obligation of receiving that Fire onto someone else. By blaming someone else, we no longer need to take accountability for our impassioned mistakes, our angry outbursts, or when we act out from a young, wounded place. Think for example of the stepfather lashing out at his stepson and blaming his angry outburst on the son because he "baits" him.

Blame temporarily gives us space from our Fire. But, without taking responsibility for how we feel, including our emotional outrage when we have been disrespected, our Inner Fire can run wild. It can spill over into other areas of our life. We paint our story on others then tell ourselves that it's their fault that we feel this way. In our state of painful lack of accountability, our behavior becomes the fault of somebody else.

Blame takes time to develop. It starts with being hurt by someone in the past who got away with abusing you. These villains of our past showed us that "life is not fair" and thus cannot be completely trusted. Knowing that there are people who will not hold themselves accountable, and may never be held to account they haven't been caught, puts those who do maintain accountability at a disadvantage. It's as if there are two sets of rules: one around personal accountability and another set of rules where "anything goes" because accountability is trumped by the pain of past betrayals.

Those who struggle with addiction often resort to blaming others for their behavior because they struggle to take responsibility for their Inner Fire. They don't trust their Fire because it has gotten them into trouble in the past. Infidelity, habitual emotional abuse and physical violence require an unconscious Inner Fire that is not held in personal accountability.

The way out of Blame is to take ownership of your own Inner Fire. Rather than pushing your Fire onto someone else and waiting for that person to apologize or rectify things take ownership of your anger, your infidelity or your addiction. By expressing these emotions, you will be able to break free from the scripted abuse of the relationship and open up the opportunity to hear the deeper truth of the situation. Own any mistakes you have made - they are all part of our learning process on this journey. It is when we deny that we have made a mistake, that blame has a chance to shift the power of our Fire away from our center and make it seem dependent upon another person's actions.

It is *your* Inner Fire, your personal spark of life. It's worth having, even when it disrupts your predictable day. It makes life more vivid, clean, and fulfilling in the present moment. By releasing the blame, the power and onus of the Inner Fire comes back home to you.

In order to clear your Inner Fire from past harsh experiences you need to take responsibility for its care. This next exercise can be repeated often, especially if you can feel a strong stream of Inner Fire coming to the surface, but you are still building trust with it.

Expressions of Fire

To understand our Inner Fire, we must often unearth it from all the past dumping it has endured. Because the Fire often gets smothered, it builds up in pressure. When we share our Fire with others without first clarifying what it is telling us, it can come out as an eruption of misguided anger. This raw Fire can be dangerous as people can be physically or emotionally hurt when this unrefined form of Fire is unleashed. When old anger is held onto for too long, it can cause splash damage. This is when people who were not involved with the original event that incited the anger take the brunt of it. This often happens when hurt, angry children become new parents. They may find themselves screaming in anger at their own children, but the people they really want to scream at are their parents, yet their children become the targets of the unexpressed rage.

Fire is meant to flow, and when it is stifled, we grow angry. When we are not seen, or heard, or when we don't receive the empathy that we feel we deserve, our fire transforms into anger as a force to break through resistance, injustice, and oppression.

But when our fire is allowed to flow, it has a whole spectrum of expressions. Fire can be passion, that enjoyable and invigorating flow of fire when we are creating something new. This could be a piece of art, embarking on a new relationship, or expressing ourselves in a dance class. Our Inner Fire is the sexual passion when we are "making love". Because most people associate fiery expression with splashy anger or hurtful memories, it is easy to forget that our Inner Fire encompasses a full range of expressions that can be enjoyable and life affirming.

Hindering the free flow of our Fire will result in us feeling depressed and struggling to appreciate our lives. Celebration will seem like a luxury or a birthday obligation where you are just going through the motions, yet not entirely feeling the full joy of the moment. When our Inner Fire is hampered, we will yearn to feel more alive!

When we are in survival mode, our Inner Fire becomes reserved as the fuel behind our fight and flight responses. It is our protective energy that seeks to protect our body physically and the energy that attempts to shield us from judgment and rejection in social interactions. To ensure our continued financial security, our Fire becomes the very drive that fulfills our daily tasks and work assignments.

Transforming Your Inner Fire

When we first reopen a wound, as in Realization #4, many emotions pour out. Among those emotions are variations of anger such as resentment, frustration, and even rage. These "hot" emotions are only the initial expressions of what our Inner Fire can become.

We are conditioned to fear our Inner Fire as something that will get us into trouble. You may have experienced judgment or punishment in the past when expressing resentment about an unfair situation at home, leading you to bite your tongue, when you were in actual fact very angry. This kind of constant repression can erupt in ways that are hurtful and lead to further wounding, if time is not taken to clarify your Inner Fire. It can be said that an immature Inner Fire, one that has not had enough time to be heard and understood, can lead to forms of anti-social behavior such as law breaking, physical and emotional violence, and acts of revenge. This is commonly seen in teenage acts of vandalism. Having the tools, means and guidance to direct you in how to express your anger in an uncensored way, to get messy with catharsis, can lead to a safer, more controlled form of anger.

Because the expression of Fire is so repressed in most societies, the natural maturation process from unconscious anger and resentment to a clearer, more conscious expression of Fire is often interrupted. This leads the Fire being stored up, building up an internal pressure that might just feel like stress at first. When that pent-up fire is finally released, its power can be surprising. But when we allow our Fire to move, it transforms into a cleaner, more exuberant expression. It leads us to understand why we are angry... and also what makes us feel passionate.

Three Waves of Fire

**Reopening an old wound will bring
forth three major waves of release.**

Emotional Catharsis: This is the first and messiest phase of release and is the outpouring of all the emotions connected to the past hurt stored inside the wound. The emotions will feel authentic, but it may be hard to identify the cause of them. The Inner Fire will be the anger, resentment, and frustration embedded in a stew of emotions including grief, fear, guilt, regret and shame. This part of the process requires high amounts of empathy to create a space outside of the wound that draws the feelings out of it. The meaning of the wound is usually not revealed in this early stage of the release. The Inner Fire will express itself through resentments that are just beginning to unveil themselves. Anger can be overt, but it may be hard to find the words to express the hurt and it may be heavily focused on making accusations about past conflicts and placing blame on other people for what happened in the past. The anger may sound like an unfocused rant that isn't fully connected to the real reason that you feel upset. It may even switch between anger and other emotions like fear or sadness, making the story hard to track at first. But, with ample expression of all emotions, clarity will come eventually.

When we reopen an old wound, as we did in Realization #4, there are three major waves of fiery release from a wound. The first wave of release is the initial Emotional Catharsis. This is the messiest because such a variety of emotions come out of the wound. The emotions may feel true, but it's hard to recognize why you are feeling this way.

The next wave is the Transformational Fire, which represents a clearer telling of your anger. The reasons why you are angry and why you want your life to change becomes known. This more mature expression of your Inner Fire comes with the belief that you have a right to feel angry about what has happened to you.

The third wave is the Awakening of Passion. You no longer only feel angry. You also feel a passionate form of love in your relationships. You remember what true celebration feels like.

Transformational Fire: This wave represents a clearer telling of your anger and begins with the expression of anger and rage during catharsis. The Fire transforms from a repression of rage to blaming or venting about what other people did or did not do. The Transformational Fire can clarify by shouting your rage or doing therapeutic exercises to release rage. One healing modality that excels in helping to embrace your Transformational Fire is Core Energetics. Developed by psychiatrist John Pierrakos M.D. in the 1970's in New York City, Core Energetics uses emotional cathartic exercises to radically release trapped Inner Fire.[18] Releasing the Transformational wave of fire burns away the emotional residue inside the wound, clearing a path to the other side of the wound. You can tell when you have reached the Transformational Fire when you are able to clearly identify why you were hurt and that you have a right to feel mad about it. It is the step when you start taking a stand for who you really are, outside of your imposed role in the script. By expressing your Transformational Fire, you take your power back from the wounded past and assert your worthiness of respect, thereby attaining a more matured expression of your Inner Fire.

Awakening of Passion: This is where the other expressions of your Inner Fire are given the space to be shared. During this wave the focus of your Inner Fire shifts to deciding what you want to do to take charge of your life. Expressing how you were hurt is no longer enough and with that comes the realization that you will need to change your life in order to

---

18   Pierrakos, J. "Core Energetics: Developing the Capacity to Love and Heal." Core Evolution Publishing, NY. 2005

feel at peace again. During this wave, the Inner Fire shifts from a justified personal outcry to a more refined expression of passion centered around your Innate Gifts. Anger passes, passion is regained, and you remember what true celebration feels like.

These three waves passing through the wound have a crucible effect that burns away the old and transforms you from the inside out. Cleaning out the wound will help you discover your emotional fortitude and resiliency. As each wave passes through the tunnel of the wound, an open pathway to your Innate Gifts will reveal itself. Your refined passion leads you to those gifts.

Reclaiming Ownership of Your Fire

Feeling hesitant about expressing your anger, frustration or resentment, is a sign that you are not completely claiming ownership of your Inner Fire. In the same way that we must own our wounds to move through the healing process, so too must we claim ownership over our Fire in order to change our lives.

To reclaim ownership of our Inner Fire, we must unravel who it is who may be demanding that your Fire serve them. Without us being consciously aware of it, your Inner Fire may be serving or even being taken advantage of by a boss, partner, family member, or even a friend to meet their personal goals and needs. While there are healthy expressions of our Inner Fire that can be done cooperatively as part of a group, what I am referring to is the disempowering relationships where you don't have complete say over your Inner Fire. It is when someone else is gaining from our Inner Fire without permission or without our conscious consent that the power struggles begin.

Let's clarify where the energy from your Inner Fire is going.

Exercise: Who is Your Fire Serving?

- Take a few deep breaths and feel for any pressure or heat inside of your body.
- Out loud, invite your Fire to come to the service.
- Breathe and notice any feelings that arise without getting attached to the emotions. These are the things that are stacked on top of your Fire. Just notice them as they pass through you.
- When you feel the sensation of your Fire, it may feel like heat, tingling, vibrancy, even nausea in its early stages. When you feel the opposite of bored, your Fire is moving to the service.
- After you feel your Fire, use your other senses to get closer to it: What color is your Fire? What does it smell like? What does it sound like?
- Once you have made a meaningful connection with your Inner Fire, ask it: Who are you serving?
- Write down all the names that pop into your mind, along with any bits of stories or imagery that come up with each name. Many may arise in rapid-fire fashion. If this happens, write down all the names as fast as you can, then revisit each name one at a time. Say the name aloud and listen to and watch what your Fire shares with you.
- Now review the list that you made. How many people is your Fire assisting? Did your Fire describe any scenarios that feel disempowering to you?
- Ask your Fire to temporarily release its efforts to these other people, knowing that you can resume any efforts that you choose to continue after the exercise is done.

- Witness your Fire in its natural state, free from expectation or exertion. Describe how it looks, feels, smells, etc. Has it changed in any way from when you first connected to it in the beginning of the exercise? If so, how?
- Take a moment to thank your Fire for revealing itself. Honor it.
- If for any reason, you were not able to make contact with your Inner Fire, then journal about how it felt to not be able to reach it on your first attempt. All the emotions and judgments that are written down are connected to the blocks that are sitting on top of your Inner Fire. Even being able to name what is connected to the block is progress.

Putting our Fire into Empowering Service

There is a difference between service and servitude. Service is chosen. Servitude is imposed.

When we live most of our lives by the script, our Fire is obliged to serve the roles that we are given. We do what we "gotta do" instead of doing what fulfills us. Because the script was created before we were born, we weren't allowed to craft it cooperatively, according to our true gifts, along with our families.

The most evolved families will encourage a family member to follow their dreams, but this does not mean that they have the skills or awareness to help that family member to unburden what has been passed onto them. The unburdening process helps to clear a path for our gifts and passions to emerge consciously.

It is not enough to just break the script by choosing a different path to our parents and grandparents. We need to uncover our Fire so that we can feel that passion. That's how our Fire speaks to us. It gets angry when we are not following our own path and illuminates into warm streams of passion when we are in the flow of our chosen path.

By feeling our passion, we have a direct link to our Fire. With a solid link, we can hear what wisdom it is trying to tell us. As the heat flows upwards in our body, visions can even arise in the form of vivid daydreams that show us what we long to do next. If we long to move to a new place that would better support the next steps of our lives, we will envision us living there to try it out. Ideas can flood up in moments of inspiration about what we want to initiate or create with others. We may see a future romantic partner coming our way, one that brings the qualities that we most value.

So often I hear of how people are afraid of the power of their Fire. They are concerned that if they feel it all the way, that they will fall back into self-destructive behavior. If they claim their sense of purpose with unapologetic passion, it means that they are seen. Being seen can be scary, because you are no longer able to hide from the judgments of others. But remember that the Inner Fire is here to protect you. Letting it out all the way can empower you to stand up for yourself and to break social conventions that would otherwise keep your from speaking your mind.

Judging the Inner Fire

All of us, men and women, are taught to judge our Inner Fires, including the various expressions of it are constantly misunderstood by the outside world. Expressing anger can lead to being labeled as an "angry person." Enjoying and expressing sexuality can lead to being shamed as "slut." Civil Rights protesters are labeled as "troublemakers" when protesting against injustices. In many cultures around the world, women are more vulnerable to these judgments than men, and are often on the receiving end of not only social shaming, but physical punishment as well.

We have all seen those people who spray their Fire all over the place. The drama queens who demand and command the attention in a room, the politicians and powerful television personalities who act with a flagrant disregard for how they affect other people, and the sports superstars who are always landing themselves in trouble with their outbursts. Yet they entertain millions with the passionate expressions of their physical prowess.

And they often get away with their explosive behavior with minimal reprimand.

So many people wish to claim the power and passion that comes with owning their Inner Fires that deep down inside, we secretly envy those who just let it all come out. Those who embrace their Fire are rewarded for showing up 100%. They are seen, they are heard, they make lots of money, and they live with invigoration. Fiery people do make mistakes, and at times they are even held accountable for those mistakes, but they have a way of rising to the top despite the negative judgments that attempt to bind them up again into a socially acceptable way of behaving.

Giving free reign to our Inner Fires may not always be wise, as in the case of anger - but nor is bottling it up. While being able to contain anger is a life skill that has its place in an adult world, bottling up anger without giving it a healthy outlet, can eventually lead to a harmful, dangerous explosive situation and people who commit aggressive crimes are often sent for anger management therapy. Locking up our anger into solitary confinement and throwing away the key is a mistake.

But there are those who use their Fire in ways to belittle others in order to remain in control of social situations and family lives. These are the charismatic dictators in life. It could be an alcoholic parent who leaves no room in the room for others to express their emotions. The moment they feel outshone, they erupt in fire displays that are meant to intimidate others into submission. They yell and wound in order to maintain their status of the twisted king or queen of the family. They are the abusers who invade the peace in other people's lives, and in order to keep everyone in submission, they have to have the loudest voice in the room. They do whatever it takes to "win" control in every situation.

Witnessing such awful abuses of power can lead to the development of a negative stigma around "fiery people." The child of a domineering tyrant or a relentless drama queen, will be left with some deeply instilled beliefs about their own Fire. In not wanting to be like the parent, the child will view the Fire as being "unclean" and will shy away from it. If the child views the Fire positively as the parent always seemed to get what they wanted, they will already know how hurtful that lashing out can be.

But our Inner Fires are not defined by how the people in our families behave. It need not be molded by the expectations of our families and communities. Your Inner Fire belongs to you alone. Whatever vitality that Life has granted you, however many years that your body may live, it is your life and your Fire.

Embracing the sovereignty of your Inner Fire enlists it as a healing force that will burn away the scripts that no longer fit who you are becoming. You need not lash out in the way your elders did to you. But that doesn't mean that every time your raise your voice to speak your truth that you are harming another human being. Even if they are startled by the power in your voice, you are not harming someone by speaking your truth. You are challenging them to hear their inner truth every time that you speak what is true to your experience.

Non-violent Fire

Expressing anger is essential to discovering our truth. Sharing your anger does not necessarily mean that you are being violent. Nobel Prize

Winners Mohandas Gandhi, Martin Luther King Jr., and more recently Malala Yousafzai, all expressed their outrage at oppression. They never resorted to violence, nor did they demean those who were causing the harm. They expressed their anger masterfully, even eloquently, in a way that was consistently non-violent.

Non-violent expression of anger occurs when we simply tell others how we are feeling without demeaning or shaming them for who they are or what they have done. You can even raise your voice and still express your outrage in a clean way. People may even be frightened of your voice or feel challenged by what you are saying. But anger itself is not harmful. How you direct that Fire and the intention you express through the Fire is the difference between violent and non-violent communication.

Sharing your Inner Fire shines a light on the truth of injustice and inequality. It captures the attention of everyone's busy minds and creates a path through all the competing thoughts so that truth can be heard. It can be harnessed to motivate mass change without belittling the challenge.

Trusting Your Fire

If you can begin to see your Inner Fire as a force that clears a path to truth, then you have already begun building trust with it. Almost everyone has their first intense experience of their Inner Fire early in our childhood during our "terrible two's." That Fire typically expands even greater in our adolescent years when rebellion and hormones perspire through our skin like heavy cologne. But by the time we become adults, we have a whole list of inner judgments and societal rules about when we can throw tantrums like a toddler or behave like horny teenager. Obviously, I don't suggest that either of these behaviors happen during a business meeting in a boardroom. But the other extreme is to never express these parts of ourselves, even when they need some type of cathartic release.

Invisible Burdens act as a cork for our Inner Fire. As long as we hold the burden in silence, our Fire will push against it from underneath, creating an inner pressure that we may experience as stress, neck pain, back pain, or even headaches. That pressure builds until we name the burden and express how we feel about it. Our Inner Fire lets us know when a burden no longer suits our life and when it is time to let it go.

If we choose not to consciously listen to our Fire, it can build up in this way for many years and erupt in unpredictable ways. We can become passive aggressive, anxious, or even have surprise outbursts when the pressures of daily life, combined with the burden we are carrying, weaken out ability to contain our Inner Fire. But the Fire itself is not to blame. Neglecting our Inner Fire creates this situation.

When I worked with clients who had been released from prison, it often emerged that they had an adolescent Fire that was never heard or respected. They would bottle up and save it for fights or rebellious acts like stealing. They were sent to anger management classes, which saw anger as a dangerous thing and directed them away from making a genuine connection with their Inner Fire. But without a safe place to express the anger without judgment, they had no way to release it. They never learned how to build trust with their Fire.

Those suffering with addictions, chose drugs, alcohol or even food to suppress their Inner Fires. Emotional eating, and the momentary coma that comes after gorging on food, suppresses anger and sexual expression. Alcohol can be used in a similar fashion in the beginning although it eventually suppresses impulse control and results in the anger splashing out uncontrollably. Such a person is often labeled as an "angry drunk," as opposed to the alcoholic who drinks to pass out and escape emotions completely. Some use uppers and speed to tap into the fire in one invigorated rush. It is even possible to use marijuana or sex on a daily basis to escape your feelings, in particular unexpressed anger. These are all different ways of controlling the Inner Fire that does not lead to greater self-understanding.

When you learn to hear your Inner Fire clearly, it's blatant and impeccably honest. What is "bad" or harmful about fiery expression is how it is shamed and judged. When we look at a blazing bonfire, there is no mistaking what it is. It's a great big Fire. It's powerful and it needs to be tended with care. If we do that, it keeps us warm. The Fire is innately clean. Now when we dump dried manure onto the bonfire, naturally a big stinky cloud of smoke will emerge that will choke our lungs and burn our eyes. Is the Fire to blame? Or is the problem that someone just dumped dried dung onto the bonfire?

The burdens that we have already inherited already contain a fair amount of fermented waste. When people dump their opinions on our Fire, when they shame us for being passionate or gifted, the problem is the toxic dumping, not the underlying passion. Enlisting our Fire as a healing ally is the first step to reclaiming it. Doing so helps us to clear it off so that we can see our clean Fire.

Fearing the power that comes from freeing your Fire is part of the process of trust building. When we claim our Fire, we light up the room and expand into a more passionate and capable expression of ourselves. For many, this may feel like they are on the spot or a target for criticism. What people say about us when they are envious or fearful is not of consequence. What is most important is our inner dialogue. What do we think about expressing our Fire? How does it feel to let it out?

Creating a supportive inner dialogue, with open-minded beliefs about outwardly expressing our Inner Fire, is the next step to recovering a trusting relationship. It helps to label the opinions and judgments that you have accumulated about your fiery core. Many of these harsh beliefs you will have heard from other people. They either said it about themselves and you followed what they modeled for yourself, or they may have directly inflicted them on you. It is even possible that in a depressed or disempowered state, you thought up new judgments of yourself and have absorbed them.

Core Practice: Letter Burning

Ancestral Dialogues can happen in the form of reading a prepared letter. For this exercise, you will need a fireplace, barbecue, or other safe place to burn the letters that you will write. It's fine to move the ancestor table to a new location or make a smaller version of it to accommodate fire safety. The point of this exercise is to move through the catharsis wave of fire and attempt to claim your right to be upset with your family. Every human being has been mad at their family at one point in their life. If you look at the disempowering events in your current life, you can always find an example that goes back to when you were growing up. Rather than judge yourself for having anger, embrace it as a healing force that might bring you new clarity.

In the previous exercise "Who is Your Fire Serving?" you may have begun to recognize when people have taken advantage of you for their own personal gain. Take a look at your family tree again and see if you can identify a form of neglect or abuse that makes you feel mad. You may even be able to see how this abuse was inflicted on other generations or family members as well. The repetition shows a pattern of abuse passed down the family tree.

Once you have chosen an event where you feel that you were wronged, collect your thoughts by writing down what happened to you in your journal. Choose a family member to write the letter to based on who you need to confront about the past abuse or neglect. Who harmed you and what was the lasting impact of that harm that still affects you today? Why did this abuse anger you? Write it down and address it to a deceased person who you think would have supported you in life. Tell them about the abuse you endured and be sure to be clear with your anger.

Once you have this completed, perform the following at the ancestor table in a confidential and private space. This is a great activity to do with your program buddy, trusted friend, or therapist.

- Set the intention for a safe ancestor (the person to whom you addressed the letter) to come forward as your trusted witness to the letter you are about to reveal aloud. You may have known them in life or may only know them by name. What's most important is that you feel trust with them. It is also acceptable to ask for someone who is not blood related to you, as long as you trust them. You may find that you need to write more than one letter.
- When you feel a connection to this person in your heart, ask them to support you as you share about what angered you.
- Now, read the letter about the past event out loud to the ancestor table.
- Feel your body after revealing why you are upset and breathe out the heat that your body has summoned.
- If you feel an overwhelming amount of Fire coming up, sit on the ground and scream into a pillow until the rage subsides. The pillow ensures that you do not trigger fears about other people

overhearing you. The most important part is that you feel the scream move through you and allow the Fire to heal you.

- When the wave of catharsis has passed, burn the letter in a fire safe container. While you burn the letter, claim your right to be angry about what happened to you. Affirm your self-respect aloud. For example: "Grandma, I have a right to be angry about how my uncle hurt me. I deserve respect and I won't stay silent when a man hurts me like that again."

- Thank your safe ancestor for being your witness and set a clear boundary about when you will make contact with them next if necessary. Close the work at the ancestor table by verbally saying, "This piece of the work is complete."

- Drink water, recover, and journal about the experience.

The 5th Birthright

Passion

We are meant to re-create ourselves. When we take a break from work to enjoy ourselves, we call it recreation. The word recreation literally means re-creation, as our rest time allows us to catch up with ourselves and rediscover who we have become. When we are on vacation, in addition to going on new adventures, we often do what we feel passionate about. If we love singing, we do karaoke or an open mic performance. We'll go dancing, sailing, or capture beautiful moments with our cameras. In the same way that our physical body is constantly repairing our tissues with new cells, our sense of identity also evolves by shedding the past to make room for a fresh expression of who we are in the world. As our sense of identity evolves, we bring along some of who we are with us, but we also make room for who we are on route to becoming. To make that space, we leave behind the experiences and labels that no longer fit our current identities.

Passion is the fire that remakes us. It's the emerging aspect of our Inner Fire that leads us to a more authentic expression of who we are in the world. What we feared to embrace about ourselves in our younger years can become a powerful self-acceptance as we mature. When we no longer care what the critics think of us, passion rises up to take the center stage in our life. I think of Passion as the most invigorating and unbridled expression of what makes us want to live. It is the very life force that we shine into the world. Passion implores us to seize the moment and taste a new experience. It connects us to the outside world in a way that leaves our personal impact upon others and leads us to taste life in new ways.

When we are in survival mode, recreation is seen as an unnecessary indulgence. When we carry numerous burdens, they can hamper our creative expressions. When we allow ourselves to feel the emotions that are waiting inside of our wounds, we slow down our minds enough to give our Inner Fire a chance to surface. When we finally go on vacation, we can finally catch up with our fatigue and feel what we have been holding inside for a long time.

The Creative Process is the Healing Process

The creative process and our own internal healing are inseparable. As we clean out the wounds from the past, they have space to mend and repair. In doing so, we reweave who we are and grow more resilient. Seeing the gifts that shine through our wounds reveals new reflections of whom we are becoming, that person we long to be. As we express those gifts into the world, we create new works of art, new performances, and new shifts in our lives. By understanding our creative process more clearly, we will also see how it is linked to healing from the past and being a more truthful version of ourselves.

There is a special relationship between our Inner Voice of Truth, our Inner Fire, and our Innate Gifts in the creative process. The Inner Voice of Truth tells us who we are meant to be through our longings. The passionate movement of our Inner Fire is the propellant for our longings to manifest into the world as a new reality. As our Inner Fire fuels the expression of our Innate Gifts into the world, we generate a product into the world. So, as we express our Truth through our Gifts, that flow is facilitated by our Inner Fire in the form of Passion.

Passion happens when our Fire is expressed through our innate gifts in a way that fulfills our deepest longings. It is the sheer desire to express our gifts into the world. Our longings are not just composed of what we wish to get out of life. They are also what we long to give to the world. Some would even say that we are meant to share certain gifts with the world.

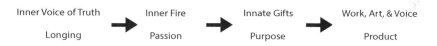

Inner Voice of Truth		Inner Fire		Innate Gifts		Work, Art, & Voice
Longing		Passion		Purpose		Product

Figure 10. Inner Dynamics of Producing Art

If purpose is the mission, then passion is the jet fuel that makes it happen. Without passion, we run out of gas. We go through the motions. We work for the sake of paying the bills, for the sake of survival. Survival can be a powerful motivator, but it alone does not lead to thriving. Passion helps us remember why we are alive. It reconnects us with pleasure, curiosity, and our thirst for living. It helps us to forge new creative and intimate relationships which enhance our experience of life.

Let's take a closer look at how passion moves energetically. It begins with a longing. The longing can either pull something towards us that we have always desired to receive, or it can pull something out of us that we feel drawn to share. In the case when we have a longing to receive an unmet need from others, like validation. For instance, our longing will draw us to the people who we sense can provide that validation. We will feel excited when we are around this person, not only because we might feel attracted to them (romantically or platonically), but also because we feel an anticipation that they will give us something that we need. This pulling out of our normal routine is beneficial because it brings us out of our old script where we can potentially have a new experience.

When we have a longing to share a gift or change something in the world, we propel that longing from inside of our body to the outside world. We try to match that externalized longing with relationships and opportunities where the longing can be fulfilled. Longing is the first extension of passion. It sparks our fires, creating the motivation to fulfill some kind of mission or purposeful exchange. Once the longing establishes a direction, our Fire has a direction to flow towards.

Passion can bring us together to forge new relationships. The creative fires are our sexual fires. The friction between personalities can feed the Inner Fire, making it rise up and push through old emotions that are connected to our past experiences. This is how the conflicts of our lives inspire change, by stimulating the Fire to move to the surface. Passion is the fuel that fulfills our longings to connect and our sense of purpose.

Recovering our Fire

In order to reclaim our full creative power and our ability to manifest our most fulfilling relationships, we need to recover as much of our Inner Fire as possible. So often, we look to what we produce in our work and creativity into the outer world and ignore the transformational forge inside of us that powers that production. We rarely look inside to check on our own inner energy levels until we have hit extreme burnout or physical distress. When the passion fades in an intimate partnership, we are conditioned to blame the other person or outer circumstances for the loss of chemistry. There will always be demanding family members, work deadlines, and emergencies in our life. Most of these situations are beyond our control. But what is always in our hands is to tend to our inner flame. By being aware of what is making us angry in a conflict, we can express it and realign our flow in passionate connection to our loved ones. By understanding when we have felt shamed in a way that has dampened or covered our Fire, we can ask for help in releasing that past experience. To understand what help our Inner Fire needs from us, we need to feel it on a regular basis.

Phases of Fire Recovery

If our Inner Fire was allowed to grow from childhood to adulthood, with careful guidance and protection from abuse, we would grow into a sense of power without hindrance. As infants, our spark of life would be an unbridled cry into the night and an infectious smile during our happy moments. Going through our terrible two's would bring us independence and teach us about the word "no" in an empowering way, without shaming or abuse. We would form fond memories in our teenage years, enjoying a balance between the pleasures of our hormones and a sense of responsibility. Teenage prom meltdowns would happen with the patient guidance of parents and grandparents. As adults, we would choose a vocation and partnerships that allow long-term passion to flow. As elders, we would pursue the pleasures of life, making our bucket list dreams come true while also serving as sacred witnesses for the younger generations.

The vast majority of people don't grow up with this smooth transition from one phase of life to the next. It is far more likely that you either grew up like a hot, splashy mess, or you had to learn to box your fire inside, like a bomb waiting to explode. You may be somewhere in between, striving to find a balance point between these two extremes, but it's very likely that you lean towards one side or the other. Honesty in your current starting point is essential to helping your Inner Fire mature into a state of empowerment.

As the hidden elements of our unexpressed family stories attract us to people who help us relive those family stories, we will eventually discover how the repeating story poses a challenge to our Inner Fire. Even after we have released our burdens, we must reclaim the power to direct our own lives. After carrying burdens for so long, we learned to behave according to the script. The Inner Fire is what helps us dissolve the deep impressions that the scripted portions of our lives have left on us.

In essence, by breaking free from the script, we recover the Inner Fire that wants to be free. The following Phases of Fire Recovery can be seen as general snapshots of how an obstructed Fire can move towards a more free and sustainable expression. It assumes that some type of generational dumping has occurred in the past.

Just because you have endured abuse in the past doesn't necessarily put you at Phase I. It takes repeated bombardments to reach the state of Phase I. In your past inner work, you may have discovered an empowering connection to your Inner Fire, but you didn't necessarily have the word or framework to understand what you have already accomplished. These snapshots are meant to help you gauge your progress, not rigidly define how "evolved" you are as a person. There are no PhDs or martial arts black belts in Fire Recovery.

Phase I: Complete Repression of the Inner Fire

Wounding from the past, in the form of betrayal, abandonment, and shaming, has forced you to hide your Fire completely. There is little to no trust in your Inner Fire. It is seen as a problem or an unclean force that will get you into trouble. Complete restriction of sexual expression, anger, and personal desires are characteristic of Phase I.

Very often, you will feel depressed. The world seems like an old black and white movie and you won't be able to really taste your food. Phase I is always coupled with being in some form of survival mode. There is considerable effort to stay low and not stand out. You hide to protect yourself from further rejection or invasion at all costs. Hope is seen as being a false experience and all dreaming is cut off to prevent future disappointment. Phase I can also come with suicidal thoughts and a misguided belief that death may be the only way out of this depressed state. It may be hard to even get out of bed, as all of your inner resources go towards avoiding your anger and repressing your Fire. People in this Phase often use addictive substances or excessive work to avoid feeling their Inner Fire. Controlling the Fire as a way of staying safe is the strongest motivation.

Phase II: Fire in Servitude

This is the do, do, do Phase, where you will be busy all of the time. Phase II happens with a more highly functional form of survival mode where everything is about being productive and having something to show for your efforts. Celebration or enjoyment is devalued. In this phase, your

Inner Fire is devoted to the service of other people so that you are valuable to them. Constantly achieving goals or making money is the driving force in your life. A sense of self-worth is built around what you *do* rather than who you *are*. The Inner Fire is only allowed to flow when it is focused on a work task or in brief moments of venting or having sex.

One way to recognize if you are in Phase II of Recovering your Inner Fire is when you are on vacation. Do you squeeze in work when you could be enjoying the moment with your friends and family? Do you pack so much planning into the trip that there is little time for rest and free flowing exploration? Are you afraid to slow down and feel your exhaustion because it may impede your brain's ability to get things done? If this sounds familiar, consider that you have successfully learned how to channel your Fire very efficiently into work, volunteering, or a sport. But the other aspects of your Fire may not have much room to be expressed.

In this Phase, there is a heavy emphasis on accumulating external proof of your self-worth. An athlete may skip going to prom and vacations to train as an Olympic athlete. A child may be completely obsessed with their online rankings of a video game to show that they have mastery and control over that fictional environment. An executive will work tirelessly for a promotion at the sacrifice of having meaningful relationships with their family, friends, and romantic partners.

Phase II comes with desires, goals, and aspirations, but celebration and exploration are curbed because there is general mistrust of the Fire being expressed outside of these very focused tasks. Sex must fit into the busy work schedule and it's not uncommon to return to checking work correspondences shortly after the act is finished. There is minimal basking in the afterglow, and the mind ramps up again to work on all the things on your checklist. The motivation behind this Phase is to feel powerful by proving your self-worth to others. The constant *doing* keeps you safe by being a moving target which limits the opportunity to be judged or rejected by other people. If you do good in the world, it's hard for others to say something bad about you.

The majority of financially successful people reside in this state of Fire for prolonged periods of time to achieve their status and wealth. There are many benefits to this way of being. But the long-term cost of prolonged highly stressful forms of performance, without the necessary relaxation, can be detrimental to our physical and emotional health. We may earn a lot of accolades and money but have little revelry and few people to genuinely celebrate the fruits of our labor with. This is why many highly successful people eventually reach a point where they leave their prestigious jobs and the corporate culture to pursue their own consulting businesses, provide freelance services, or simply take sabbaticals away from their highly stressful responsibilities. To do so often requires some kind of decompression and fiery expression that occurs in the next phase. Because Phase II is often glorified in many societies, it can be very scary to break away from the disempowering servitude that comes with the personal successes.

Phase III: Personal Rebellion Against the Script

It often takes some kind of Catalyst Event, either positive or negative, to reach Phase III. It could be embarking on a new relationship that invokes strong feeling of chemistry that proves to you that there is more to life than just service and achievements. Or, it could come in the form of some type of appalling crisis: the death of a loved one, a divorce, or repetitive abuse that brings you to your breaking point. While it is possible to make a conscious decision that you have earned enough to safely enjoy your life, most people must be forced into facing their Fire in order to move from Phase II to Phase III.

Hitting Phase III means you enter into a personal rebellion. It comes with recognizing just how much of your life has gone according to the expectations of others, and how few of your personal dreams have come true. A voice deep in your gut will say, "I can't take this anymore!" As the Fire surfaces, personal feelings that are trapped in the wound are also released. It's the Inner Fire that helps push them to the surface. In Phase III, you begin to value other aspects of your life outside of your formal obligations. You begin to pay attention to your sexuality, creative expressions, hobbies, and interests in travel.

This phase is characterized by an outpouring of resentment and outrage about how you have been expected to behave in a certain way by others. You rebel against the restrictive expectations of your family and society. Phase III is when the glue of the script really begins to melt, as you rebel against dynamics and expectations that are unfair and one-sided. It is common for people going through this phase without guidance and support to do impulsive things like suddenly quit their jobs without having a safety net. The impulses to change your life will be incredibly strong and it's important not to rush into decisions while experiencing your Inner Fire come up this strongly. Take time to get to know your Inner Fire. Give it time to clarify before you end a relationship or move to another country. Your Inner Fire is still clarifying itself as the catharsis clears the path of the Inner Voice of Truth. The first angry expressions may have a degree of truth to them, but they can be muddy with shame, judgments, and the desire to seek revenge for how you have been hurt. The more the emotional catharsis is allowed to flow, the more refined and clear the truth behind it becomes.

During this phase, you can move through large amounts of catharsis and reach the Transformational Fire that asserts your right to be angry and clarifies what you want out of your life. You'll realize that the past has been disempowering and the current state of your life is limited by the familiar scripts of the past. Personal liberation becomes a greater priority than living the life you are expected to live.

You do not need to lose your livelihood, become homeless, or fire all those friends and family members who have hurt your or disappointed you in the past in order to embrace your Inner Fire. It is healthier to be with your anger in order to understand what is telling you about relationships before you make major changes.

The motivation of Phase III is to express the unheard hurts from the past to validate what you have been through. Revenge can be tempting during this phase as a way of bringing people to account for what they have done to you. As your Fire burns away your reactions to past abuse, you become more in touch with your Inner Voice of Truth. Instead of revenge, the Inner Voice of Truth will guide you to what you need to do next to set the record straight. If you were the victim of a crime, you will have the motivation to address what has happened to you. You may feel the need to confront your parents or other family members for past offenses and moments of neglect. In your personal relationships, you will feel the need stand up for yourself in conflicts. There is no perfect way to act in this phase, but those who spend time feeling their anger and getting to know their Fire tend to make decisions that they can trust.

Phase IV: Owning your Passion

When rebellion has helped you to break free of the scripts that kept your Fire restrained, you will notice that the Transformational Fire leads to the Awakening of your Passion. As this more mature expression of your Inner Fire surfaces, it will feel invigorating and enlivening. You will once again dream about what you want to do with your life. Your yearning to see other places will re-emerge. You will taste the full flavor of your meals and sex will feel passionate and exploratory. Life will feel as if you are living in a full color adventure, where you are the hero on a journey.

If you fall in love while your Fire is expanding in this way, the playful courtship of the relationship will last longer than usual if the other partner is also reaching the same phase. The freshness and excitement of the relationship will sustain for many years as you help each other to recreate the relationship, making is fresh and stimulating again.

This is when you come into the full realization of what you are truly passionate about experiencing and what you really want to do with your life. You explore your long-neglected talents, and tap into new ones, with a sense of play and satisfaction.

Phase V: Owning your Power

Phase V is when you begin to understand how powerful you really are as an individual. This inner power is not about your family's influence in the world or about job titles. It's a deeper understanding that you are the most powerful person in your life. You have the power of choice over your major life decisions. When you reflect on your life in this phase, you know that all the people who coerced you and convinced you to repress your Inner Fire in the past could only have done so with your participation. You had the final say in the matter.

As you move through Phase IV, you realize that you move from a victim perspective of "life is not fair, and the world is unsafe," to "I own my part in this, and I take responsibility for expressing my Inner Fire."

Further empowerment comes after the catharsis of how we were hurt by others by seeing the power that comes with self-responsibility. If we are responsible, then we have the power to change how we live our lives and how we relate to our Inner Fires.

This is the phase where you not only explore the gifts that you feel passionate about, but you also commit to making your passionate expressions a significant part of your daily life. You make the changes that are necessary in your relationships in order to be surrounded by people who understand and support your passion. You make changes in your romantic relationships so that you feel empowered to explore each other again.

Phase V can be considered as the most crucial step in the maturation of our Inner Fire. Your rebellion, which disrupted the unhealthy scripts, has grown into a more developed self-awareness of how capable you are of changing the direction of your path. You are no longer the hostage of a hijacked ship. You are the empowered captain who owns past mistakes and charts a new course for your life.

The motivation of this phase of recovery is to reconcile with yourself and to unify with your Inner Fire. By owning your participation in the oppressive scripts that you colluded with, you reclaim ownership over your Inner Fire. You apologize to yourself and others for your part in past hurt. You courageously face the feelings that come with making amends to yourself and others. Like a crucible, your Fire dissolved guilt, shame, and fear away so that it can flow more fully. Only the purest elements are left behind, making you a channel for the clear expression of your Inner Truth.

When you have laid the inner fight between the life you "should be living" and the life you feel passionate about living to rest, sharing your Fire will feel empowering. Your Inner Fire is no longer in servitude to the expectations held in the script or to the obligations of work. True service is when you share your Inner Fire because you want to make the world a better place, not because a scripted life demands it.

Exercise: Cleaning Your Fire

To take inventory of the muck that is stuck to your Inner Fire, try the following exercise.

- Set the intention to connect with your Inner Fire. Feel for any pressure, heat, or tingling inside your torso.
- In your mind, envision yourself expressing yourself in very passionate waves. Give yourself permission to be over-the-top, flamboyant, irreverent, and even inappropriate in your vision of yourself. What are you doing? Dancing? Screaming? Singing Karaoke? Having sex outdoors? Smacking your boss across the face? Whatever you envision, allow it to happen.
- Now write down all the judgments that arise up in your mind as you watch this movie inside your mind in which you are expressing your Fire without hesitation.
- Once you have a list of judgments, question each one: "From whom did I hear this judgment before?" Write down as many names, institutions, and sources of judgment as you can for each one - it's more than likely that you've heard the same message from more than one source.
- Once you have completed the list, notice how many of these judgments about your Inner Fire came from other people.
- Now turn your attention to the number of judgments that you had a hand in creating yourself. You may have just tailored judgments you heard from other people to fit something about yourself.

- Ask yourself if any of these judgments somehow protected you? If so, write down how.
- Now ask yourself which of these judgments you are ready to release.
- Write them all down onto little, separate pieces of paper. Using a candle in a fire safe environment or a fireplace, burn the judgments that you are releasing, saying out loud, "I release the judgment that I am _____." After you burn each piece of paper, say aloud, "I honor my Fire as a source of healing and passion."
- Don't worry if there are judgments that you are not ready to let go of. Just being aware of them is healing because you have illuminated what has been stuck onto your Inner Fire and earmarked it for future work.

The Dance Between Fire and Empathy

Although we have learned how catharsis happens when a wound is first opened in Realization #4 and how the Inner Fire expresses through the wound in Realization #5, we have to be aware that when a wound opens up, a mix of emotions and angry truth can come up all at once. The process does not always happen this neatly in the moment, but it does help to separate the various feelings that are experienced after the catharsis has happened.

There is often a dance between Empathy, the ability to feel what other people are going through emotionally, and our Inner Fire which wants to be the one who is heard and seen. Empathy for another person and the full expression of your personal Inner Fire does not happen at the same time. They take turns. When you are the one emoting, especially when the Inner Fire is speaking your truth, you need other people to be empathic towards you. If you try to be empathic to another person while you are expressing your own feelings, you change the direction of the energy flow in your heart. Rather than energy coming out, you are now taking in someone else's experience empathically. This obstructs your full ability to emote.

To help us make sense of the back and forth movement between Empathy and our Inner Fire, lets look at how we experience Empathy and Inner Fire in our bodies. The heart is the center of our empathy. While it is possible to have an empathic response in any part of us, the heart is where empathy is often felt the strongest. The hips are the center of our Inner Fire. While we can feel fire in any part of our body, including inside our passionate hearts, our vital fire is strongest in our hips when it is allowed to flow in an unrestricted way. It often flows up to our hearts in a way that attempts to clear out the blocks in our hearts so that when it arises to our mouths, it helps us to express our Truth.

When we over-empathize with others, we will take on their clouds of hurt into our hearts. We will imbibe their feelings and if we aren't aware of where the emotions are coming from outside of ourselves, we will mistakenly call them our own. When we do this, we lose our center and overly identify with the sad story of another person. This takes the attention away from what we need to feel about our own life experience.

As we take on the woes of another person and confuse them with being our own feelings, their clouds of hurt begin to fill our inner space. As the inner space of our hearts fill up, there is less space for our own emotions to rise up and be expressed. When we are overly empathetic to others, we essentially keep our own emotions repressed because we give away the space to other people. We de-emphasize the importance of our own feelings, which devalues what we have been through, and places too much emphasis on what others are experiencing.

Taking on the heavy emotional exhaust from another person can lead to fatigue. Whereas only a few moments ago, before we came into contact with that other "moody" person, we were feeling very at ease, we may suddenly become irritable. This is commonly experienced when one feels drained after listening to someone vent about the difficulties they are experiencing. As the emotional clouds fill our inner space, we become frustrated and annoyed. These feelings are early indicators that our Inner Fire is pushing back against the emotions that are clouding the heart. When empathy is out of balance, it gives too much space away to others, so the Inner Fire rises up, like an emotional immune system. It attempts to protect the body and mind from being drained or infiltrated by the heavy moods of others. Again, empathy is a gift that is necessary to heal ourselves and the world. But the Inner Fire is its dance partner that must take steps forward in order to preserve a healthy balance in our relationships. They work together to establish a sustainable give and take in a relationship.

The problem that many highly empathic people encounter is they are judged when they respond in a way that is "fiery," and that is unexpected as they had always formerly assumed the role of "the shoulder to cry on." These judgments can come in the form of comments about your "attitude," or in the form of body language that recoils or withdraws from you as you express your annoyance, and even being labeled as being "bad," "angry," or "a problem." These comments may even have been made in the past and may have left you with a judgment that you've absorbed.

For instance, Linda and Wendy had been lifelong friends. When Wendy's husband committed adultery, Linda would be the person she would turn to for support and advice. Wendy, however, returned to her husband after each incident and would carry on the charade until the next time. After one too many evenings of hearing the same story over and over again, Linda suddenly felt irritated and lashed out at Wendy for not taking ownership of her own situation. Being empathetic towards Wendy for so many years had left Linda drained and as if she had no space in her own heart to deal with her own life and challenges. Their friendship had become unbalanced and because of her nature, Linda was being weighed down with Wendy's sadness. Wendy could not understand her friend's sudden change in attitude and accused her of being a bad friend.

Harsh judgments push the Fire back down, preventing it from rising up to defend the inner sanctum. But the irritation is a good thing. It is the first rumbles of that protective fire in your hips rising up, like a hot geyser deep beneath the ground. You can hear it before you witness the full power of its expression.

When the Inner Fire is expressed vocally, it can more effectively protect you. Sometimes, a clean expression of anger is all it takes to back someone off who may be dumping their stuff on you. The anger sets boundaries with other people. Too much empathy with others eclipses self-empathy, meaning, and having enough space to feel your own feelings, including anger.

On the flip side, people who are overtly expressive of their anger and passions in a narcissistic way, often lack empathy. Their capacity to relate to another person's struggles, including the harm that they have personally inflicted, is very limited. There is no internal room in their hearts to feel what others are feeling. Their Inner Fire is overactive, like a constant allergy where the immune system constantly overreacts to everything it encounters. Emotionally, they are overprotective of themselves and express their Fires in ways that maximizes personal gain.

People in this state walk into a room like a superstar, commanding attention, and have little awareness of how they are impacting others. They are often labeled as being "selfish," though they are often rewarded for their behavior with success. But underneath their external, fiery display, they have very thin skin when it comes to criticism or disapproval. Very often, they were deeply betrayed in the past and learned to keep their hearts closed, relying on their Fires to protect them from people getting too close again. Without their heart reopening, empathy isn't possible.

The most satisfying and complete healing experiences come when both Empathy and the Inner Fire are given enough room to dance with each other. Neither of them steals the show. You have your chance to share your story in an uncensored way and also listen to others in a heartfelt way that is mutually supportive.

Robin's Purge

Robin was a 50-year-old Caucasian woman from southern California. She came from a long line of alcoholics and got sober shortly after having her son. Her mother died early due to a painful autoimmune disease, as well as the unhealthy lifestyle of an active alcoholic. Determined not to repeat the same mistakes as her mother, Robin vowed to herself that she would be healthy and be present for her son. She eventually married and created the safe, stable home life that she never had growing up. She maintained her emotional and physical health due to a combination of support groups, yoga, therapy, and healing work.

Her peaceful world was disrupted when two major family crises happened while she was bedridden after a hysterectomy. Her son was away at college and was admitted to hospital because of a ruptured appendix. Shortly after, she received a phone call from her brother telling her that her niece had died because of a drug overdose. Flat on her back, Robin naturally wanted to jump on a plane and rush to her son's aid. If she had been able to walk, she would have done so, and then planned to fly to her niece's funeral to help her family grieve. But the stitches had only been sewn hours earlier and it was physically impossible for her to do anything but receive updates by phone.

When our healing session began, Robin was relieved to say that her son was on the way to making a full recovery from his surgery. But the grief of losing her niece was still fresh, as was the tender recovery from her recent hysterectomy. After years of advancing endometriosis, she decided to have the surgery. This perfect storm of crisis mixed with a very invasive and painful medical procedure squeezed this normally placid woman to have severe gastric reflux and pain.

After scanning her body, I shared that her Inner Fire had been repressed inside her uterus for many years. When the uterus was cut out during her hysterectomy, it ruptured the emotional storage container of those emotions. Now, her anger was rolling up from her hips to her stomach, trying to find a release for all the past abuses, including childhood sexual abuse, from her body.

Because Robin had been in therapy for years, she felt like she had done enough emotional work to be free from pain. The eruption of the gastric reflux was disrupting her life, impacting her ability to eat and even sleep in the same bed as her husband because she needed to be on an elevated surface. She suffered physically and emotionally each day. Both her primary care physician and her gastroenterologist confirmed that the reflux was stress-related.

I helped Robin to see that the Inner Fire, however disruptive it was to her daily life, was a healing force. She felt "burning" sensations, first in her uterus when she had endometriosis, and now the burning in her stomach from the gastric reflux. I lead her through an exercise to breathe into the physical pain to feel the heat trapped inside her stomach. As she breathed out, she could feel the burning grow more intensely. Then she realized that the burning was anger. Eventually, the red clouds of anger released out of her stomach area.

In a follow-up session a week later, I directed her to write letter to the people who had angered her. She wrote two letters. The first one was to her brother, who had been an active drug addict for many years. Venting her rage at the premature death of her niece, she expressed to her brother in her letter how he had neglected his daughter. Robin had warned him that she needed help so that she did not die young the way their mother had done. But he didn't listen to her and now her niece was gone.

The second letter was to her still living maternal grandmother who had abused her mother growing up. Robin had helped manage her grandmother's finances, however, she avoided being around her because she was a lonely toxic person who insulted everyone she met. In her letter, she vented to her grandmother about her brutal emotional treatment of her mother. Robin could see that the abuse that her mother had endured at the hands of her maternal grandmother had contributed to the alcoholism that contributed to her early death. That abandonment and emotional ridicule also impacted on Robin, because while she wasn't ridiculed in the same way by her mother, she felt a deep abandonment by the emotional distance of her constant intoxication.

Both letters helped her purge her hatred for her grandmother and the way her family had treated the younger generations. As her Inner Fire released from her body, I asked her to listen to what it was telling her to do regarding her relationship with her still living brother and maternal grandmother.

She decided that she was going to return the responsibilities of the finances back to her grandmother. As she put it, "If grandma can buy jewelry from television infomercials, then she can write three checks a month to pay her own bills." She made an agreement to tell her case worker that she would no longer be available to assist her grandmother and she passed that responsibility onto the case worker. Because of how extreme her grandmother's recent verbal abuse had been, she decided that she would say goodbye to her grandmother and not be in contact with her anymore.

Robin also decided that her addict brother was not able to hear what she needed to tell him. He didn't heed her warnings about her niece's need for in-patient drug rehabilitation and he was not able to hear the truth of how she felt about his neglectful parenting. Because she didn't want to be responsible for triggering more depression or drug use by calling him out on his failings as a parent, she decided to spend the next week or so venting and journaling about her anger towards him. Eventually, it became clear to her that her concern for her now deceased niece was the only reason she had tried to maintain a relationship with her brother. She didn't feel close to him, and while she had moments of empathy for his grief, she didn't have a reason to be in his life. As she released that relationship, she also released the burden of being the voice of reason to her drug addicted and alcoholic relatives. Her contribution to her family would be her own longevity as a mother to a well-adjusted son.

Like Robin, we all need to make tough decisions about the relationships in our lives. When the initial anger has been expressed, our Inner Fire helps gain clarity about which relationships are healthy, and which need to be changed or released. Such big changes can often come with social pressures to stick out toxic relationships and can even result in family or community punishment for making such potent choices.

But a toxic relationship will not change on its own if both people are stuck in the script. It only requires one person to wake up, listen to their Inner Fire, and then express their truth to shift a relationship.

When you identify a toxic relationship in your life, your Inner Fire will direct you to make a choice, such as talk to the person about a conflict or stand up for yourself in a work meeting. It may direct you to release the relationship completely, which may happen after a direct conversation or with a conscious falling out of contact.

Exercise: Purging Toxic People

You will notice repetitive patterns in the Letter Burning practice. What repeating themes emerged in those letters? How were you disrespected or hurt in the past? As you begin to see the cyclic patterns of abuse in your lineage, you can begin to examine your current life to see if any of those disrespectful scripts are repeating themselves.

For this exercise, we need a recent community map done within in the last two weeks. If you have already noticed a lot of recent flux in your relationships or it's been more than two weeks since your last Community Map was completed, please do a fresh one. Then follow these steps:

- Take a few deep breaths and allow the energy in your head to drop down to your heart. Put your hand on your chest to help you feel your heart.
- Take a few more deep breaths and bring your attention to your solar plexus just below your chest bone. Put your hand over your diaphragm and feel your breathing.
- When you feel like you have a good connection to your gut, scan the Community Map with the intention of locating toxic relationships. Without analyzing whether or not the person is toxic, write their name down. Do this for as many names that come up.

- Now think about the people who might not show up on your Community Map, but who you encounter in other areas of your life. This may be your child's teacher, an acquaintance in your gym class, or a co-worker. It might also be an old friend who has resurfaced, or a family member who has been involved in a recent conflict that has impacted you. Write these names down on the list.
- Now go through each name one at a time. Ask yourself the following questions and write the responses down:
  - How does this person make me feel? (Write down both physical sensations and emotional responses)
  - Why am I upset with this person?
  - What does my Inner Fire tell me to do about this relationship?
  - What agreement can I make with myself to change or leave the relationship?
- Once you have done this for each name that appeared on the list, set reasonable timelines for the agreements that you have made with yourself.

Listening to your Inner Fire takes practice. This fiery voice inside is trying to protect you. By understanding how it is trying to look out for you, you can find a sense of empowerment in your relationship choices.

The agreements you make with yourself are self-promises to respect and protect yourself. Our Inner Fire helps us determine what's right for us in moments of conflicts. When we make agreements that re-establish our self-respect, we empower our Inner Fire as the source of authority over our relationships. We no longer behave according to the socially acceptable scripts. We do what we feel is healthiest for ourselves. This is not being selfish, it is being self-aware of what we need to feel respected, healthy, and clear in our relationships.

As eager as you might be to re-establish respect in all your relationships, it is important to set reasonable timelines for the heart-to-heart talks, work stand offs, and uncomfortable confrontations. If you have multiple toxic people in your life, pace your agreements so that you can recover your energy after an intense conversation. Don't binge purge.

Traps:

Blaming Yourself

One way of repressing the Inner Fire after it has surfaced is to redirect it towards yourself. Instead of owning the Fire in a healthy and productive way by expressing it aloud or sharing how you feel with a trusted supporter, the anger is aimed back inside with angry self-talk. This is done with the assumption that it is better to take it out on yourself than to inflict it on another person. But you are just as valuable and important a person as another human being. Inflicting verbal and physical abuse against yourself is still harming a sentient being.

People who are highly masochistic not only neglect to take responsibility for their Inner Fire when they hurt themselves, but they often put the responsibility of taking care of the after-effects of self-punishment on their loved ones. This is done in the hopes that someone will value them in a way that they cannot or will not do. This can place the burden for their emotional and physical well-being on the shoulders of another person who cares for them greatly. This dynamic can be likened to the masochist punching himself in the eye, and then complaining that he was not even offered a pack of ice for the bruise he inflicted upon himself.

As you come to know your Inner Fire, recognize self-destructive behavior.

The Undertow

The Undertow is a seductive pull that keeps people in their place within a family. It is often built around seniority, where the older family members have more of the authority, although not always. It's easiest to recognize when we have return to our family home after being away for a while. When we fall into its pull, we come back into the fold. We assume the expected role, we dust off the old scripts, and we tone down anything "different" about ourselves. It can feel like a warm, familiar bed to some or like a lushly padded and stifling coffin for others. The Undertow is not inherently bad, as it creates a gravity that brings a family together. What makes it feel differently to people depends on what roles they are expected to play.

Among survivors of sexual abuse, there can be an alluring pull back into old patterns of abuse, no matter how much pain they may have endured as a result of the abuse. There is a hypnotic haze that encases them when they are in the presence of their abuser. Only an inner repulsion, a fiery defiance, can help them break the spell and pull away.

As we defiantly pull away from whatever script we inherited from our families, we begin to feel the unsavory side of the Undertow. Just like the undertow in the ocean, it can feel pleasant as it quickly and smoothly pulls us out to sea. We need not paddle our arms at all, yet we are in motion. But the moment you try to move in the other direction, you feel the scary pull and massive strength of it. As you try to walk to shore, the shell pieces cut like glass and your legs are pulled out from under you. If you tire, you can drown.

The first-generation survivors of the Holocaust often tempered their zest for life, as if the very ghosts of the deceased were watching them. They didn't want to celebrate because it felt as if it may be interpreted as insensitivity to those who had perished. They remained subconsciously connected to their fallen loved ones. Their children and grandchildren were taught to minimize their celebration and fun out of respect for the dead. The message was; *keep your head down, don't stand out, and remember the ones who didn't make it.* That grief painted a shadow on every moment of their lives. Even those Holocaust survivors who didn't necessarily believe in an afterlife, they still behaved as if the ones who didn't make it would somehow know. To many, it was safer, and more loyal, to lay low.

That Undertow drew them in. Because the family missed the deceased, because they loved them and longed for them to be alive, the magnetism of their love often disguised the undercurrent of the heavier emotions. It was the force that pulled people back into the expected scripts and kept family members who had never even been to the camps, in a suppressed state of being. When involving the deceased, the Undertow was illusive, a tug from some mystical source that analysis alone did not seem to break. It all centered around the lost family members, those who had perished among the anonymous victims of war. No funeral. No closure. No clear goodbye. It was a recipe for being perpetually haunted by the past.

Repressing Hatred

When our Inner Fire becomes tangled in numerous scripts, the limiting beliefs can stifle our expression of it. These scripts can be religious, cultural, racial, and those that are unique to your family. These scripts can even be personally created based on your own experiences. For instance, if you were robbed by a man or woman of a certain race, you may be suspicious or overtly racist towards other people from the same background. This is based on your personal experience, not necessarily what a racist grandparent told you, although it is possible for both the personal script and family script to overlap. Any discriminatory script based on race, gender, creed, or other distinguishing characteristics can restrict the Inner Fire so completely, that the fire festers and takes the form of hatred.

Hatred is the most powerful unconscious expression of our Inner Fire. Unlike the conscious expression of justified anger, which is directly expressed to the offending individual who caused you pain, hatred takes over the free will of the person feeling it. Without bringing awareness to the hatred by tracing back the original source of the hurt and anger, hateful scripts will assume control of behavior like a robot programmed by software.

A further hindrance to healing hatred is to judge it as being "bad" or "wrong." It's true that a hate crime is morally wrong and should be addressed by legal means. Acting out of hatred is wrong. But feeling hate is neither immoral nor unhealthy. Feeling your hatred allows you to get close to it and understand why you feel that way. It allows you to sort through the scripts you are carrying and trace your way back to the original wounds that helped create the hatred. It's not wrong to feel how you feel; it's wrong to act upon it in an unconscious or intentional way. Feel your hate and allow yourself to get close to it. Doing so brings consciousness to your Inner Fire, enabling you to transform hatred into a more productive form of energy.

Our Inner Fire is the driving force behind our creativity, sexuality, personal empowerment and our vitality. It is also the healing force that opens our wounds and reveals our Innate Gifts that our wounds helped us to discover.

Our Inner Fire is fully realized when our passion is expressed through our Innate Gifts. The act of repeatedly expressing our passion through our gifts leads us to constantly experience the truth of who we are inside. It is the Inner Voice of Truth that pulls us to our Innate Gifts, wanting us to discover our most authentic expressions as a way of embracing our deepest identity. The Inner Fire has burned a clear path for us to claim the Innate Gifts emerging from inside the wound.

The 6th Realization

We All Have Innate Gifts that Give us Purpose

Vision for Realization #6

We sat together on the shore. I held her hand as the waves of fire and emotions rippled through her. She couldn't believe what she had just done. It was invigorating and scary. There were moments of laughter and relief. These were followed by salty tears of regret at having to leave her family behind. She felt both free and uncertain.

"What am I doing?" she screamed. She had lost everything familiar to her. Breaking away from her scripted life felt liberating, but she also feared the unknown path that she had chosen.

In the distance, she could still see her family treading water in the distance. The pull of guilt made her fantasize about swimming back to them. I had watched other Catalysts in the panic of an identity crisis, return to their family in the ocean. They tried to fit into the mold again, but they had grown too much to resume their old role in the script of the family theater. No longer having a script to follow, she needed a new way to direct her life.

Her gaze turned to the shimmering waves of the ocean. Memories of ballet and childhood plays surfaced in her mind. Her family, always too overwhelmed by their jobs and personal struggles, never came to watch her dance. They didn't recognize her passion. They couldn't understand her need to express herself through dance. Alone in her room at night, she would dance before the mirror in front of an imaginary audience.

She rose from the sand and began to dance. She pressed her wrists together as if they had been bound together. Her body contorted in pulses as if she were trying to break free. Her hips twirling, sliding her body across the beach in powerful circles. With speed, she launched into the air, her wrists freed and legs extended in opposite directions. In the ruby light of sunset, her body soared free. The rush of fulfillment and celebration filled her form. It felt right to finally dance again.

"You have a gift," I said to her. "You tell stories through the movement of your body."

Tears streamed down her face, those tears of gratitude when you finally receive the acknowledgement of your talent. She had been waiting her whole life for her family to witness her gifts. When she danced, she felt like she was being herself. It was who she was in her purest form. This was why she had broken away, so that she could embrace her gifts and share them with passion. She was no longer just surviving. She was beginning to thrive.

Claiming Your Innate Gifts

Our passion leads us to our Innate Gifts. These shining gifts are what make us brilliant, unique and needed in our communities. They are the next reward that we receive for passing through our wounds and facing our greatest fears. They are the light at the end of the tunnel that helps us define who we are becoming.

By Realization #6, we switch our source of identity from our shared family wounds to defining who we are based on our unique talents and strengths. We no longer hide in our assigned roles according to the script, rather, we claim the personal sovereignty to define ourselves. Our gifts light the way to this self-discovery.

A Catalyst who becomes a professional singer will no longer define herself by her wounded past. Instead, she will use her past hurt as inspiration to create music that reaches deeply inside of her. Those rough experiences of the past become ways of relating to other people on a human, feeling level. But it's that inspiring rush that she feels when she courageously shares her gifts with the world that will help her recognize her true identity. Our Innate Gifts, ignited by our passion for sharing them, are a deeper source of our selfhood than our family story and the wounds we have inherited.

When a past abuser wounds us, they are giving us a beneficial offering in disguise. This doesn't make how they disrespected you in the past right. They harmed you and they should be held accountable for what they have done. But by this stage of the healing process, you can see how all the hard work of healing that wound that they inflicted has brought you a greater self-awareness.

The past abuser is now a clear mirror to reflect back who you are and unconsciously helped you discover your hidden strengths. This is why you don't place your identity in their hands; because they are caught in the unconscious, repetitive wounding of others. They can't see who you truly are inside. But now that you have passed through your wounds, *you* can begin to see you by embracing the gifts of that painful past.

Inherited Gifts and Personally Unique Gifts

Our gifts can take numerous forms - some may be inherited talents while others may be unique to us as individuals. You may have the same artistic prowess as your grandmother or the ability to carry a tune like your father. Or you may have a gift that your family hasn't seen before, or at the very least, not been seen in your lineage for a very long time. Most families in countries with large immigrant communities, like the United States, forget their lineage past a few generations because the family was often escaping from horrible circumstances.

The distinction between inherited gifts and personally unique gifts is important when it comes to validation. If you have the same talent as a recent family member, you are more likely to receive some type of acknowledgment for the gift, because it is known to your family. People will say to you, "you remind me of your grandfather. He could draw too." You may even experience some favoritism or encouragement, because you remind your family of the previous person who had that gift.

You may also have certain expectations placed on you based on what your elders see in you. In traditional Iroquois society, you carry a Native name that was carried by a deceased person. If you have the same gift, it is likely that you will be given a name with the expectation that you carry a similar role. For example, young women who demonstrate strong will and leadership abilities early on will be groomed to be a Faith Keeper or Clan Mother, two important authority roles in traditional Iroquois society. In Westernized society, we may be named after an elder who had similar talents and personality traits. In both cases, we will be expected to serve the family in a similar way to the deceased elder, because we also carry their name.

A gift that is unique to you, meaning a gift that hasn't appeared in the family in the lifetime of the oldest elders, will more likely be misunderstood or undervalued by your family. These gifts are off the current script of the family, so there may be little encouragement to develop the gift. It would take a very observant and supportive parent or elder to give validation for uncommon gifts.

Having a unique gift can make you feel like an alien within your family, even if that gift is the intellectual capacity to see outside the small world mentality of your upbringing. You may experience more discouragement than validation if your talent is deemed to be "weird." One benefit of having a unique family gift is that there are fewer pre-existing expectations placed on the gift, there is also a freedom to explore it without your elder family members trying to exploit it for their own relief or gain.

I make this distinction because it's important to recognize all our gifts, even those unseen or misunderstood by our kin. Unique gifts are off the script. Because these unique gifts often come with less burdens, they can be harder to discover, because the gift doesn't necessarily have something to push against. There's nothing for your Inner Fire to rebel against. Claiming these gifts often requires someone outside of the family, like a teacher or coach, to recognize your potential and encourage you to pursue it.

While there may be less burdens associated with unique gifts, these untapped talents are often brought to the fore by some type of sounding. Many great musicians and artists discover their gifts, in part, by enduring suffering of some kind, which almost always ties into their childhood family story. They turn to their gifts as a way to relieve their emotional agony. Without a script and burden, it can feel like the gift is left in a vacuum without a witness to call if forth or without an adversary to push against it. These gifts must be discovered by having enough space to play and explore what is inside of you, combined with enough relationship conflicts to bring the wound to light.

A good example of this is Martin Luther King, Jr. inheriting his father's ability to speak with charisma, which they both used as preachers. Both were intelligent men who were reliable leaders in service of their communities. However, in addition to having these shared gifts with his father, Dr. Martin Luther King Jr. was a visionary in a way that reached beyond his father's work as a local community leader. His powerful ability to receive a vision of racial equality in America was a gift beyond what his family had known before. He combined those oratory and leadership abilities with a courageous fire that took non-violent resistance to the next level. Dr. King also had an uncanny gut instinct that helped him to lead people through the spontaneous challenges of the Civil Rights movement protests. His deep connection with his own inner voice of truth was enhanced by him knowing and sharing his innate gifts. So, King Jr. had both inherited gifts and unique gifts that he utilized to change the way the world views race.

Martin Luther King Jr. was actually born Michael King, but like his father he changed his name, after the great religious reformer Martin Luther who stood up against the abuses of the church during the Middle Ages. The young Dr. King, Jr. struggled with what profession he would pursue, so he followed the known script of his family and went to the seminary like his father. It was there that he learned about the work of Gandhi resisting oppression in South Africa and India. Gandhi was a catalyst and inspiration to Dr. King Jr. It inspired him to go beyond the expected obligations of a pastor who ran a church, and to be a pillar in the community as his father had chosen. He was meant for more, and soon began walking his own path after the historical catalyst event that saw Rosa Parks refuse to give up her seat on a Montgomery, Alabama bus because she was a black woman. Martin Luther King Jr. was chosen to be the community organizer of the Montgomery Bus Boycott which was a historic victory of the American Civil Rights Movement.

Multiple Intelligences: The Domains of our Gifts

Educational Psychologist Howard Gardner created a splash in the news when he advanced the idea that human beings have more than one form of intelligence.[19] The Westernized education system is built upon the intellect. The average curriculum is clearly dominated by rational, mathematical, and linguistic forms of thinking as tested in the S.A.T. college entrance exam and the G.R.E. graduate school entrance exam. Other forms of intelligence such as art, music, and physical education are built around rational and linguistic competence in most Westernized education programs. While music education and certain art forms are still celebrated by many institutions, job offerings in more logic-based professions far outnumber those in the creative arts. So, when Harvard Professor Dr. Gardner advanced his idea that there are multiple forms of intelligences beyond our intellect, he immediately validated the many forms of Innate Gifts outside the intellect. The public had to embrace the possibility that human beings were more than just nerds, band geeks, starving artists and jocks.

Westernized societies in general need to see a broader spectrum of our human abilities. For the first time, those who went into other fields

---

19   https://www.niu.edu/facdev/_pdf/guide/learning/
      howard_gardner_theory_multiple_intelligences.pdf

of study that were not completely dominated by physicality (professional sports) or intellect (every office job) received acknowledgement for what made them special. A ship captain who hated the confines of a classroom could finally be appreciated for their spatial intelligence, that ability to gauge distances and direct the vessel through a field of icebergs. This form of intelligence also includes the ability to navigate the vessel in relation to the constellations of the stars. Monks of many traditions are trained in rational discourse and literature, as well as mindfulness training, which gives them a greater awareness of their inner realm, thus enhancing their intrapersonal intelligence.

Dr. Gardner laid out nine forms of human intelligence with the acknowledgement that there may be more. It further specifies our intellectual forms of intelligence as verbal/linguistic and logical/mathematical. It expands intelligence to include those who are gifted in interpersonal relationship-building like agents, public relations specialists, and politicians. Athletes and dancers have bodily/kinesthetic intelligence, while artists and theoretical physicists must rely on their visual/spatial intelligence. Musicians have musical/rhythmic intelligence. Park Rangers and Environmental scientists who work intimately with nature possess a naturalistic intelligence. Yogis and meditation instructors who concentrate on developing their self-awareness develop extraordinary intrapersonal intelligence. These forms of intelligence are summed up in the figure 11.

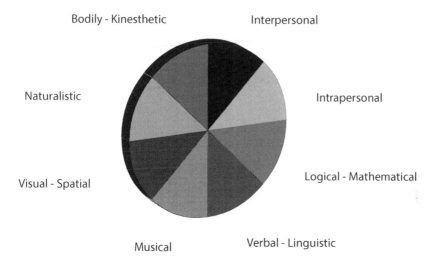

Bodily - Kinesthetic

Interpersonal

Naturalistic

Intrapersonal

Visual - Spatial

Logical - Mathematical

Musical

Verbal - Linguistic

Figure 11. Multiple Intelligences Chart

As seen in figure 11, there are 8 main types of intelligences based on Dr. Gardner's work. Bodily - kinesthetic intelligence refers to body control as seen in an Olympic gymnast and the ability to do hands-on work like a carpenter or mechanic. Interpersonal intelligence represents the ability to understand feelings and needs in relationships with other people as seen in real estate agents and mediators. Intrapersonal intelligence is about understanding interior feelings and thoughts in a clear way as seen in an experienced meditation teacher. Logical - mathematical intelligence is often tested in standardized university tests and represents the ability to rationalize and calculate numbers as seen in physicists. Verbal - linguistic intelligence is also tested in standardized exams to gauge the level of reading comprehension and mastery of one or more languages as seen in a United Nations Interpreter. Musical intelligence is the ability to analyze, compose, and perform music as seen in classical composers and modern day concert performers. Naturalistic intelligence entails understanding the way nature works and the ability to classify living creatures based on their perceived similarities to other living beings as seen in conservationists. Visual – spatial intelligence is the ability to envision, interpret, and create visual images as seen in artists and architects. 18

Exercise: Owning our Innate Gifts

Return to the Innate Gifts that you discovered from the previous Family Tree Scanning exercise. Make the following chart to help you develop a greater understanding of those gifts. Start by entering in all the gifts you discovered in the first column. Then consider which of the intelligences best describes that gift. Don't worry if one of the intelligences doesn't match perfectly. You can change categories at any time. The point of the exercise is to validate that your gifts are a legitimate form of intelligence. It is also fine to include more than one form of intelligence for a gift. The point of this step is to validate that you have a unique form of intelligence that your schooling may not have recognized.

Gift	Type of Intelligences	Vocations
i.e. Painting	Visual/Spatial	Graphic designer, gallery artist
i.e. Nurturing Heart	Interpersonal	Social worker, Healer

Table 2. Gifts to Vocations Exercise

The last column is for vocations that will allow you to express your Innate Gifts. As you consider the vocations that could be a potential expression of your gifts, ask yourself what you have always wanted to do in life. You may be doing something similar for work now, but perhaps you have been considering a shift to a related field or a complete career change. Let this process help you clarify that shift by allowing yourself to daydream about what work would allow you to express your gifts. Refer to the following the Career Chart to help you find the words to match your specific gifts.

Interpersonal	Intrapersonal	Logical-Mathematical	Verbal-Linguistic
Mediator	Actor	Physicist	Language
Therapist	Monk	Accountant	Teacher
Community	Energy Healer	Mathematics	Translator
Organizer	Philosopher	Professor	Interpreter
Public	Poet	Civil Engineer	Comedian
Relations	Writer	Computer	Historian
Agent	Thought	Programmer	Writer
Talent Agent	Leader	Economist	Reporter
Real Estate	Theologian	Bookkeeper	Librarian
Agent	Consultant	Financial	Trial Attorney
Teacher	Silent Retreat	Analyst	Speech
Wait staff	Facilitator	Clinical Trial	Pathology
Promoter	Entrepreneur	Manager	Speech Writer
Trainer	Intuitive	Epidemiologist	Politician
Group	Reader	Real Estate	
Facilitator		Attorney	
Human		Banker	
Resources			
Manager			

Bodily-Kinesthetic	Naturalistic	Musical	Visual-Spatial
Gymnast	Park Ranger	Soundtrack	Architect
Dancer	Ecologist	Composer	Cartoonist
Surgeon	Ergonomics	Piano Teacher	Painter
Personal	Equine	Sound Editor	Pilot
Trainer	Therapist	Songwriter	Ship Captain
Yoga Instructor	Conservationist	Voice Coach	Truck Driver
Physical	Landscaper	Conductor	Urban
Therapist	Veterinarian	Music	Planner
Mechanic	Assistant	Therapist	Interior
Fireman	Environmental	Professional	Designer
Physical	Attorney	Musician	Car Designer
Education	Wilderness	Recording	Contractor
Teacher	Guide	Engineer	Graphic
Construction	Geologist	DJ	Designer
Worker	Nature	Jingle Writer	Theoretical
Skydive	Photographer	Wedding	Physicist
Instructor	Dog Walker	Singer	
Stuntman/			
Stuntwoman			

Table 3. Career Path Chart

Keep in mind that these charts are only examples of how a vocation fits with a form of intelligence. They are by no means meant to be complete lists. In the event that you have a vocation that does not appear in these lists, go back to the original descriptions of the intelligences, and assign one that feels right to you. It is also possible to have a career built upon more than one gift and vocation. You may be an artist/mother/teacher. Include all that feels relevant.

By completing this exercise, you are self-validating that you have Innate Gifts. Give yourself permission to dream big when exploring how you will share your gifts with your communities.

Intuitive Gifts

Intuition is often described as a sixth sense, suggesting that it is a supernatural ability beyond our usual five senses. It has been overly romanticized by Hollywood and almost completely discarded by mainstream scientists. Though it is possible to validate information that is discovered through intuition, science has neither definitively proven, nor disproved the existence of intuition. As studies continue, each individual must evaluate its validity based on personal experiences.

The truth usually resides somewhere between the extremes. At one extreme, intuition can be believed to be a mystical, wizard-like ability that allows the receiver to be all-knowing. The other extremes are to see intuition as either witchcraft or complete fantasy.

Mother's intuition is a very prevalent phenomenon that may help a woman steer their child away from harmful people. There are many mothers who just know when their children are in danger, even in the absence of a phone call or any other logical source of information. How did they know that their children needed them? But just because a mother is able to sense danger through her gut instincts doesn't mean that she's a psychic that can pick the winning lottery numbers (if such a thing is even possible).

Rather than looking at intuition as a sixth sense, think of it as an extension of our normal human senses. Intuition can then be seen as a heightened sense of perception that comes from listening to our normal senses more intently. Instead of listening to the mind noise of compulsive thoughts in our heads, we need to tune into another radio frequency by focusing on one of our senses with greater concentration. For example, if we are tuning into our bodily sensations, our body can tell us what feels safe and what feel dangerous by feeling the reaction in our guts. These are our gut instincts, the same sensations that help us determine whether to take a job offer or not.

The voice of our heart sounds different to the voice of our brain. Thinking about someone fondly isn't the same as feeling a surge in your heart because you are madly in love with someone. This is why so many romantic relationships defy all logic. But if you have been deeply in love with another person, you will know that feeling in your heart that says, "this is the one for me!"

Both the believers in intuition, and the skeptics who demand proof, seem to expect that intuition be accurate 100% of the time. But if you view intuition as an expansion of your normal, fallible senses, then you can embrace the possibility that you may get extra information with the use of your heightened senses.

In recent years, intuition has been formally studied with more seriousness. Neuropsychologist Simon McCrea, PhD, published an impressive study on intuition that brought together several scientific disciplines including neurology, psychology, linguistics, and sociology. In his study, titled *Intuition, Insight, and the Right Hemisphere*, he defined, "Intuition is the ability to understand immediately without conscious reasoning and is sometimes explained as a 'gut feeling' about the rightness or wrongness of a person, place, situation, temporal episode or object."[20] Even though some studies point to intuition being one of the emerging higher functions of our intelligence, it is up to each individual to determine their own beliefs

---

20   McCrea, Simon M. *Intuition, Insight, and the Right Hemisphere*,
      Psychol Res Behav Manag. 2010; 3: 1-39.

about intuition. These beliefs may start off as inherited beliefs from your religious and societal upbringing, however life experiences are also valid when determining what you personally believe.

Intuitive senses can be seen as the extension of our five basic senses. Clairvoyance literally means "clear sight," an extension of our normal sight to see beyond the veil of our normal limitations. Clairaudience is "clear hearing," and clairsentience is the ability to clearly feel what is happening on another level.

Intuition can also be understood as a flow of information from our inner depths. As our self-awareness grows, so does our relationship to our guiding Inner Voice of Truth. Our ability to interpret that information depends on our confidence and ability to use those gifts most closely associated with our senses. While each person has potential instincts, it doesn't mean that everyone has the same intuitive abilities. Nor does it mean that everyone can access their intuition in the same way. Some people are more visual while others are more auditory. Others are very empathic and are able to sense the anguish another person is experiencing without knowing the details of their problems. An exceptional massage therapist is likely to be more tactile and will be able to sense the area of pain without the client telling them anything.

Two children receiving the same guitar lessons, for example, will progress at different rates and one may excel beyond the other. While some may possess the talents to be like Jimi Hendrix, others will make excellent baseball players. The same goes for intuition. It can be developed by anyone who wishes to have greater access to their senses, but it's fair to assume that intuition operates like any other ability, in that we all have different starting points.

Many people learn to use their intuition in high-risk situations because of the dangers they have experienced and been exposed to.

Children who grew up in a violent household, a sniper who has to be on constant alert in a conflict situation, and teenagers who have had to be on the guard on the streets because of rife gang violence, will have learned to tune in to their instincts. Those who are able to interpret their intuition in a survival situation have a much higher chance of breaking free than those who only hear the repetitive societal scripts in their minds. For the sniper perched on top of a building, hearing that instinct may warn him of a hidden danger, thus saving his life. But a sniper in the same situation, who only believes in what he can see, and ignores his deeper instincts, could end up dead.

A workshop participant shared this story when we asked the group about their beliefs surrounding intuition. He started off by saying that he had been unsure if intuition was real, until he had personal experience of it. He had been waiting to board his plane, and while sitting outside of the gate, he had this terrible feeling about getting on the plane. He had trouble determining if he was feeling sick to his stomach or if it was something more emotionally-based. The inner turmoil was so strong that he chose not to board the flight. Instead, he canceled his trip. When he got home, he learned that the plane had crashed. That was his defining moment that convinced him that intuition does indeed exist.

For the sake of this work, we openly acknowledge the existence of intuition as a way of accessing deeper reserves of information and past family experiences. This information may come from memories stored in the body or can come from some type of energetic exchange between family members or workshop participants. When speaking about intuition, it's important to realize that the intellect is not the creator of this information, rather our conscious intellect is the observer that interprets the messages, much like a radio tower receiver unscrambles radio waves. Intuition is not the same as imagination. It is not made up, rather it is deciphered.

Core Practice: Finding Inherited Gifts in your Family Tree

In the previous *Family Tree Scanning* exercise, we focused our attention on the discovery of what burdens we've inherited from our family. Now let's look at it again to focus on what *gifts* we have inherited from our family. Sharing it with a friend, partner or therapist will enhance the benefit of this exercise.

1. Scan your family tree with the intention of locating gifts that you inherited from family members.
2. Share what you know about that person. Allow the story inside of you to be told.
3. Share why you admire that person. What qualities do they have that you also wish to embody in your own life?
4. Do the same for as many family members as you feel is necessary.
5. Write down the gifts you discovered and reflect on each gift with the following focus questions: How do you feel about sharing the gifts from your family members? Do you have any resistance towards being like them? What expectations are associated with the gift you carry? What do you long to share with the world? Journal about each of the focus questions and allow them to help clarify your relationship with your gifts. We will use your answers as part of your next Ancestral Dialogue.

Core Practice: Thank a Supportive Ancestor for a Gift

If you discovered one or more inherited gifts that you share in common with someone else in your family tree, consider this optional Ancestral

Dialogue. Many past participants have shared that it brought them a sense of belonging to their family in a way they hadn't felt before.

To help you further honor your Innate Gifts, return to the Ancestors Table with your list of gifts from the *Finding Inherited Gifts in your Family Tree* practice. We can expand how we look at our Innate Gifts as not only being a gift that we share with our community, but also as a gift that can help us grow personally. By feeling a sense of sharing gifts with past family members, we can feel less alone in our families as we transition to our own path.

Go over the list of Innate Gifts and recall the people who also share those gifts. Take a moment to thank each of them aloud for anything they did to support you in discovering your gifts, even those you discovered for yourself through the earlier exercise. If there were people who saw your gifts while they were alive, be sure to thank them as well, even if they didn't share the gift with you. By allowing gratitude to flow to others, it also allows gratitude to flow inwardly for being the carrier of these Innate Gifts.

The 6th Birthright

Purpose

Innate Gifts Lead to Purpose

Many of my past clients practiced some form of the healing arts. They were physicians, therapists, acupuncturists, and body workers who all had a thirst for learning the art of healing. One of the most valuable offerings to them has been the inspiration they gained from me sharing my own story of how I became a Healer.

After graduating from Cornell University, I worked at two hospitals in their new Integrative Medicine departments. As a research assistant, I was able to witness how cutting-edge science was expanding the services offered to patients, in addition to standard medical care. As a recent college graduate, these were my dream jobs as it placed me alongside scientists at the forefront of the unconventional healing practices that I felt passionate about.

On paper, my life was perfect. The thoughts in my head told me that I was on the right track. At that time of my life, I fully expected to go to medical school after gaining valuable work experience and sterling letters of recommendation from established physicians. As exciting as these jobs were to me, it felt as if something was still missing.

After nearly four years of working in the field of research alongside premier physicians, I realized that my perfect life on paper was not feeding my deeper Innate Gifts. I no longer looked forward to coming to work. I no longer daydreamed about becoming a physician. As perfect as it all seemed, I was living according to a script that didn't allow enough room for my Innate Gifts to bloom.

That script was forged from a combination of my own self-expectations that I change the world, and by my family's expectation that I bring them pride. I had convinced myself as an adolescent that becoming a respected and exceptional physician would be the way that I could make those big changes happen. When I shared my dream of going to medical school with my family, they believed that I could do it, especially since I was the first member on both sides of my family to go to college. My father would often walk through our house saying, "my son the doctor! He's gonna cure cancer!" I had formed a large part of my identity as a young adult around this notion.

In a moment of self-honesty, I finally admitted to myself that I didn't want to be the physician in the white lab coat studying the methods of the Healers who were caring for the patients. I wanted to be one of the Healers giving direct care. I longed to put my healing hands on the bodies of those in pain. My intuitive gifts were stifled by the protocol-driven life of the physicians I witnessed each day. I needed to express my deepest gifts and my plans to go to medical school didn't leave room for me to pursue them in the way I truly longed to do.

My decision to break with my future plans and to not apply to medical school forced me into an identity crisis. Leaving that script meant that I was sacrificing family approval, leaving a prestigious career in a respected field, and would need to endure ample skepticism and woo-woo jokes about my new career path. I unapologetically hung up my shingle as an Intuitive Healer.

My career change was inspired by my Innate Gifts. Though it felt like I was risking it all, I was comforted by the joy of exploring my favorite talents. My ability to forge empathic bridges with people allowed me to use a variety of intuitive gifts to help people in ways I couldn't have predicted. Those intuitive gifts helped me to see their strength and the latent abilities that were emerging from the rawness of their wounding.

I held onto my Innate Gifts through each life-altering decision that showed me my purpose of being the developer of this generational healing work. By becoming a Healer, I've disappointed many people by not becoming a famous physician. I've even endured the ridicule of shortsighted people who could not value my gifts. Yet, the choice to embrace my Innate Gifts led me to align with a true sense of purpose. It's a remarkable feeling to have touched so many people, so deeply; an experience only made possible by sharing my most treasured innate abilities in a way that helped them find personal healing.

Knowing your Innate Gifts will lead to finding a fulfilling sense of purpose. By becoming clear about your gifts first, and making life plans second, your purpose reveals itself in the most direct way possible. It's in the process of sharing our gifts that we start to understand the details and personal missions that we carry inside. Our past wounds help us to learn about what we want to change about the world, and our gifts tell us how we'll do it. From these past experiences, we develop missions on how we will change the world to make it a better place for all.

Types of Purpose

Think of purpose as having three main categories: personal, family and world missions that we feel called to complete in our lives. These are the tasks that motivate us from behind the scenes.

Personal missions are normally the things we put on our "bucket list." They are the places we wish to visit, the accomplishments we wish to achieve such as graduating from a school program, and the meaningful events that feed our soul. These tasks fulfill an internal longing that may not always make sense to others, but the bright feeling of personal satisfaction truly makes doing them worthwhile.

Family missions are often carried by several generations and can take more than one family members' lifespan to fully address. At best, one family member can move the mission along through a few steps. These missions always involve some type of cyclic pattern. When this type of mission goes unfulfilled, it causes the family some type of repetitive pain or consequence. For instance, when no one intervenes to stop a pattern of repetitive physical violence against women, children live in fear, the abusers live in shame, and the abused live with the emotional and physical scars of the abuse.

In humanity's current state, these missions are rarely fulfilled in one generation, though it is certainly possible. An example of a successful family mission that happens in one generation would be a young daughter being the first woman in her lineage who did not die from breast cancer because she took proper health precautions for prevention. In a family where so many generations face the same disease and die early, having a woman survive to raise her children is a major accomplishment that benefits many generations of the family by having a healthy mother.

Another common family mission is finding a home by immigrating to a new country. It takes a few generations for this transition to happen. One generation must courageously initiate the immigration to another place. The next generation must help the foreign-born generations to learn the new customs and language in the new place as well as seek out new educational or work opportunities. The third generation often inherits the unfulfilled dreams that come from immigrating and must face the residual impacts of any shaming or hostility their family may have endured for being immigrants.

Our world missions entail sharing our gifts with our larger community to help change a problem or condition that we feel passionate about. This might be publishing a dissertation that educates the public about a cause close to your heart, such as plastic pollution, or founding a youth recreation center as an alternative to the pastimes of drug use, which then becomes an intentional community. World tasks could also include resisting oppression and the liberation of a particular community or culture, like the U.S. Civil Rights Movement sparked by the brave protest of Rosa Parks. It may be the resolution of an age-old conflict or the championing of a new cause. Our world missions tend to be those most closely aligned with our greatest desires of how we want to change the world for the betterment of humankind. Embracing this mission usually takes the most courageous inner dialogue and also requires help from others in order to complete it. It is possible that the work may encompass many generations from various families to be completed.

It is possible for our family missions to overlap with our world missions. Very often our family missions can hold a strong cultural component, which may resonate with many others who are from a similar cultural background, thus affecting people beyond our family unit. Our cultural background can be part of our greater contribution to the world, especially in addressing racial and political issues. In the case of Matriarchs and Patriarchs, their family work may in fact be their work in the world, thus fulfilling both a family mission and a world mission simultaneously. The benefits that the future generations receive from that family shift will benefit the world ten-fold.

How Wounds and Gifts Create our Missions

Our missions are first informed by the wounds that we have been exploring in the previous realizations. Our past experiences of being wounded point to problems in the world around us. For example, a girl who grows up hearing that she will never fulfill her dream of becoming a renowned scientist because she's female, her skin is too dark, and her family is too poor, will have a problem with being seen for her true potential. Conflict will arise because of the clash between her inner desire to become a scientist and the discouragement from society because of her background.

Our Innate Gifts are the agents of change that we apply to these problems. We can, for example, use our linguistic abilities to speak out against the ignorance about the abuse we have endured, and in this way develop our ability to reach people with our words to help change how they think.

Your wounds expose the problem,
your gifts are used to address the problem,
and your mission is fulfilled by living with purpose.

Our initial wounding is necessary to help
identify where we have a problem between
our personal aspirations and the scripts
imposed upon us by the outside world.

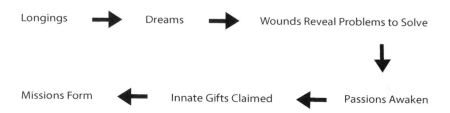

Figure 12. Formation of a Mission Steps

Exercise: My Missions

If you were to start a company, one of the first things you would do is define and state your goals and vision for the business through the development of a mission statement. The same approach works for individuals.

We are now we are going to clarify what missions would best fulfill your sense of purpose. By clarifying the problems from your past wounding, you can create an alternate vision of how you believe the world could be instead. That vision gives you a destination. How you address the problems on the way to that destination becomes the mission.

On a piece of paper, answer the following questions to help clarify a mission. It is best to focus on one dream and one problem at a time. It is perfectly fine to apply multiple gifts to address each problem (which is often the case). You can repeat this exercise many times to define your personal, family, and world missions, as we often have more than one of each type.

1. Longing & Dream: What dream do you long to fulfill?

2. Wound: How were you hurt around this longing and dream?

3. Problem: What limiting beliefs and messages did you receive about your ability to make the dream a reality? What limitations have you told yourself about making the dream come true?

4. New Vision: If you didn't follow these limiting messages, how could your life change to make your dream a reality?

5. Gifts: What gifts do you possess to address this problem and manifest this new vision?

6. Mission Statement: Based on your answers to the previous steps, how will you use your gifts to make the new vision your new reality?

7. Goals: Set tangible goals to make the new vision happen. Set deadlines to the goals. Share the new vision, mission statement, and goals with a trusted witness as a way of reinforcing self-accountability.

8. Reflect on the mission statement and ask yourself whether this mission is personal, family-altering, or world-changing in nature.

It's possible that a personal mission may expand to change your family, community, or the world at large, so there could be a link between personal and larger missions. It is also possible that your personal mission is so specific to you, that it won't necessarily be part of your work in the world or have a direct influence on other family members. Let the clarity of the mission emerge without trying to make it fit into set expectations.

This Old House

Sometimes our invisible burdens come with physical symbols that help us recognize the stories that we are carrying. By clarifying the burden, we can more easily recognize the Innate Gift connected to that unfinished story.

Devon was a young man in his late 20s who was studying to be an architect. Originally from Colorado, he moved to Santa Fe, New Mexico, after inheriting money from his now deceased father. He used it to buy a house.

Devon's inheritance of the money, which he used to buy a home, was both a gift and a burden. It was a gift in that he was given a home that somehow connected him to his deceased father. He knew that this house had some bearing on the direction his life was taking, but he needed more clarity on why this was all happening. Even though his father's death and the inheritance of the house wasn't a part of his original plans, he was approaching his new circumstances with curiosity. But the house was also a burden in that it came with many responsibilities, such as repairing the leaky roof and updating the appliances and electrical system.

Devon entered the adobe house for our healing session with a prominent smile and a nervous air about him. It was his first time working with me and he wasn't sure what to expect.

"Wow, you're so young," he said as we shook hands.

"I get that all the time," I replied with a chuckle.

"You sound so much older on the phone. I guess, I was expecting someone who looked like a wizard from Lord of the Rings!"

"Ohhh. Can I be the evil wizard?" I quipped. We laughed.

"It's the fixer upper," Devon said as he began to tell me about his newly-acquired house. "I liked the idea of working on it and really getting it to where I wanted it to be. It reminded me of my childhood home. For instance, it's a one-story house and my childhood home was the only one-story house on the block. My father was always working on our home when I was growing up, because it gave him a sense of pride. He liked the challenge too, so I guess I'm a lot like him in that respect. He was the one who always made sure that we were provided with a good home."

"You must really miss him," I said softly.

"I do miss him," he replied, wiping away a tear. "And yet, I don't feel like he is so far away, because here I am swinging a hammer just like him in the house that I chose to take on. I take on big projects... just like Dad. But the house is a constant worry for me. The roof is leaking, a pipe burst open last weekend, and I feel like I've gotten in over my head. My new home even has the same leaking sound as the one I grew up in."

Along with the responsibility for his leaky house, there was a burden of grief around his father having passed away so young. As we talked about his father's passing, I could see the dark clouds arising from his chest and stopping at his throat. Before he could claim the Innate Gift underneath the burden, he needed to allow the grief to move.

"Can you feel all that heaviness that you have been carrying?" I asked Devon.

"Yes!" He was sobbing now.

"This is good. Just let the grief pour out." The sobbing lasted nearly a half hour. When the waves of streaming tears and dark clouds had finished pouring out of him, we talked about what was happening.

"You inherited these feelings of fear and grief from your family," I shared. I had an instinct that the early death of his father was not a new story in their lineage. Suspecting that this was repeating story, I asked Devon, "Did your father also lose his father when he was young?"

"Yes, his father also died of a heart attack. It's one of the mysteries of our family, because my father ate healthily and worked as a carpenter, so he always had plenty of exercise. His doctor said it was stress that gave him a heart attack," said Devon, while wiping his face with a tissue.

I explained that it's possible to hold feelings of grief and fear in our body for so long that they become chronic conditions. Some people hold the emotions in their stomachs which can lead to gastric reflux and ulcers. Others may hold the feelings in their chests, causing high blood pressure which can contribute to heart attacks. Some hold it in their heads and suffer from insomnia. Devon had taken on his father's grief and nervous feelings that dated back to when he lost his father to a heart attack.

"The story of your family seems to be repeating with the heart attack. Also, your new home seems to have the same problems as the home you grew up in, which can be a stress on its own. You seemed to have put yourself in the same overwhelmed circumstances that your stressed father was in."

"I think about that every day," Devon replied. "There are things I like about the house, because they remind me of my father. But I don't want to relive the same story as my father and grandfather!" he replied with conviction.

Like his father, he had a passion for building homes. They both shared a work ethic and sense of fulfillment in the work they did. But in addition, Devon had the rare Innate Gift of vision. The same ability that he used to envision blueprints before constructing a building was what also helped him to see the bigger picture of his family's repeating tragedy.

By the end of the healing, Devon was able to see that the men in his paternal line held their stress inside their hearts, and never asked for emotional support for the grief and fear they harbored there. Devon's father lived in fear of an early death, so he ate healthily and got plenty of exercise. Yet, he didn't address the stress which he had been holding onto in his chest, the reason his physician gave for the early heart attack.

By asking for help, Devon received emotional support for releasing the grief in his chest which was not part of his family's script. When he swung a hammer on a fixer-upper house like his dad, he was still walking in the same footsteps as his father. But his gift of vision would both inspire his career as an architect as well as help him step out of the pattern of holding the "stress" (fear and grief) in his chest. The simple act of crying and releasing his fear gave him the relief that the men before him did not allow themselves to experience.

Traps to Realization #6

Fake Humility

So, after all this hard work of emoting, journaling, baring your tender heart to others, and deep self-reflection, the gift of your wounding experience is now clear. Of course, the next natural step is to rebury that gift, hiding it from public view, and forgetting that you ever discovered it in the first place. After all, you don't want people to think of you as being arrogant, right?

Being gifted does not mean that we are arrogant, nor does it mean that we are better than anyone else. To be gifted is to be human. We all have innate gifts that we long to share with the outside world. Becoming aware of those gifts and discovering the courage to express them to our community is a necessary part of understanding who we are as individuals.

Many indigenous communities that I have visited still have their naming traditions where children and adults are given indigenous names that somehow describe their qualities to their communities. This time-honored tradition has been lost in most Westernized societies that have completely abandoned their Celtic, Germanic, Norse, and Basal roots. But people have not lost their need to be seen and to have a place in their community.

Much of our place in society is still decided by our bloodlines, which determines the class we start in, as well as our ethnicity, faith, and nationality. As humanity continues to shift more towards a gift-based sense of self-awareness, our place in communities is more likely to be determined by the individual qualities we bring to our communities. Seeing Innate Gifts as a clearer path to our self-identity is not only internally liberating, but also creates a shift in how we function in the outer world, including our vocation. As more and more people claim their Innate Gifts and publicly share them, the chain reaction will result in us defining *our own* places in society - and in so doing, will disrupt oppressive systems of power as laid on us by pre-determined scripts.

So, hiding our Innate Gifts after we discover them is selfish. In doing so, we rob others of the inspiration and encouragement that happens when we courageously share our Innate Gifts with the outside world. Fooling yourself into believing that you are somehow being humble by throwing away all your hard work and hiding your shine is a delusion. It's fake humility. True humility is realized by "how" you share your gifts with the world, not whether or not you choose to share those gifts with the outside world. Hiding your gifts is about self-protection because you're afraid that once you shine, you will become a target for the criticism of others. True Humility is realized when we clear all obstacles out of the way for our Innate Gifts to be shared with the world.

From Purpose to the Inner Voice of Truth

By sharing our Innate Gifts and focusing on the missions that fulfill a sense of purpose, we are put in direct connection to our Inner Voice of

Truth. It's the force of inner knowing that has been directing us through this whole process all along. It begins to speak to us through our longings. As we follow those longings, we come into increasingly clearer expression of our Inner Voice of Truth. Our intuitions become sharper and more recognizable. Our personal challenges come with a greater sense of which choice feels "right" to us. Passion and purpose become more powerful drivers in our lives as we courageously make decisions that make them a priority. Those we ask to be our supporters are chosen by that inner knowing of who feels like they are genuinely present for us.

The 7th Realization

We Have an Internal Source of Wisdom Called the Inner Voice of Truth

Vision for Realization #7

When the dance on the sand was over, she was very still. The passionate expression of what she felt inside had cleared the way for a deeper truth to surface. As she looked around at the beach, it felt right to be there. She belonged on the sand. A peace washed over her. She didn't need to worry about drowning anymore. No longer did she need to wonder about what she was supposed to be doing with her life. The steadiness of the sand and the natural flow of her dance had made everything clear to her.

"I can see now that I was meant for more than just being a caretaker of my family," she finally said. "It was almost as if taking care of them was some

sort of training. Taking care of my family taught me how to reach people, how to anticipate what they were needing and feeling. It helped me to learn empathy and how to make a deep connection with another human being. But their neglect taught me something too... it taught me that I need to be seen by others. It also forced me to see myself firsthand. I am a dancer. To feel alive, I must move from a deep place inside of me and share that gift with others. My hardships with my family prepared me for what I am going to do next with my life."

She looked down at her footprints on the sand and realized that she was the first of her family to make those marks on firm ground. She was no longer following in the footsteps of the family members who came before her. She was off the map of what her ancestors had known. It felt scary and exhilarating all at the same time. A voice inside of her affirmed that she was exactly where she needed to be, right there, right then.

When she looked towards her family still swimming in the ocean, she could feel the undertow of their pull. She could feel their needs, and the residual guilt that made her want to plunge back into the water to save them. But now that her feet were planted in the sand, now that she knew what it took for her to get there, she knew not to just jump back into the water. That voice inside of her was stronger now and it told her to stand in who she is and to be patient.

That voice had been there all the time, but she needed to learn how to listen to it over all other voices, including those of her elders. She needed to find the courage to follow it. That voice led her to the shore. It told her to dance. It reminded her of who she truly was inside.

Some of the swimmers saw her dance. Captivated by her movements and inspired by her expression, they swam closer to the shore to watch her. While many stopped short of coming to the shore, a few broke away from the pack. She called out to them, encouraging them, guiding them to the safest path through the rocks and jetties. Her Inner Voice of Truth was being expressed to people who were ready for her help. Her voice was clear and strong.

Instead of rescuing people haphazardly, we worked together. We grabbed each others' hands and formed a lifeline. The approach was different now. We were a team. Our efforts were focused on those who saw the dance, who heard the call, those swimmers who were ready to meet us half-way.

She called out for help, to other people who were on the shore. Soon there were two more people on the shore. Then there were four. Our lifeline was growing. As our team grew, so did the number of swimmers who saw us on the shore. When they were ready, they too came to the shore. As more and more people made it to the shore, our one lifeline became two lifelines. The more we expressed our encouragement, the more people came to the shore.

Our collective truth was simple; there was room for all of us on the shore. All of us could live together as a thriving community, sharing our gifts and speaking our Truth. We were there to help each other. One day, there would be more people walking on the shore than there were swimming out at sea.

The Inner Voice of Truth

Our Inner Voice of Truth has been there throughout the entire healing process. Through each previous realization, this voice has sought to reach us, to guide us. What changes as we grow in awareness is our ability to perceive what the Inner Voice of Truth is trying to tell us. The more we trust it as our source of inner authority, the less dependent we become on the validation provided by others and the less affected we are by the ridicule of envious people. Furthermore, we stand in our leadership more firmly when we are attuned to that inner source of guidance.

When we walk through the fear of being alone and wean ourselves off the need to be validated and liked by others, we claim autonomy for choosing our own lives. The scripts that we were raised with no longer give us comfort and no longer bring meaning to our lives. A necessary part of claiming this autonomy over our lives is to allow our mentors and elders to come off their pedestals - to recognize their limitations as human beings and to release them from the responsibility of being guides over our paths. They may still be honored, but coming off the pedestal means that you no longer need their help in the same way.

The Inner Voice of Truth is our ultimate source of our sense of identity, because it comes directly from our own essence, the part of us that is truly unique to who we are inside. How can outside sources define who we are on a personal level? At best, our trusted supporters can be clear mirrors that reflect what is inside of us. This reflection and validation is at the heart of true friendships, and will echo what the Inner Voice of Truth has already been trying to tell you.

When we can clearly hear our Inner Voice of Truth in a consistent way, we often feel called to speak it. Expressing that Inner Voice of Truth into the world is how a Catalyst reaches their full potential. When we look back at the luminaries of history, each one of them expressed their truth into the world in powerful ways. This often involved speaking that truth through speeches and writing, and very often this came at great personal cost and with sacrifice. When we hear those speeches and read their written legacies, it serves to inspire us on our own journeys, to act from that place of awakened truth when it is our turn to express ourselves.

When we speak our truth, we are not only fulfilling a sense of purpose, we are also being who we are in the most brilliant way possible. We stop hiding and we share our shine without reservations. Showing up so completely has its own deep satisfaction that feels like we are fully expanded and energized. In this state, we wonder how we could have been anything else but a shining, brilliant being. Once expanded, there is no way to return back to the cramped confines of a limited script. We are the authors of our own stories, the painters of our own canvasses, and the conductors of our own symphonies.

Gandhi called his approach to speaking truth without violence *Satyahgraha.** In Sanskrit, the word can be broken down into *satya,* which means truth, and *graha,* which means to grasp or seize. Gandhi saw his process as 'seizing truth,' implying that we actively engage the process of knowing our truth.[21] The word for truth, *satya,* contains the word *sat,* which means 'being.' One way to view the process of knowing truth is to say that our truth originates from our deepest being, and we must actively engage with that being (essence) to know what truth it is speaking to us.

The Inhale and Exhale of Truth

The first part of the work in this realization is hearing the Inner Voice of Truth speaking to us. At first, this process happens with the encouragement and validation of our trusted supporters and mentors. With practice, we gain confidence in not only hearing the Inner Voice of Truth, but also following its guidance.

The work further extends to others when we express that Inner Voice of Truth to others. Not only do we follow its guidance for the decisions of our personal life, such as which relationships to focus on, but we also express that voice into our communities. Catalysts are fully empowered agents of change when they express their truth into the world on a regular basis.

Just as the wounding process has an inhale and an exhale, so does our experience of our Inner Truth. Once we have passed through our wounds,

---

21   *M. K. GANDHI, *An Autobiography or The Story of My Experiments With truth,* Ahmedabad; Navajivan Trust, 2003, 254.

we can inhale directly into the core of our being, the very essence of what makes us unique. To hear the Inner Voice of Truth, we must go inwards, like a monk on a silent retreat, learning to concentrate on the voice that is connected to our truth.

As we express our Inner Voice of Truth, we exhale the truth of who we are into the outside world. We take the confidence of recognizing our Inner Voice of Truth from our introspection and apply it to expressing our Innate Gifts to fulfill our purpose. This breathing cycle alternates between moments of going inwards to hear our Inner Voice of Truth, then shifting to moments where we express our truth to others, inspiring their next inhale. When they are ready, they exhale their next expression of their Inner Voice of Truth.

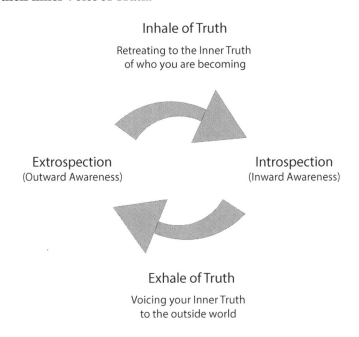

Inhale of Truth

Retreating to the Inner Truth
of who you are becoming

Extrospection
(Outward Awareness)

Introspection
(Inward Awareness)

Exhale of Truth

Voicing your Inner Truth
to the outside world

Figure 13. Inhale and Exhale of Truth

Figure 13 shows how retreating inwards brings you into a state of introspection. By meditating, doing yoga, being in nature, or free form dancing, you actively engage with the inhale of truth. When you creatively express yourself to the outside world, when you speak out about what you believe in, you enter into a state of extrospection. In this state of being, your awareness of your environment and relationships becomes the focus of your attention. When you share your gifts and passions with other people, you actively engage with the exhale of truth.

The inhale is the "being" of our truth. It's easiest to feel when we meditate or go out into nature. We go inwards to just *be*. We make contact with our essence by just *being*. We let go of the thoughts that are running their scripts in our head and feel the buzzing vibrancy of who we are without words. We often need to go into retreat, pulling away from a busy work schedule and socializing in order to really connect with the truth of who we are without having to do anything in particular. Like an infant, we just *be*.

The exhale is the "doing" of our truth. It's what Martin Luther King called "Love in action." This happens when something deep inside moves us to express our truth in a way that transforms the world. Many prominent monks, like St. Francis, ensured that their followers didn't just retreat into being solitary monks in the monastery. They reached out to their surrounding communities and offered service. They didn't just pray and contemplate. They also repaired old churches and provided other services to the outside world. We don't break free from the limiting scripts of our lives just so that we can completely escape from our responsibilities and relationship conflicts. After long periods of introspection, the exhale of goodness into the world is a natural reflex. Putting our *love into action* happens when our Inner Voice of truth motivates us to share our gifts in a purposeful and passionate way.

369

The *doing* and being aspects of our truth both lead to a greater sense of self-awareness. Our essence tells us when it needs to breathe in and needs us to just be present with it. It also knows when it can no longer hold back what needs to be done or said to change the world for the better. As we express our true voice into the world, we shake loose all the things that we carry which are no longer true of our identity. As we go inwards and make space to feel who we are underneath the scripts and burdens of our lives, we feel renewed, as if our essence becomes quenched by our captivated attention. Both "being" in the truth of who we are and initiating action from a deep center of our truth are necessary to "know thyself."

Both the inhale and exhale of this process feed into our self-awareness. It's much like the yin-yang symbol where neither aspect can exist without the other. For the sake of focus, we'll begin with the inhale, the "being" with the truth of who you are, then explore how voicing that truth, the exhale, moves from that deeper source.

The Inhale of Truth: Being

To know our Inner Voice of Truth, we need to go inwards to perceive it. Now that we have cleansed our wounds, these areas of our body are open doorways for our introspective inhale. Going inwards puts us directly in touch with our inner dialogue. The work of this realization begins with determining which inner voice is speaking your truth.

Everybody has their own way of going inwards. Some people meditate on a regular schedule. Others need to be hiking, surfing, climbing, or photographing nature. Whatever your discipline may be, turn your attention inwards to observe what is happening inside of you. Take stock of your inner environment.

From this place of being present with ourselves, we realign with our center. Before we do something with our wisdom, before we exhale our truth into the world, we need to be sure that we are in touch with the Inner Voice of Truth. This is the inner voice that knows who we are actively becoming. It knows how we can become fully aware of our inner identities. It guides us to our next projects, new relationships, shifts in our careers, and the adventures that help us to consciously catch up with what the Inner Voice of Truth has already recognized, and in a way periodically rediscover who we are becoming. This inner reflection, the inhale, alternates with us expressing our truth, the exhale, through our missions. Who are we without our survival mode or the family scripts that we were born into? How has embracing our Inner Fire and Innate Gifts enhanced the expression of who we are? Our Inner Voice of Truth is the constant guiding force that helps understand our transformation. Our job is to learn how to consistently recognize it and make decisions based on its guidance.

Three Aspects of the Inner Voice of Truth

At a Harvard University graduation speech, Steven Spielberg said the following:

...at first, the internal voice that I needed to listen to was hardly audible, and it was hardly noticeable, kinda like me in high school. But then, I started paying more attention and my intuition kicked in. And I want to be clear that your intuition is different than your conscience. They work in tandem, but here's the distinction. Your conscience shouts 'here's what you should do', while your intuition whispers, 'here's what you could do'. Listen to that voice that tells you what you could do. Nothing will define your character more than that.

Spielberg was helping us distinguish different aspects to our Inner Voice of Truth. In my work with clients, three major aspects to the Inner Voice of Truth have consistently emerged in our work together. Each aspect works hand in hand with the other. These aspects are our conscience, our intuition, and the deeper insights we receive through an epiphany. Each aspect feels different when they speak to us, but they all convey a new awareness of our truth.

Our conscience is a voice that tells us a deep sense of moral right and wrong. It also tells us whether an opportunity or relationship is right for us. People often relate that this voice comes with visceral sensations in their gut that feel different to the emotional stirring connected to the mind noise. The sensation of our conscience comes from a deeper place than our emotional fantasies or worries in our heads. This expression of our Inner Voice of Truth is the aspect that can scream above our noisy thoughts. When we have witnessed a crime, it will speak up, motivating us to consider doing the moral thing. If we are offered a job that is just not a good fit for us, it will speak to us loudly even though our heads tell us that the title and salary increase would be good for us. Our conscience is also the voice that can tell when someone is lying to us. It is the 'push comes to shove' voice that tells us what is right and wrong for us.

Intuition is our heightened ability to perceive information from the outside world. Intuition needs to first inhale a sniff of information through our senses (sight, smell, feeling, hearing, taste,) and through our empathy. After the inhale of information, our intuition processes that sniff and then communicates an interpretation of what was inhaled. It can communicate that processed information through words, symbols, nighttime dreams, or even visions.

We can apply our intuition to determine what is potentially possible in our lives; such as if a person we just met would be a good fit for a long-term relationship. Intuition is the way our Inner Voice of Truth plugs into our senses to raise our awareness of our life's path.

While both our conscience and intuition can bring fresh wisdom to our conscious mind, there is a deeper, more intense expression of our Inner Voice of Truth that rapidly downloads an insight into our consciousness. This aspect of our truth can hit us unexpectedly and can be triggered in various ways, from seeing a painting to relaxing into a calmer state of mind (giving us the impression that it just hits us). Epiphany is when the light bulb goes on above a character's head in the cartoon. It's when a stroke of brilliance strikes a composer like a lightning bolt and the musician is able to compose a song with a profound understanding of great wisdom conveyed by the music. Sometimes, just reading a book can align our mind in such a way that we receive an insight and our Inner Voice of Truth expands into our waking mind with a new awareness. However, the epiphany hits you or wherever the insight came from, recognizing the truth of the moment when an epiphany arrives is what is most important. We can focus to access intuition and conscience at any moment; however, epiphany is beyond our control. It arrives when it arrives. However, by cleaning out our wounds, we create space for epiphany to find us more frequently.

Conscience is the most self-focused of the three aspects of the Inner Voice of Truth. It not only tells you when something is wrong, it also tells you what you personally need to do about the wrong. It is the voice that speaks "your truth," which may not be a completely universal truth for everyone you know.

An example of when conscience is deeply personalized is when that voice tells you to leave a romantic relationship. People who want the two of you to stay together, may encourage you to stay. But even in the absence of validation and at the risk of social ridicule, your conscience tells you that you must move on in order to grow. Leaving the relationship would be an instance when your truth is different to what feels right to everyone else. Given time and a clear expression of your conscience, others may be able to see the truth of what you have chosen after their grief of the parting has passed through them.

But our conscience can also be personalized while aligning with a truth that is universally relevant to all others. For instance, when Rosa Parks, the catalyst for the Civil Rights Movement in America, refused to give up her seat to a white man, she was simultaneously acting from a place of personal experience but was also part of a much larger expression of truth. It didn't feel right to give up her seat because of the color of her skin. She was tired of the discrimination and she stood up for herself. But in doing so, she stood up for people like her and inspired many other African Americans to galvanize into the American Civil Rights Movement. In this example, it was essential that the inequality of race in America be directly addressed by the minority because power had to be claimed by the disempowered. Conscience is connected to a more universal truth, but operates in the most personalized way of all the voices.

Intuition can also be self-focused when we direct our attention to "reading" ourselves. We can listen to our bodies intuitively and discover what a pain or sensation in our body means. We may be holding an emotion there that gives us physical discomfort. When we tune in, that area of our body tells us the unfinished story that we are holding onto. It may also help us recognize a symptom of an illness that we would have otherwise tried to numb or ignore.

Intuition needs conscious direction. We need to aim it at something, much like a GPS that gives us directions to a destination when we enter in an address. When we set an intention, we are giving our intuition a destination. When we aim our intuition to something outside of our bodies, like reading a person whom we've just met, intuition becomes less personalized. It brings us information about what we are focusing our attention upon. This information comes through more clearly if we don't project our own feelings and stories on top of it. In essence, intuition can bring us much greater awareness when we don't overly personalize it, rather, we just let it come through in its raw form. When we don't corrupt or warp what our intuition is telling us, it connects us to a greater sense of truth that can also be truth to other people.

Epiphany brings us to our most universal expressions of truth. When Archimedes took a bath, and discovered that the water displaced equally to the mass of his body entering into it, he shouted "Eureka." Apparently, he then proceeded to run around the streets naked, his mind blown by the epiphany that just found him. This experience led to the theory of water displacement that has been proven over and over again. While running around town in your birthday suit may be a very personal experience, the universal truth that when we put our bodies into a bathtub, the water will move in proportion to our weight is true for everyone. The same holds true for equal rights for all human beings.

Emotions and the Inner Voice of Truth

All three aspects of the Inner Voice of Truth will feel clean when they speak to us. However softly or loudly these voices speak to us, they each come with a sense of steadiness. The pace of the voice will be unrushed, a direct contrast to the more speedy and frantic movement of the more surface thoughts. The tone of voice, while maybe lower in volume, will be pervasive, as if the voice is gradually bubbling up from a deep place inside and expands when it rises to the level of intellectual awareness. Once it comes to your head, it can expand to reveal pictures, visions, words, or even a deep knowing, that feels different to the more tense and compact thoughts of the mind noise. Learning what each aspect of your Inner Voice of Truth sounds like, requires discipline and self-trust that can be built with consistent practice.

Even though our Inner Voice of Truth tells us what is real and what feels right, this doesn't necessarily mean that we always feel immediately soothed by what it tells us. The truth of what it tells us can trigger an emotional response, especially if it is telling us that we need to make a drastic change in our lives that other people might not understand. Whatever reaction you have after hearing the voice for the first time, your Inner Voice of Truth always represents what is best for your long-term well-being, even if those changes come with discomfort or sacrifice.

Emotions are not the voices of our intuition, conscience or the insights that come to us through epiphany. Emotions are the reactions to what our Inner Voice of Truth tells us, and the reactions to what is happening in the outer circumstances of our lives. If your Inner Voice of Truth is telling you to leave a partner that you have been with for years because you need your freedom to grow, this realization may trigger a flood of anxiety, grief and angry thoughts. It is possible to lose track of your Inner Voice of Truth after it has spoken, because it becomes eclipsed by the urgent feelings that emerge.

When we focus on our emotions and express them with sincerity, it can lead us through the mind noise to the truth of our experiences. Crying brings clarity. Screaming brings catharsis and empowerment. Feeling our shame and allowing it to move through us will clear the pathway so that we can access our Inner Voice of Truth more readily. Once we have processed these emotions, we can focus on hearing the wisdom of the matter, including 'why' we are going through the challenge.

Exercise: Cleaning House

Before we can definitively identify the Inner Voice of Truth, we need to clean house. Here's an exercise designed to help you distinguish the thoughts inside your head so that you can gain proficiency in labeling them.

- On three pieces of paper, put the following titles at the top of each page:

  Page 1: The Mind Dump

  Page 2: The Loudest Voices

  Page 3: The Truest Voice

- Page 1: Write down every thought that you hear inside your head. Don't censor anything, even if you are using harsh language or pointed judgments. Just honestly write every thought, crappy or cheerful, onto the page. Give yourself up to 10 minutes to do this section.

- Write all your thoughts down until you either feel a sense of relief or notice a slowing down of your mind. It's fine to write the same thing more than once. The point of this step is to exhaust the scripts in your head.

- Now take ten steady breaths. Rub your heart with your hand and detach from your thoughts. Feel the buzzing of movement in your head without getting too caught up in what it is saying to you.

- Page 2: Make a note of which voices in your head were the loudest during Page 1. Write these voices down on Page 2. The Loudest Voices are not necessarily the truest voices. They are just the thoughts that grabbed the most attention.

- Now put your hand on your gut and ask yourself if any of the Loudest Voices were your Inner Voice of Truth. If any of the

377

Loudest Voices were your Inner Voice of Truth, write what was said on Page 3. If not, move onto the next step without writing anything.

- Once you have vetted the Loudest Voices from Page 2, rub your gut with one of your hands. Take in ten steady breaths and focus on feeling your solar plexus.

- Once you feel that you have established a connection with your gut, ask your Inner Voice of Truth to share a piece of guidance with you.

- Page 3: Write down the guidance that was shared with you. Read what you have written and feel inside your torso. Do you feel a resonance inside of your body as you read what you have written? Many people describe it as a sensation inside of their bodies that feels like a ping, a bell ringing or some type of harmonic vibration. If you don't feel a resonance of some kind at this stage of the exercise, return to the first step and repeat. It is possible that there is more mind noise that needs to be purged before you can focus on the Inner Voice of Truth.

Don't feel discouraged if you don't feel the resonance during the Page 3 writing on your first try. Just continue to practice the exercise until you have cleansed enough of the mind noise to hear your Inner Voice of Truth. This exercise is meant to be repeated daily, so don't feel discouraged if you don't feel like you have mastered it the first time. If you have any doubts about whether or not you have heard your Inner Voice of Truth on Page 3, then repeat the exercise again, this time doing Page 1: The Mind Dump, for an additional 10 minutes. This exercise is also good for coming out of survival mode.

The Cleaning House exercise gives us an opportunity to hone the crucial skill of determining what voice we are hearing. If we follow the wrong voice, it can lead us down a painful path that does not further our growth and healing. Think back to how many times you said to yourself, "I knew that was going to happen. I just didn't listen to it."

What you may have noticed in the exercise is that the first voices you heard weren't necessarily the truest. There is a reason that so many meditative practices are built on the foundation of breathing and observing your mind. The process of detaching from your thoughts makes it easier to observe them. As we come out of our heads and sink into a deeper presence, the inner voices become slower and more calming. An echoed voice from your nagging mother will be a stark contrast to the velvety, measured tenor of your deepest voice. In short, the Voice of Truth will make you feel more peaceful. The other voices will either trigger distress or pull you into a whirlwind of analysis.

Becoming consistent in hearing our Inner Voice of Truth is not about perfection. It isn't about willing ourselves to achieve a state of enlightenment or attaining inner peace as fast as possible. If you find yourself rushing the experience, then you need to spend more time on the Page 1: Mind Dump to discharge the emotional energy inside that you don't want to feel. Feel those emotions and write down the emotionally-charged statements that you hear in your head, including self-judgments or judgments about how this exercise makes you feel.

The Difference Between Beliefs and Truth

If a belief is not always true, then how can it be an eternal truth? For instance, if we believe something negative about ourselves, such as "I am ugly," we will identify with being ugly, along with all the associated emotions of shame, low self-confidence, and self-disgust that go along that that self-belief. But it is not the truth of who we are inside.

Very often, I encounter people with a deeply seeded belief that it is never safe to ask for help. With this limiting belief comes a lot of fear of being rejected and shame about needing help when your past requests were dejected. As long as you believe that all people are unsafe, you will never ask for help as an act of self-protection. We all need help sometimes, especially when we are breaking free from abusive patterns and need validation.

Beliefs can be recited in our heads, but the voice speaking may not be the same as your Inner Voice of Truth. Once you get attuned to how your Inner Voice of Truth sounds and how it makes you feel inside your body, you can then ask it what it has to say about your current beliefs.

Many beliefs are taught to us as if they are absolute truths that should never be changed. However, changing your beliefs based on your own personal experiences and the inner guidance provided by your Inner Voice of Truth can be an absolutely empowering experience. This is especially clear when a negative belief about your abilities and potential has held you back from pursuing your dreams. Being diagnosed with Attention Deficit Disorder as a child, for example, can lead to negative and limiting self-beliefs when teachers attach labels like disorganized, disruptive and incapable to the diagnosis. Yet many well-known successful personalities, from trailblazers like Richard Branson to historical figures like Winston Churchill have proven otherwise. To change racist scripts that we inherit often involves challenging the beliefs about the supposed inferiority / superiority /stereotypical traits of people from other races and cultures. Interacting with people across color and cultural lines, can dispel these ingrained beliefs and inspire us to change our beliefs for the better.

Perceiving the Inner Voice of Truth Chart

We are now learning to perceive our Inner Voice of Truth, despite the distractions in our minds. This ability will become more consistent with practice.

During the process of working through each of the previous Realizations, our Inner Voice of Truth was expressing itself. It was that resonance when we first learned the truth about carrying burdens on behalf of others. Unburdening thus becomes an act of unearthing our Inner Voice of Truth.

While many may experience their Inner Truth as a voice, we all have different ways of perceiving it. As our truth bubbles up to the surface, it will signal its presence to us in different ways before we are able to connect with it directly. As it makes its way from deep inside the core of our being, it touches upon whatever sense it can use to reach us. The more we recognize the truth behind each sensation, emotion, and inner signal, the more clearly we are able to understand the truth of our situation. While it is possible to hear, feel, see, or otherwise detect our truth at any moment, the following chart may help you to gain a closer grasp of how your Inner Voice of Truth is trying to speak to you during each Realization.

Let's look at how we may perceive the Inner Voice of Truth at each of the previous steps in the Path of the Catalyst.

Realization	Perception of the Inner Voice of Truth
1st Survival Mode	Shock, an abrupt event interrupting the script and creating space for pause. This brief pause allows us to perceive outside of the script, although the Inner Voice of Truth may not necessarily be heard clearly.
2nd Invisible Burden	Pressure and Heaviness indicating that we are carrying something. Awareness of Truth comes from becoming aware of what burden is being held.
3rd Unburdening	Pain and Relief
4th Wounds are pathways	Emotions, feeling usher the Inner Voice of Truth to the surface.
5th Inner Fire	Inspiration, Fun, Passion, Power surge
6th Innate Gifts	Longing, Truth comes from Creative Expression and meaningful connections with other people around gift sharing.
7th Expressing Our Truth	Clarity, Alignment, Spaciousness, Vibrancy, The Inner Voice of Truth is Heard directly and clearly

Table 4. Perceiving the Inner Voice of Truth

8th Forgiveness: In a state of complete forgiveness, our Inner Voice speaks to us without interference from thoughts, emotions or repetitive stories from the past. We find the most direct path to reconciling the past so that we can move on in the most wholesome and empowering way possible.

The 7th Birthright

The Exhale of Truth: Doing

Identity Crisis

"What am I doing!?" This is the question that often surfaces when rapid transformation and intensive self-awareness have pulled you out of your script. A state of limbo ensues as you learn to release the old scripts that used to define you, while simultaneously learning to trust your Inner Voice of Truth as the new director of your life. During this intense transition time, large ripples of energy flow through you, completely at odds with your once predictable, scripted life. At the same time, the external circumstances of your life also begin to shift as you start no longer fit into the roles that feel too small for who you are becoming. Add in the major relationship shifts that happen when you break free from abusive dynamics, and suddenly this accelerated growth can feel like an identity crisis.

More accurately, what occurs is an identity *shift*, your sense of self transitions from a more surface image of who you thought you were, to a deeper knowing of your true identity. To know your truth requires that you surrender the familiar image of who you were told you are by the script. Even though the wise part of you knows that the transformation is leading to a more authentic life, your personality may go into panic mode as where you anchor your identity changes hands from the script to the unscripted Inner Voice of Truth. Before you can "do" something with your new-found awareness of your truth, it's best to finish passing through that threshold that happens just between the inhale (introspection) and the exhale (resurfacing to share your new-found truth with the world).

It's in that in-between state between the inhale and exhale that we pass through that threshold and experience the actual identity shift. As I was passing through many core wounds and just beginning to claim my tingling gifts, I remember hearing from friends, families, even colleagues who were also Healers, that I was having an identity crisis. They gave this feedback partially out of concern for my well-being. They were worried for me because they couldn't grasp the transition I was going through from their own personal experience. They couldn't relate because they hadn't done the inner work yet. By breaking the restrictive scripts in my life, I was also disrupting those same scripts that were present when those relationships were forged. I was going beyond what they knew, a place outside of their comfort zones that they couldn't follow. It's not egotistical to acknowledge when you are taking a step beyond your supporters, rather it is essential to embrace the truth of the matter so that you don't get stuck in an apologetic and guilty state of limbo between the script and your Inner Voice of Truth. The people who really care about you will understand that sometimes you need to do things that they don't understand. But they can still respect your decisions when a clear effort is made to communicate the shift that you are going through. It's also important to understand that you might not have those words at the time that the shift is happening. Very often, the explanation comes later after you've had a chance to re-anchor your identity.

My "identity crisis" label also came with some emotional stickiness. Some loved ones tried to convince me that I was making a huge mistake by exploring my life outside of the scripts it was assumed I would follow. There was an emotional tug to their pleas. They were scared to lose me, because they weren't ready to cross their threshold and they didn't want to lose the comfort of the scripted exchanges that we used to have. They knew that by claiming my gifts in an earnest way, my life would be taking me in new directions and taking me to faraway places that would limit their access to me. Sometimes, I was even shamed for making changes that felt authentic to me. According to the people who wanted to hold me back, I was wasting a perfectly good life situation, the relationships, neighborhood, and expected routine of my existence. But something inside of me squirmed at the idea of working so hard on myself to reach this exciting threshold, only to turn back for the sake of comforting frightened loved ones. It became clear that they wanted me to come back to the them and say, "you were right. I was wasting the last several years of my life meditating, going to Healers, delving into therapy, and journaling my nights away. What was I thinking?" But doing so would have brought me right back to the scripted behavior that made me feel tired, resentful, and trapped.

Once I realized that their guidance was more about them holding onto me, rather than witnessing a very important turning point in my life, the decision to follow my Inner Voice of Truth became easier to make. This doesn't mean that having that clarity made breaking away and walking my own path easy in any way. It is hard to leave people who had otherwise been good supporters up until the threshold. They weren't bad people; they were just scared and needed more time before they could relate to my choice. Recognizing their manipulations did help me decide that there was no turning back from who I was becoming. The process was too far along to pretend that I would be happy in the mold from which I had just broken free.

A prolonged identity crisis happens when the release of our scripted image happens more quickly than our ability to hear and trust our Inner Voice of Truth. We release the image of who we were through the "doing" parts of the process such as the expressing emotional catharsis, actualizing career changes, and initiating conversations in our relationship shifts. But if we don't devote enough attention to looking inwards, to the "being" part of the process, then we will not recognize the new expression of who we are to fill the vacuum that the script once occupied. There will be a gap in our understanding of who we are and a lack of self-acceptance because we haven't devoted the time to our rediscovery. A prolonged identity crisis is often a sign that we are constantly *doing* and not just *being* with ourselves enough. Go for a hike, take a vacation, go on a silent retreat, or go surfing if you find that the identity shift is taking a long time. Recreation is how we recognize how we are re-creating ourselves.

Being Seen: Validation

I will never forget the first time that I met Carol, my most significant Healer and mentor. I was still in college when I first sought her help. Her office was on the basement level of a little house on Long Island, NY that served as a real estate office. I descended the stairs and passed by the shingle that said "Carol Abramowitz, Holistic Alternatives." The warmth of her office was palpable. Just sitting in her waiting room made my whole body tingle.

What made my first session with Carol so memorable was that she saw two important things about me. She witnessed both my struggle and my unique shine. Without me saying much to her at all, she was able to see that my heart had endured a lot of hurt. She could see that my heart was undernourished and that it was holding a lot of grief. She was also the first person who saw me as a Healer. "I don't say this to many people, but you got it. You have the gift to be a Healer."

She gave me validation for the silent suffering that I had endured in my heart for many years. I always ensured that other people received what they needed first, and whatever emotional support or nourishment that was left over, I received for me. Her seeing my deep need for nurturing and a trusted provider filled my heart with care. When I got off her table, I remember feeling whole in a way that I hadn't experienced before, like I could feel my chest again after it had been numb for so many years.

By seeing who I was beneath my brooding defenses and heavy grief, I felt truly seen for the good person that I was underneath my hardships. Each of us has a light inside that sparkles through when we are truly witnessed. Once Carol had seen that deep shine that I had learned to bury and protect, I remembered that it truly existed. It came to the surface more fully in a way that I could see when I looked in the bathroom mirror after the healing session.

Validation feeds our inner being. When someone sees the real us, that truth expands and becomes more visible. We inhale that validation, which strengthens our connection to our Inner Voice of Truth. When we feel seen, it is easier to get in touch with the truth of who we are because a deeper part of us is welcomed into the outer world by the witness.

To shift from the "doing" mode to a "being" mode, we need to take an inhale. Validation by others and self-recognition are two ways to take that inhale and become introspective. This shift gives us a chance to catch up with ourselves and listen intently to what the Inner Voice of Truth is telling us about our new sense of identity. It's important to recognize that when people validate who we are, they are not telling us who we are or defining who we are becoming. They are merely reflecting back to us what is already emerging. By conveying what they see in us, they are echoing what the Inner Voice of Truth is already saying to us. By feeling the resonance inside of our bodies when validation "sounds true," we are being helped to track that internal voice on which we need to focus our attention. The truth of who you are is already inside of you. Our true supporters are the ones who are able to witness that and respect it.

Exercise: Who Sees Me?

- Write the following question on a piece of paper: Question:

Who sees me for who I truly am?

- Put one hand on your gut while allowing names to just splash onto the page. Don't analyze the names, just let them come onto the page.
- Now read the names aloud and see how your body feels as you read each name.
- Go through each name again and ask yourself the following question for each name and write a response next to the name:

What does this person see in me?

- By now, your list should look something like this:

388

1. Mike: Sees my passion for children, my big heart
2. Julie: Understands my sense of humor
3. Sandeep: Sees the warrior in me
4. Uncle Bo: Admires my accomplishments, is in awe of my skills

- Go through each name on the list and read aloud what they see about you.
- Now feel your body. What reactions do you have towards recognizing how people see you?
- Now write down one more question and answer it while looking in the mirror.

What do I see when I look at myself?

- Write down the response and read it aloud. How does it feel to acknowledge these things about yourself?
- Journal about any discomfort or struggles that you encountered during this exercise. It helps to share it with someone you trust.

This exercise is particularly powerful for getting in touch with your Inner Voice of Truth. The more you feel seen, and the more that you see yourself for who you are, the more energized your Inner Voice of Truth will become. It vibrates more strongly. As it buzzes, it can kick up more blocks which will show up as voices in your mind. Instead of immediately hearing the wise voice of Truth that accepts the validation given by your trusted supporters, you may hear voices of doubt, embarrassment, and resistance. That is part of the process. As the truth comes to the surface, it clears off whatever is left over from the work you have been doing up until this point. It may take a lot of practice before you feel comfortable with receiving the admiration of those who have already seen you and love you for who you really are inside. Repeat this exercise daily until you finally start to let the goodness in.

Seeing Yourself

Most people need to receive validation externally before they are able to give it to themselves internally. In this way, our most trusted supporters teach us how to do it. When we are children and just learning how to speak a language, we ask our elders if we said the word correctly. "Toy?" we ask. "Yes, 'toy,' that's right."

By receiving validation from others, we know what it feels like. Once we know what it feels like to be seen, we can look in the mirror and see who we are beyond our survival mode, our burdens and our internalized self-judgments.

Giving honor, love, respect, and witness to yourself are all part of what nourishes that inner being which holds the truth of who we are. There comes a point where validation is primarily an inside job. We can't rely on others to see all of who we are because we each need to be able to perceive ourselves firsthand. The validation we receive from others gives us strength and support in our self-discovery. Once we are strong enough, we no longer ask others to validate whether we are saying the word "toy" correctly. We know firsthand that we are.

Even when you feel lonely, it doesn't always mean that you need people around you - in fact you may be surrounded by them. It means that you need to be seen, to be heard, and to be understood. You are qualified to do this.

Identity from a Deeper Source

Healing is the process of becoming more self-aware. As we progress to living a more authentic life that is informed by our Inner Voice of Truth, our sense of identity comes from a deeper place within us where the voice originates. Looking back at each Realization, we can witness how the depth of our self-awareness grows. Our sense of identity is constantly coming from a deeper place inside as we embody each Realization.

Because we can re-enter survival mode based on our life circumstances, and because we have multiple burdens, wounds, and gifts to explore, we can pass through these levels of identity numerous times. It's as if we have many holes within that we need to pass through in order to see all the sides of our inner being. It may seem like you are back at step one when you discover a new burden or wound, but in actuality, you are just adding a more 3-dimensional awareness to all the facets of your being. It is impossible to explore them all at once, so going through each Realization is normal. You are accumulating more self-knowledge and more rewards each time you pass through those pathways to reconnect with your Inner Voice of Truth.

Realization	Source of Identity
I am in Survival Mode	My identity comes from the script, which is only momentarily interrupted by crisis or brief, intense moments of pleasure such as an orgasm. I am the image of how my inherited scripts define me.

I am carrying a Burden	My identity still comes primarily from the script, but the realization of my burdens and where they are coming from creates gaps in my mind. This space creates room for my emotions to begin to flow. With these feelings, a hope for a different path is just beginning to emerge. I am a feeling being who is carrying burdens on behalf of other people.
I am releasing my Burden	I am breaking the rules of the script by letting go of responsibilities and feelings that are not mine. I stop identifying so strongly with the stories of other people and begin to explore my own needs and desires. What I want for myself begins to matter in my life. I am a seeker of my own path.
I am feeling my Wounds	Rather than listening to outside expectations as my primary motivation, I feel my own inner experience more deeply. Through the emotional pain, I reconnect with my heart and a sense of empathy. I recognize that I have been hurt. I am a feeling being with a good heart.
I embrace my Inner Fire	I speak out against oppression and toxic relationships. I protect myself from overt and subtle forms of harm, because I am someone worthy of care and safety. I am a passionate being and I have a right to express myself.

I am discovering my Innate Gifts	Instead of solely following the scripted expectations of what I should be doing with my life, I explore my favorite innate talents and abilities. My motivation comes from sharing my gifts with people who will "get it". I am a gifted person who identifies with my chosen craft, interests and passions (designer, conservationist, teacher, baker, yogi, masseuse)
I am a unique being who speaks my Inner Voice of Truth	It is true that I am a feeling being, full of innate gifts and passion. I am here to inspire others and to make important changes in the world. I speak my Truth. I see myself for the unique being that I am. I am a Catalyst who inspires others to claim their truth. I am an empowered co-creator of the world that I wish to live in.

Table 5. Sources of Identity

Exercise: Head, Heart, Gut Check

Because most people devote too little attention to being with themselves during the inhale part of discovering their truth, I've developed an exercise that can be done before you take action on important decisions. It is essential to take a big introspective inhale before making any major life decisions. This exercise ensures that you are clear about your decisions before sharing your Inner Voice of Truth with the outside world.

Since the head is involved with almost every decision we make, I ask my clients to also feel their hearts and their gut, one at a time, in order to access their intuition and conscience. For instance, when a client is having a relationship struggle, I will ask them to put their hand on their heart and ask their own hearts questions about what to do next as a way of getting in touch with their intuition. Likewise, I also ask them to repeat the process with their gut to help them double-check decisions with their gut instincts.

As each voice arises, we sort through them to process the emotions and glean the insights that can fill in the blanks in your head. Think of this as a process to ensure that your brain has all the puzzle pieces, some of which are provided by our conscience, intuition, and any epiphanies, so that you can make the most complete choice.

1. Write down the problem or conflict that is causing your distress. If there are numerous conflicts or problems, mind dump them onto the page into a list and address one problem at a time with the following steps.

2. Formulate a clarifying question about the problem or conflict. *For instance, should I quit my current job to pursue my career as a writer?*

3. Place your hand your head and ask the clarifying question aloud. Write down all that comes up until your head voice has said all that it needs to say.

4. Place your hand on your heart and rub it in a circular motion. Take several deep breaths until you feel like the energy in your head finally settles down into your chest. Then ask your heart the same clarifying question. Write down all that your heart voice tells you, including how you feel about the conflict or problem at hand.

5. Place your hand on your solar plexus, which is your belly area beneath your rib cage. Rub this area in a circular motion and breathe deeply into your diaphragm until you feel like your

attention is fully focused on your belly. Once you are there, ask your gut the clarifying questions. Write down your physical sensations, such as tightness, lightness, spaciousness, tingling, pain, etc... The response of the gut often comes in sensations that can be interpreted. For instance, your gut contracting or hurting may mean a "no" response, while an openness or pleasurable excitement may be a "yes" response. You may also get clear words or images, as well as emotions that need to be heard. Write everything down.

6.   Now review what your head, heart, and gut voices have shared with you. Ask your Inner Voice of Truth to sum up what your decision will be regarding the choice at hand. When your head, heart, and gut voices are saying different things and they don't seem to be in total alignment, even after several attempts to find inner consensus, then go with the gut voice. The gut instincts keep us safe when we over-analyze things in our head to no avail. The gut also helps us to make important relationship decisions when our heart is hung up on the wrong person for us. In other words, if your gut tells you to leave your job or a romantic relationship, even if we love our co-workers or we are still in love with someone who is no longer good for us, listen to it. Once you give the gut voice the emphasis it deserves, then you can prepare your heart for the impending change and you can enlist the power of your head to figure out the best way to go about the change.

Expressing your Truth

Vocalizing your truth and being heard is one of the most powerful ways to gain trust in your Inner Voice of Truth. When you speak the truth in your relationships, you catalyze powerful change in those who hear you. But verbalizing your truth through speech it is not the only way to express your truth.

Just as each of us has our own gateway sense (sight, hearing, smell, taste, feeling, empathy), we all have unique ways of expressing our truth into the world. Some "speak" their truth through dance. Others express their truth through a painting or sculpture. Others play instruments or sing. How you communicate your essence to the outside world is unique to you as an individual. So, *voice* doesn't always literally mean vocalizing through your mouth. It can refer to any expression that feels authentic to you.

There's a story about the Buddha doing a teaching where he simply held a flower before his disciples without any verbal instruction. All but one of his students became flustered by the lack of verbal instruction. They didn't get his lesson. But their teacher was intentionally pointing to a truth beyond words. Only one student smiled with contentment as he stared at the flower and recognized the larger lesson. He understood the simple beauty of the moment that the Buddha was pointing to by being present with the flower. This story reminds us that there are a number of ways of experiencing and conveying truth.

Exercise: Expressions of Truth

On a piece of paper write the following:
1. Primary Expressions:
2. Secondary Expressions:
3. Tertiary Expressions:

Other Ways of Expressing my Truth:
- On a piece of scrap paper, brainstorm about all the ways that you feel that you express your truth. Once you have a list, begin to write down the expressions from your scrap paper into the above headings. As you write down the expressions on your scrap paper, ask yourself "Is this my primary way of expressing my truth?" Say each expression that you have written down out loud and feel your gut as you say them. Do this for each heading. Note: it is possible to have more than one expression per heading. It may look something like this:
  1. *Primary Expressions: Singing*
  2. *Secondary Expressions: Writing*
  3. *Tertiary Expressions: Surfing*

  Other Ways of Expressing my Truth: Dancing

As you look over your results, were there any surprises? Share the results with someone you trust to enhance what you have witnessed about yourself.

Sonia Hears Her Truth

Hearing your Inner Voice of Truth can save your life. Let me share a client story to explain how this can happen.

Sonia was crying on the plane that was still on the tarmac. This 21-year-old woman was scared because she was waiting to take off to a place that she had never been: The United States of America. This was the first time that she would be leaving her birth home of Chile. Her family felt toxic to her, leaving her feeling desperate and alone, as if she was an alien in her own homeland and a stranger to her own family. Sonia was about to leave everything that had been familiar to her.

In her pocket, she still had the pills that would have ended her life if she had stayed. Suicide was her back-up plan and the idea of staying in Chile made her fantasize about swallowing those pills. Her plan to move to the U.S. was the only thing that seemed to give her hope. Though getting on the plane and going to a new land was the more frightening and unfamiliar option to her, she heard a voice inside of her that told her to "leave this place. Go to America."

This voice was not the paranoid doubts that constantly cycled through her head. She wasn't listening to the deeply depressed thoughts that had sought a way out of suffering through self-harm. Underneath the head noise and the lonely ache in her heart, there was another voice, one that was more serene and clear. This was her Inner Voice of Truth, a simple and deeply caring voice that told her what to do next.

Most people leave their homeland because of an extreme external crisis, such as a financial collapse of a country or a famine. But for Sonia, it felt as if her family had alienated her and betrayed her throughout her young life. They didn't see who she was, and she couldn't relate to the people that lied to her so often. The Inner Voice of Truth emerged gradually to help her break free of her depressing family situation.

Now at the age of 41, Sonia was coming to me because the depression that she had felt for most of her life was surfacing in a way that eclipsed her hope. America had become her home for the past 20 years, and she was fast approaching the anniversary of the day she made the courageous choice to get on that plane.

The resurgence of her depression left Sonia feeling confused, because she had been married for 20 years and had two young teenage girls. While she still struggled with issues around work and voicing what she needed, her life had drastically changed from the 21-year-old young woman who had once considered suicide. But her struggles to find hope and direction were alarming enough for her to decide to book a session.

"Why did you leave Chile when you were 21?" I asked.

"I just couldn't take it anymore," Sonia said. "The lying. Everybody cheating on each other. The people that I grew up with measured how good a friend you were by the weight of how many secrets you could keep about them. I knew that I wanted a family, but I didn't want to raise my children in that environment. I didn't want them to learn how to lie like that. Everything seemed to be a lie."

"So something inside of you felt that this was wrong with the way your family lived and you wanted to live another way?"

"Yes. I couldn't take all the secrets anymore. I felt like I was suffocating. I didn't want to lie for other people, so I just didn't talk much. But it also made me feel like I didn't belong with them. I didn't belong where I grew up."

"Go back to that day when you left your first home. You were 21 years old. What was going through your mind when you sat on your seat in the plane?"

"Oh, I was terrified. I didn't know what was going to happen next and felt so much dread. But I knew I had to leave. Something inside of me told me to get on that plane. When I called my sisters after I landed in America, they made it sound like they were having a party there, like things were better than ever now that I left. It made me feel like I was the problem all along, that I just needed to leave and then my family would be happy."

"Is it possible that they were hiding how they really felt to cover up how they really felt about you leaving?" I challenged.

"Yes, that's possible. I just felt so ashamed."

"It sounds like you felt rejected because they never expressed how they missed you or didn't acknowledge how you felt about the family."

"Yes, I felt rejected...like nobody cared that I was gone. I felt so alone," Sonia said.

"But in truth, it was you who was rejected how the family lived. You weren't rejecting your family members; you were saying no to the whole system of lies that your family followed. The cheating on each other and the talking behind other peoples' backs were acts that didn't fit with your integrity."

"Yes, I can see what you are saying," Sonia said. "I wasn't rejecting them. I just wanted to live differently. But why is all this loneliness coming up now? It's been almost 21 years since I left and I'm still feeling this way. I have a family now that is so much different than the one I grew up with, but I'm still feeling these same emotions."

"You are approaching the 21st anniversary of when you made that leap from your old home to your new home in America. Once you hit that point, you will have lived more time in America than in the homeland where you were raised."

Sonia broke down into tears. The sadness, the gnawing heaviness that was resurfacing from her past was finally named. She could feel the strong fear and sadness of the 21-year-old woman as if she were sitting next to her on the plane that brought her to her new home.

"You're revisiting that day to see how the Inner Voice of Truth had steered you in the right direction. Did you your mother, or sisters, or father see you off at the airport when you left?"

"No," she sobbed. "I was all by myself. I felt paralyzed by all my fear."

"But you still did it. You listened to that Inner Voice of Truth even though you felt terrified to get on that plane and leave everything that you had known."

"Yes, that voice told me that I had to get on that plane."

"What did your courageous choice bring into your life now nearly 21 years later?"

"I have a good husband and two wonderful girls," she said with a wet smile.

"Is the family that you made like the family that you grew up with?"

"Not at all. We don't lie to each other like that. I always wanted to raise children without all the lying and hurt."

"Sonia, are you really alone now?"

"No, I'm not alone. I have a beautiful family now."

"By listening to your Inner Voice of Truth, you were rewarded with an honest and loving family. Because you chose to get on that plane and not take your own life, look at all the goodness that Life brought you for being courageous."

"Yes. I am very grateful for what I have now. I didn't realize then that I was being brave because nobody saw it. But I can see it now for myself now. It was brave to move away."

Two weeks after our session together, Sonia sent a quick note about how she was doing.

Our last session was deeply transformative. I have not felt depressed nor sad since that day. My mind is clear, my body lighter and I have not said a single bad word to myself. I've slept great and I'm able to focus on the beauty around me.

Traps to Realization # 7

Believing Your Limiting Beliefs

"*Argue for your limitations, and sure enough they're yours.*" Richard Bach[22]

Everyone has been betrayed. After a deep betrayal, many people begin believing that "I gotta do everything myself." In this defensive state, it can appear safer to do things on your own, because you don't need to worry about people disappointing you or rejecting you by saying no to your request for help. By refusing to ask for help, you minimize the drama that comes with being vulnerable with other people. But without supporters, life can be more difficult. Without the clear reflection of people outside of ourselves, our self-awareness process can also be slowed down because we lose the mirrors that reflect back who we are.

This prevalent belief is a prime example of how a limiting belief can seem like the truth. We can gather many examples of all the times we were disappointed, rejected, abandoned and outright injured as if we were building a case against Life in general. This limiting belief keeps us safe in the short term, but ultimately, it starves us from the nourishment and support that would help us evolve in the long term. This can put us at risk when we truly need outside help, but we have isolated ourselves from potential supporters.

We carry many other limiting beliefs. These beliefs are almost always received from some repetitive script and they are often tied to our surface

---

22   Bach, Richard. Illusions: The Adventures of a Reluctant
     Messiah. Delta: Reprint edition (2012), London, UK.

qualities. Social status, financial class, race, religion, and nationality can all become points of attachment that our self-defeating and demeaning beliefs hold onto.

These beliefs can only stick to us if part of us still believes them. The voices inside that validate these beliefs are not connected to our Inner Voice of Truth. These voices compete with our inner wisdom for our conscious attention. When we have built up enough self-awareness, listening to these beliefs becomes a choice, not an automatic response.

Follow the Energy

When all else fails, follow the energy. If you have done all the exercises, talked about your major decisions with trusted supporters, and you still can't find that clear inner voice that feels like your truth, then feel for which fork in the road holds the most energy for you. By following the invigoration, you give your Inner Voice of Truth more opportunities to make itself known to you. The path that feels the most alive will be the scariest and most unknown path of all. Feel your fears and walk that path anyway. Seek out that challenge that brings you to your edge. It's completely acceptable to need additional experiences to develop a more substantial conversation with your truth. Applying yourself in this new way will take you out of your comfort zone and bring you opportunities for self-awareness.

Remember, self-awareness is the one thing in life that you can't lose.

The 8th Realization

Forgiveness brings us Shared Peace

Vision of Realization #8

 She wasn't sure if the day would ever come, but she always wished that it would. It was years until she had last seen her mother, but she never stopped hoping that she would see her again, even though their separation had been so raw. The hardest part of breaking free from her former life was that she had to leave her mother behind.

 Her mother was still treading water, out at sea, afraid to leave the life that she had always known. She missed her mother, a mix of guilt that she had to leave her behind to live her own life and a genuine fondness for the woman that she loved.

She saw her mother swimming to the shore, a sight she didn't fully believe at first. When the shock wore off, she screamed out to her, "Momma!" She ran into the ocean.

"Mom, over here!" she yelled.

They embraced in the chest deep water. Tears of joy mixed in with the lapping waves that slapped their faces. Mother and daughter were finally reunited. She had been a lifeline to so many people, but none of them had been her mother. The day she dreamed of pulling her mother on to the sand had finally come.

"I'm sorry," her mother said. "I'm sorry for what I said to you when you left. I knew that you had to go. It's just..." Her mother choked on her sobs, but still tried to talk. "I just didn't want to lose you. And I didn't know where you were going. I was too scared to follow you."

She could see the pain and struggle that her mother went through, that inner battle which prevented her from coming to the shore sooner. The honesty of her struggle and the sincerity of her mother's apology warmed the hardened edges of her heart. The last remnants of resentment burned through her hot tears as she surrendered to the relief of embracing her mother.

"It was hard for me too, Mom. I didn't want to leave you behind. I just knew that nothing would change if I stayed. This is where I belong. Every time I pulled in a woman who reminded me of you, I hoped it would actually be you the next time I took someone's hand."

Forgiveness made room for their hearts to flood with the gratitude. They were both speaking their truth. They were both truly listening. Sometimes, that's all that is needed for forgiveness to happen.

Forgiving My Father

It was the first time that I was going to see my father in a long time. After years of uncontrolled alcohol and drug abuse, and a stint of homelessness,

406

Dad had entered into the work rehabilitation program at the Salvation Army. We had fallen out of contact when he hit rock bottom, but something inside of me told me to give him a call. He had been sober for a year, was in charge of running the sobriety meetings at the Salvation Army, and most recently had been promoted to manager of their store. It seemed like an ideal time to meet in person.

My father's descent into deep addiction was a shock to most of our community. He was known as the guy you called when you had a flat tire on the side of the road. He was part of the specialized environmental clean-up crew that responded to the 9-11 Attack in NYC in 2001. He wasn't in Manhattan when the towers fell, but like so many people in the surrounding areas, he wanted to help out. The #7 World Trade Center building collapsed the same day as the Twin Towers. There were concerns that fires from the collapsing buildings could spread to other buildings in the World Trade Center Plaza. [23] Dad was one of the guys risking his life to pull out barrels of kerosene and other potentially flammable materials from the remaining World Trade Center buildings in order to prevent additional explosions. It was there that my father experienced one of his proudest moments. Among the crowd of first responders and the clean-up crew, he got to shake the hand of then U.S. President George W. Bush on his visit to ground zero on Sept. 14th, 2001. [24] I remember my father coming home exhausted at night. The gray ash never seemed to leave his clothes. But meeting a sitting president at such a historic event

It was shortly after the 9-11 attack that my father descended into his addiction, a surprising slide from such a proud day of meeting a sitting U.S. President to trying to rebuild his life in rehab. Because our extended

---

23 https://www.huffpost.com/entry/september-11-timeline_n_3901837

24 http://edition.cnn.com/2001/US/09/14/bush.terrorism/

family and local community held him in such high regard, few could believe the stories they'd heard about his deterioration.

As I walked up to the entrance of the old brick building of the Salvation Army, I thought about the deep rift that had happened between my father and I. Though I had felt abandoned by my father since early childhood, I also recognized that he too was abandoned by his father. Dad had been chasing his workaholic father his whole life. Grandpa George was an orphan and grew up without a father figure. The absence of fathers was cyclic in my lineage, so this repetitive suffering wasn't unique to me. When I looked back at the generations of men in my family, I could see that we had actually progressed. My paternal grandfather had no contact with his father and lost his mother to cancer as a child. Though he was always working and had emotionally abandoned my father, Grandpa George did make efforts to take my father to Coney Island and other such special occasions. At least Dad grew up knowing his father and had a few special memories to share with him. To my Grandpa George's credit, he had a problem with alcohol in his younger years, but quit cold turkey before I was born. These efforts contributed to the healing of our lineage. I was hoping that this meeting, only possible because of my father's sobriety, might be the next contribution to the healing of my own heart as well as the healing of my lineage.

As I opened the door to the Salvation Army, my heart was pounding. I feared the unknown. I was afraid that some angry comment from either of us could derail this delicate reunion. But through the trembling, I also felt a surge of courage, like a stream of power flooding throughout my body. It radiated from my heart, telling me that something new was going to happen, something good was taking place. This was an unusual contact between men in my family that most likely hadn't happened before in many generations. The Hunter men were actually going to talk to each other in a real way.

The man at the front desk greeted me with a weathered face and a mouth that only had a few teeth left. His eyes were clear, but were devoid of enthusiasm. I could tell that this man was just getting through the day.

"Can I help you?"

"Yes, I'm here to see George Hunter."

"Are you his son, George?" he asked.

"Yes. That's me."

His deadpan eyes popped open with surprise. He gushed like he just met a celebrity.

"Your father talks about you all the time," the man said. The once stoic man became animated, his face alight with enthusiasm.

The surprise in his eyes became hope. In this rehabilitation center filled with men who had burned bridges with their loved one, he was one of those men who hoped to see his family again someday.

The man phoned my father. Minutes later, Dad strode through the spacious front lobby dressed in used clothes from the Salvation Army store. He smelled of stocking stuffer aftershave and communal soap.

"GEORGE!" he lit up. We embraced, a hug that was a long time coming. For all his mistakes and all his flaws, my father has always had a charming way about him, a genuine enthusiasm to connect. His warm heart and charisma made him a favorite at family parties.

"This is my son, George," he bragged to other men in the program that we saw along the way. His fellow workers looked at me like I was a mythic beast. They stared in wonderment at the special occasion of a family member actually visiting one of them. But their amazement was surely enhanced by the preamble of stories my father had told them for months before my arrival. Even through his darkest periods, my father's pride in me being his son was clear.

Dad and I sat down at the diner table. We nervously shuffled fat, stubby mugs of acrid coffee that had been sitting in the pots too long. The pancakes were comically large and our feeble butter knives struggled to cut through the thick slabs of mammoth-like hides.

"You know, son, I think I really went crazy," he said, referring to his drug-assisted mental breakdown years ago. He had been verbally and physically violent to the point where no one in our family would take him in anymore. Turning away a family member in need was completely counter to the way we were raised, especially considering that I was born into a tiny home that was packed to the gills with my grandparents, parents, a couple of aunts, an uncle, and a few cousins. When my Dad left the family, it was hard for all of us. But most of us just suffered in silence and never spoke about it.

Dad owned that what he had done was wrong. He didn't try to defend himself. He just simply acknowledged that he had lost control of himself and hurt a lot of people in the process. As he spoke his words of apology, I felt this influx of softness, a gentle breeze that filled my chest. The anger that I had felt in the past wasn't there anymore. I was just glad to have my father back. I knew that what was happening between us was rare. Generations of Hunter men had been hoping for that simple recognition from their fathers that they had made a mistake and that they were sorry. I felt my father's love, combined with his appreciation that I showed up.

"I forgive you Dad." The words spilled out of my mouth on their own. I didn't plan it. It just happened as a natural reflex of two men speaking from their hearts. I just followed the energy of the moment throughout the meeting with my Dad. Doing so allowed the whole conversation to unfold on its own. Something momentous had happened on its own. The greatest thing that either of us did was that we both showed up.

When I dropped my father off in front of the brick building of his Salvation Army, I gave him a bear hug. In his ear, I said, "I'm not ashamed of you anymore, Dad. Keep going." He laughed, as if my words tickled his heart on the way in. I was being honest, because for many years I had been ashamed to be called his son. But after the reconciliation that had just happened, I felt free from that past heaviness that once had a grip on me.

I got in my car and drove away with tears in my eyes. My heart was filled with heat, a fire that was melting away the old walls inside my heart. As the sensation grew, my heart seemed to expand. I'm still grateful to my father for having the courage to meet me that day. We both gave each other a rare gift, a precious exchange of forgiveness that seldom happens before the grave.

The Path of Forgiveness

To forgive takes enormous courage. In order to fully forgive someone, you must first have the willingness to feel what they have done to you. To feel the full impact of your devastation by feeling that pain, you first surrender your resistance to experiencing overwhelming emotions which can even manifest as physical pain in your body. This is evidenced by the way we feel when we have our hearts broken and the pain feels as if our chests are splitting apart, the physical pressure in our necks that lead to migraines during emotional turmoil and the more severe physical reactions of fainting and vomiting on hearing tragic news. Feeling the physical pain, albeit uncomfortable, helps us to recognize the impact that a conflict has had on us.

Forgiveness means that you give up the wound. Now that you have passed through the wound and claimed the gifts and lessons from the experience, the need for the wound shifts. Because we're already in touch with our Inner Voice of Truth, keeping an open wound serves no further purpose. To keep the wound open at this point is like conducting every step of a surgery except the last step of stitching up the gaping incisions. The wound no longer has a clear purpose and forgiveness is the process of releasing the wound completely.

Why would we be tempted to continue to hold onto a wound after all the hard work we have done in the healing process? While wounds are painful by nature, and our initial reflex is to avoid that discomfort, we ultimately want to control how we feel. So, by controlling whether or not we feel our emotions inside of our wounds can give us a sense of temporary control over our lives, especially since emotional expression and grieving can disrupt our daily routines.

Wounds can also give the wounded a certain amount of control in their relationships. Diseases and afflictions that are connected to emotional wounds can be leveraged to get partners and family members to bend around their situation and cater to their needs. Co-dependent family members give up on holding addicts accountable and just decide to take care of the addict's responsibility for them. In the short term, it's just seems easier to do that than to get into another fight. Others can use how they were victimized in the past as reasons to win arguments with people who had nothing to do with the original injury.

Having a sense of control over others can be very appealing. Many people go to great lengths to maintain that control by keeping themselves in a wounded state. Having wounds can give weight to their needs and demands. If someone was abandoned by their father, they may expect their male partner to make up for that abandonment by being immediately responsive to their emotional needs for verbal reassurance and physical presence. The moment that consistency is broken, wounds can be used to corral the partner back into responsiveness by dumping all the emotions held inside onto the partner. "You don't really love me! You're never there for me!" Meanwhile, the partner may have an excellent track record of being sensitive and responsive, but they were just fatigued from work and couldn't generate the same level of responsiveness as usual. The verbal accusations that the partner no longer cares, are really speaking to the past abandonment and are projections. But if the partner gives a lot of attention after hearing these accusations, then why let the wound go? Wounds have a way of securing extra attention, so some choose to hold onto the wounds for the sake of convincing others to keep meeting their emotional needs.

Even in the case when a wounded person does not receive some direct form of influence from their wounding, it is possible to hold onto the hurt of our wounds as evidence that Life/God/Universe/Fate has treated them unfairly. In a way, they are secretly holding themselves to ransom, and the wound is evidence that the disappointing direction of their life has nothing to do with their choices. They are a perpetual victim of circumstance. Holding onto wounds happens with the irrational hope that some karmic balance will finally kick in, because they have suffered enough. In this line of thinking, the hurt gives them rights to receive what they didn't get earlier in life.

Forgiveness requires that we give up what we think is owed to us. By doing this, we release our expectations and demands that life bring us what we have always wanted in exchange for a new spaciousness in our lives. Letting go of the demand that Life make up for what we are owed (such as a soul mate, stolen property, an apology) is necessary for forgiveness to happen.

Complete Forgiveness

When we speak about forgiveness, we often focus on specific hurts inflicted on us by other people. We may also be talking about how we hurt another and how we are seeking their forgiveness. These are the most obvious parts of a conflict that needs to be addressed.

But to completely give up the wound, we must also look at two other factors that may have played a role in the wounding. In the case of child abuse, the abuse is not the fault of the victim. The child often chooses not to tell an adult about the abuse because of fear of not being believed and the possibility of being shame. This hesitation is often compounded by threats from the abuser and misplaced guilt about lack of parental oversight. As adults, these victims may be left with conflicted feelings about their past choices, including regrets about not reaching out and seeking help at the time of the abuse, can lead to mistrust in themselves for not doing more to stop the abuse. Self-forgiveness can be enhanced by realizing that as a child, they were powerless to stop it from happening. But this part of the forgiveness process is difficult because the victims often hold onto their misplaced feelings and are unable to forgive themselves.

The other aspect of forgiveness pertains to forgiving the harm caused by forces and factors outside of human control. Communities who have been decimated by natural disasters, like earthquakes, tsunamis, hurricanes and drought and families who have lost children to illness can cause a crisis of faith. These events lead us to question how such devastation can happen in a just world. For some, this is about their direct relationship with God, the universe, or their higher power which allowed such painful wounds to be caused and this can lead to a breaking of trust in the greater forces of life.

To embody Complete Forgiveness, it helps to address each focal point to ensure that we are not still holding onto a painful story connected to our wounding. More specifically, we need to forgive those who hurt us, forgive ourselves for hurting others and ourselves, and forgive the powers of life that are beyond our control. These aspects are represented in the Triangle of Complete Forgiveness.

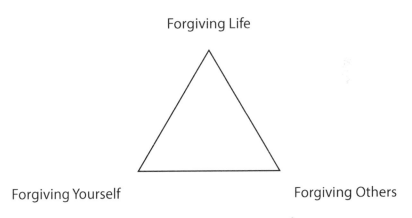

Figure 14. Triangle of Complete Forgiveness

Forgiving Other People

Emotional scarring slows us down enough so that we don't jump back into the same pattern of wounding over and over again. When the emotional scar tissue builds up, we will develop a feeling of repulsion to the cyclic patterns of suffering. If we have been hurt in the same way numerous times, we will avoid forming relationships with people who are abusive. Repetitive wounding can be part of our awakening to how we need to change our lives.

We need that pause to allow space for our Inner Voice of Truth to speak to us. Repetitive suffering gives us numerous opportunities to claim the lessons of harsh experiences. That awareness allows us to see how new people are playing old roles in our scripts. Learning to say "no" to these relationships is essential to keeping the space clear for something new to enter into your life. But once we have claimed the gifts from the wound and learned to say *no* to re-wounding ourselves, it's time to say *yes* to releasing the grievance that taught us to respect ourselves and step out of the abusive scripts. Holding onto the suspicion, resentment, and grief no longer makes sense when you have already learned your lessons.

When you leave the scripted life, you will no longer be compatible with people who continue to live by their scripts. Now that you have taken a step back, you can see their survival mode and the repetition of their scripted dialogue from afar. No longer subjected to their harm directly, forgiving them in their desperate state becomes easier, because you realize that they just can't help themselves. They are obliged to live an unhappy life until they gather the courage to face their wounds and pass through them. With the space that comes from separating, the higher wisdom of the Biblical proverb, "Forgive them... for they know not what they do," Luke 23:34 can be practically applied to ex-partners, estranged family members, and former friends.

Wounding is not about becoming a perpetual victim. Passing through our wounds is an initiation into our power. The more powerful you become, the more your tolerance for forming reciprocal relationships with disempowered people will fade. You will no longer relate to people just for their sakes. Instead, you learn to form relationships based on mutual exchange, which leads to sustainable partnerships and genuine friendships.

The act of forgiveness is a vulnerable empowerment of the heart. It starts with allowing yourself to feel any leftover emotions surrounding a wound. Grieving that these people who you care about have not done the work it takes to be in an empowered relationship, clears your heart so that

416

forgiveness can happen. When you fully surrender to your disappointment, resentment, and grief, it leaves your body and creates space for something fresh to enter.

This forgiveness happens when our self-love is greater than our need to be right. When we have said all that we can say, learned all that we can learn, and feel our desire to be free so intensely, we finally surrender the control that holding onto our wounds could grant us. We take the gifts of the experience and let go of the way we thought apologies and amends "should" have happened.

To forgive is a personal choice made in our hearts. No one can tell you when it is the right time. The shift happens when your reasons to hold onto your point of view no longer feels worth it, because you are losing that precious access to all that could be experienced in your life right here and now.

Forgiving Ourselves

To blame others entirely for our wounds can create a blind spot to our personal accountability in conflicts. Even in extreme circumstances, like child abuse where the child is a victim of Generational Dumping, it may be that an inner reconciliation still needs to happen. For instance, divorce is not the fault of the child, but this doesn't mean that the child is free from inner conflict. They may feel a need to choose one parent over the other when they separate, creating guilt that needs to be released. They may also erroneously blame themselves for the divorce, which needs to be released for healing to happen. Survivors of sexual abuse may feel betrayed by their bodies, because even though the abuse was unwanted, they may still have experienced pleasure or even an orgasm during the abuse. The body has its own way of functioning and can participate in acts that the individual does not want to experience. It's not a child's fault when the body responds in this physical way, but forgiving the body is part of the process.

In many ways, self-forgiveness can be the most challenging part of this Realization, because it requires us to see how we have harmed others and ourselves. To do this work, we must surrender our victimhood and recognize how we were the ones who caused harm, that we aren't perfect, and that we too, have hurt others and taken advantage of their trust.

Although blatant forms of inflicting emotional or physical hurt are immediately recognizable, more subtle modes of harm can be overlooked, thus delaying the forgiveness process. Perhaps you pulled away from someone who had hurt you, and rather than talking about the hurt, you punished them by shutting them out in a neglectful way for long periods of time. Even though you didn't say something nasty to them or do something physically drastic that threatened their safety, it is still possible to hurt someone through pulling away and ceasing communication. If the person is dangerous, then you might be doing it just to protect yourself. But in circumstances when you are in a relationship with someone who is trying to apologize or reconnect in a safe way, shutting people out causes harm.

You can also harm yourself by not expressing your feelings, thus restricting the Inner Voice of Truth that is trying to protect you. Keeping emotions tucked down deep inside can cause elevated stress that can directly impact your health. Emotionally, you can become depressed, which can impact every aspect of your life. While biting your tongue so that you don't harm another person with your sharp words might be necessary from time to time, keeping those venomous words inside with no safe place to release them can also be toxic.

Self-love and self-forgiveness feed into each other. When we practice both, we compound the effects of our inner healing. Both acts create a warm internal space that gives us a growing permission to make mistakes and to learn. Seeing our life as a journey of learning about people, the world, and a quest for self-awareness helps us to loosen up our rigid grips on the past in favor of a more vibrant now.

Forgiving Life

Each person has their own way of relating to the greater forces of their life. Many in Western societies have a personal relationship with a higher being, most commonly referred to as God in English, while others have an affinity with the forces of nature, the spiritual wisdoms of Buddha, and even atheists have an appreciation that because of some higher force, the earth will continue to operate as usual. If your vacation trip gets cancelled because of a natural disaster like a hurricane or blizzard, you may have feelings towards nature and the weather for ruining your trip. Some look up at the stars and marvel at how the planet Jupiter protects the planet Earth by pulling asteroids to it with its enormous gravitational field. These asteroids would otherwise hit the Earth and devastate our way of life. People working 12 step programs may prefer the term "higher power." Even atheists wake up in the morning believing that gravity, a force that they have no control over, will continue to operate as usual. In my work with clients from many backgrounds, I've met a growing number of people who are not exactly sure what they believe, but are actively exploring that in their own time.

For the sake of our healing process, Life will be the neutral term used to describe all those greater forces that are outside of our human control. However, you personally connect to Life is your choice, and you need not change what you believe to embrace the entirety of this Realization. Even not being sure about what you believe is still a workable situation when it comes to recognizing what is in your power to change and what is not.

Talking to Life out loud can be incredibly cathartic and can ultimately clarify why you may be holding onto past events that were beyond your control. To understand this, let's look at the wisdom captured in the Serenity Poem, often attributed to[25] theologian Reinhold Niebuhr.

Grant me the serenity, to accept the things that I cannot change; courage to change the things I can; and the wisdom to know the difference.

We can apply this wisdom to the Triangle of Forgiveness. Some circumstances happen because of our personal choices and actions. If we run into a wall and smash our face because we chose to drink too much alcohol, we harmed ourselves, even if it was inadvertently. If we actively harm ourselves, it is in our hands to change that. If we chose to strike someone or demean them verbally, we are liable for those acts.

Some conflicts and wounding happen to us because of the choices and actions of others.

If a frustrated parent is unhappy in their job and vents that frustration on their child, emotionally or physically, the parent is responsible for those actions. A child can't be blamed for the abuse inflicted upon them, however, the abuse they may in turn pass onto others does become their responsibility, especially as they grow into their adulthood.

Some wounding we experience happens to us because of a *tour de force* or circumstances that are completely out of our hands as well as the hands of our communities. When a hurricane hits a town, that town is not personally responsible for the hurricane hitting that specific spot on the planet. However, the aftermath of a devastating storm does involve many hands in the clean-up. The more frequent occurrence of powerful

---

25   https://www.nytimes.com/2008/07/11/us/11prayer.html

storms also prompts us to gain a more worldly understanding of how human contributions to global warming are impacting the weather.

Speaking aloud to Life helps us to discern what was in our hands to change, and what was not. By venting to Life about what we have endured, we can open all the feelings about how we have been impacted and to see what grudges and blocks we are still holding onto. Sometimes just hearing ourselves acknowledge how Life or others have hurt us, can help forgiveness to flow.

Exercise: Clarifying Forgiveness

- Chose a confidential space where you will not be overheard and you are assured of privacy. If you are doing this with a trusted friend or supporter, it is fine for them to hear what you are saying to Life and vice versa.
- Set an intention to speak honestly about the past hurts that you still need to forgive.
- Choose a reference point to represent Life. This reference point will be what you speak to in this exercise. For some, this might be a visualization of God appearing in a human form like Yaweh of the old testament, Latchmi the Divine Mother, or perhaps a new expression that you haven't seen before but feels right for this occasion. This point of reference could be the moon, the nighttime sky full of stars, or one star in particular. If you struggle to find a vision of what Life looks like for you, choose a place that felt personally meaningful to you like a favorite vacation spot or a sacred space that you have visited. Put yourself in that place and allow it to get you closer to the

cosmic forces that are at work even though we have no direct influence over them.

- Give yourself permission to speak in an uncensored way. This means that if you need to use foul language or talk about graphic things that you are not normally accustomed to doing in your daily routine, allow yourself this special circumstance to use them for the sake of cleansing the past.

- Make contact with Life using your point of reference and allow whatever feelings, thoughts, or memories, to be expressed. Remember that the Inner Voice of Truth has a way of moving the right things up to the surface to be said, which is why speaking in an uncensored way is absolutely necessary for the process to work.

- Vent about how you were hurt, how you feel your life circumstances were unfair, how you have been treated unfairly because of your appearance, culture or faith. Don't worry about offending God, some higher power, or about some karmic backlash where "God punishes" you. After facilitating thousands of these processes, I can earnestly share that none of my clients were ever struck down by a lightning bolt from Zeus. Consider that whatever grander power who is listening will not be mortally wounded or profoundly insulted by the words of one human being. As powerful as one human being can be, cursing the sky will not throw Jupiter's planet off its axis. Let it rip.

- When the streams of hurt have been expressed and there is a long pause after you speak, put your hand on your heart and feel any changes that you notice in your body.

- Journal about what was expressed as a way to assess what you still need to forgive in your life.

Focus Questions for Journaling:
1. Were you surprised by any of the hurts that you expressed to Life? If so, why?
2. Was any particular instance shared that you thought you had already forgiven? If so, ask yourself why you still feel like the forgiveness is not yet complete.
3. Do you need to forgive Life for any past event that was out of your hands to change?
4. Do you need to forgive anyone who hurt you or could have helped you in the past, but made other choices?
5. Do you need to forgive your part in any of the past hurts mentioned?
6. In the act of expressing to Life, did you discover any new forgiveness through this process?

Forgiving Our Ancestors: Getting to the Heart of the Script

When we release the wounds, we release the final footholds of the old scripts. When the wound closes, our involvement with the unfinished stories will be complete. Other members of the family may still be working on these unfinished stories. But you have done the work around this specific wound, and your part in the healing of your family will serve as a living example to the others. As a Catalyst, you will no longer be on stage as a character wrapped up in the angst of the family drama. You will be in the audience, watching it unfold, remembering what it was like to be trapped in a script that left very little room for the authentic, empowered you. This detachment is healthy. When you forgive your family, you even have the freedom to walk out of the theater completely and explore what other stories are out there.

This freedom is the ultimate motivation to forgive. Letting go of the wound, the opening that has already birthed so much new awareness into your life, allows you the personal liberty to live your own life. Living your life unapologetically also gives an unconscious permission for others to live their authentic lives.

To complete the forgiveness of your lineage, we now need to depersonalize the wounding that once felt like a personal affront. Depersonalizing the wound means that you recognize how you weren't the only one to endure the cyclic abuse from your family and community. Only you can say when the time is right for you.

Depersonalizing the wound too early will make you feel like your pain and strengths were not fully acknowledged. If you still feel a need to be acknowledged for the hardships that you've endured and still need to be recognized for your strength in the face of those challenges, it may be a sign that you missed something in the previous Realizations. When we delay the depersonalization step, you remain on the edge of the stage of your family's drama. Staying personally attached to your past pain keeps you in a disempowering limbo that drains you of your enthusiasm and sabotages new developments that want to offer you new love, respect, and opportunities to thrive. If you're not ready to let go of how you personally feel offended and disrespected, it's a sign that you are not ready to forgive, and that the wound needs more processing. To help you flush out the wound more thoroughly, return to Realization #4 to further cleanse the wound and follow each Realization on the way back to #8, focusing your efforts on the most emotionally-charged memory.

One of the most direct ways to depersonalize your wounding is to look at the bigger story of your family tree. Did your lineage leave their home country in desperation? Did your family survive a war? Was your family forced off their homeland? Did you come from an indigenous family where land, power, and rights were taken away? Did your lineage oppress less fortunate families? By taking several steps back from your specific story, you can see the greater arc of it all. Seeing that you are not alone in your suffering can sometimes make room for forgiveness to happen.

It only takes one generation to wound a lineage, yet it often takes several generations for the pattern of wounding to be healed in a family. One war can send ripples of suffering through a family for several generations to come. However, it only takes one lifetime to heal the wound in an individual family member and that one successful Catalyst gives willing family members inspiration as to what their healing could look like. Even against seemingly insurmountable odds of massive generational wounding, one individual can show the way and change the way a family treats their younger generations. One family that changes how they treat each other can be an encouraging example to their community. One reformed community can prove to other communities that change and healing are possible. When enough cities change, a nation can eventually shift as well. When an exemplary nation shows the world that a freer, kinder way of life is possible, the world listens. A prime example of how nations can change how the world operates can be seen with end of slavery in the Americas and Europe.

Many might see the wounding process as being unfair, because repetitive wounding comes from an unconscious place that spares no individual human being. Often, wounds are inflicted without anyone realizing the impact that it's having on you, because they too were harmed and hardened by the same scripted abuse. But the wounding process is certainly a fruitful one if the wounds are given enough attention. The redeeming quality of the wounding process is that it pierces us in all the right ways to reveal the gifts and hard lessons that we need to learn in order to grow. When you can embrace the rewards of the healing process, it becomes easier to forgive your ancestors who very likely both endured and re-inflicted the same wounds as you.

Emotional Debt Forgiveness

When a poor farmer from an impoverished community takes out a loan from an establishment in order to buy seeds and farm equipment, he must make loan repayments each month to pay back the loan. Hopefully he has a good crop and can make enough profit when he sells his harvest, so that he can pay the loan back. But when he is struck by drought, it puts the farmer and his crop into survival mode. With the loss of profits, the farmer must decide where he will spend his limited funds. What bills does he pay for first? Does he decide to feed his children or pay for their schooling first? Even when a farmer can't make the loan payment and feed his family, the debtor can still demand that the loan be paid back on time. In these circumstances, however, it can be immoral, and even heartless, to try collecting on the loan because the children can starve. So, the establishment may choose to forgive the debt, since the farmer did not cause the drought, nor did he intend to default on the loan.

Debt forgiveness gives the struggling farmer a chance to get back on his feet in hopes of a better harvest next year. The establishment releasing part or all of the debt owed becomes an act of compassion, as the alternative would be to let the children starve. It also allows the lender to cut their losses and frees the lender from the guilt of making the farmer's children starve.

Our unmet needs from our childhood can become demands. These unmet demands signal that we are holding an unacknowledged emotional debt. Like the poor farmer who was unable to pay back his debt, many of the people who weren't able to meet your emotional needs in the past were also in some form of survival mode and weren't in a state of mind to give you what you needed and expected.

As much as a well-meaning lender deserved to be repaid, the extenuating circumstances of the farmer were more urgent. As much as you, as an individual, deserved to have your emotional needs met while growing up, the people who were supposed to take care of you were likely just getting through the day emotionally. They just didn't have the love and attention to give to you. Or perhaps they just didn't have the courage to stand up for you. This doesn't make your needs any less worthy or important. It just means that those needs were not given attention because of a dire situation in your family, often connected to the generational wounding.

In Realization #4, we recognized that we can accumulate emotional debts from both our lineage and our long-term relationships. If you have uncovered other demands in your healing process, add them to the list. When we first acknowledged these demands, it was important to express our anger, sadness, and fears about our needs not being met at crucial moments of our lives. The catharsis makes room for the gifts and meaning of these experiences to reveal themselves. For instance, a child that was treated unfairly and neglected can grow up to be an advocate for the less fortunate. But the healing process is not complete without forgiveness. To forgive the emotional debts that we feel our families and communities owe us, we need to release them from the expectation that they meet those needs or acknowledge that they failed us.

Not every family member will get what they need when they need it. Well-meaning adults can wind up sacrificing their own needs and dreams so that their children can have a better life than they had. However, this often leads to the parents feeling constantly exhausted and leaves their personal dreams unfulfilled.

We hold onto these images of what our family *should be* so that we can value our unmet needs. It's a way of saying that we are entitled to care and deserve love, even when facing the harshest abuse and most blatant neglect. This image can even become the blueprint of the family we create when it's our turn to be in charge as adults. But even in this scenario, where you create a family in the "right way" according to what you believe you should have gotten as a child, you are giving what you never received. You receive a sense of gratification at seeing your children thrive in a way that you did not. Then you plop down on the couch, exhausted, realizing that you are still not receiving that same care that you believe you have always needed.

When the weight of carrying the demands over your family keeps you from being open to the new offerings from Life, they pinch off the grieving process. The unfinished conversation is no longer between you and the deceased or between you and your failed elders or siblings. For the expression of grief to move forward, you need to talk to Life. However, you see the greater forces that turn the tides and spin our planet, regardless if you believe in karma, a benevolent being or are a staunch agnostic, we all have feelings about what we did and didn't get while growing up. If you are still not getting those needs met today, then expressing the emotions about your "bad luck" can help you complete the grieving process. Lamenting over how life didn't go your way or wailing about how your family broke your heart are both healthy acts.

When practicing this on your own, it is essential that you do so in a space where you will not be overheard by people other than your supporters. Because these feelings can trigger so many emotions in other people, be selective with who you share this process. Therapists, Healers, and your Catalyst buddies are always good places to try something new. The process can also be done on your own, through writing in a protected diary or speaking aloud in a confidential space.

Once you release your demand over Life to provide you with the family that you never had, a new space opens up in your chest and in your mind. It is true that you didn't get everything that you thought you should receive. But it is also true that you made it this far without that checklist being met. Grieving what you haven't received doesn't mean that you will never receive love and care in the future. It means that it won't come in the way that you expected it and from the people you demanded it from. Life will bring it to you from sources that you might not have foreseen and in ways that you do not control, if you give it a chance to do so.

Releasing our demands can be a very sad process, because with it we release the dreams that came with those demands. "By this time in my life I was supposed to be happily married and have two children a girl and a boy." Or, "I finally have that family I always envisioned, but something is still missing. What about my needs?" These are two common examples of dreams that are linked to our demands. When we first let them go, it can be a very deep experience, filled with shuddering cries and even desperation about the direction our life is going in. While we are doing this part of grieving, we can feel lost, more so than we started doing this deep inner work. But what is actually happening is that we are surrendering a fictional future in exchange for the ripe, unaltered *now*. Letting go of the debts that life owes you liberates your heart and makes space for unseen sweetness to find you. You can meet someone you never thought that you would meet. You can move to a place that finally resonates with that inner song inside of you. Or it can even come in the form of an unexpected career change that was far more fulfilling than you expected.

When you finally release these debts towards Life, you make room for the loving surprises.

You truly let go and let Life steer you towards new forms of care and new supporters who validate who you are becoming. This is how the transformation happens, with moments of raw release and unexpected beams of sunshine that warm the forgotten parts of your heart. However bittersweet it may seem at first, once the work of releasing what you no longer need happens, you heart grows in ways where receiving fresh streams of love and sweetness becomes a part of your new life.

Fire and Forgiveness

Forgiveness is not only the act of releasing an offender from his or her debt. Forgiveness also releases victims from holding onto the hurt and shame of what another person has done to them. At some point, we must let go of the past hatred in order to move on. Hatred forms when the shame of how we were taken advantage of and demeaned meets the fire of revenge. The shame we hold about ourselves, when we believe it, traps our fire.

When the fire stays trapped inside because we believe the ridicule and the negative judgments about ourselves, self-hatred is born. That fire smolders, burning inside our organs, making it feel as if the hatred is eating us up inside. As the pressure builds inside, the fire seeks release in the form of revenge. More often than not, these feelings are stored up inside, waiting for the moment when you are strong enough to retaliate. This hatred can be passed onto another generation, where younger children who never experienced the direct abuse, take on the tar-like hatred of their elders. As a result of these feuds, the children of each family involved learn to shame their neighbors based on their last name because of an insult or injury that happened years before their birth. Holding onto the hatred becomes a form of loyalty to the family, even though the younger generations might not even know the details of why the feud started.

Forgiveness releases us from the old, tired fights of our ancestors. It reclaims our energy for positive construction. It releases revenge and our obligation to fulfill it. Forgiveness gives our fire room to breathe. It is cleaner to therapeutically scream and hit, than to actually re-inflict harm for the sake of revenge. A therapeutic space allows us to purge the shame and free the fire. It gives us permission to release our own hurt and claim the reward of our fire passionately flowing through the gifts connected to the wound.

Ensuring Complete Forgiveness

Because we receive many wounds in our lifetime, forgiveness is not a one-off process. Each wound gives us a new opening to get to know ourselves on a deeper level and a fresh opportunity to forgive. Forgiveness is the end of learning from a particular wound, the time when the wound closes up.

Each time we successfully heal a wound and forgive someone for what they have done, we develop a more fluid heart. We become skilled in learning how our heart works and how forgiveness can be repeated. How do we know when we have completely forgiven a past hurt and have truly given up the wound?

Let's look at the elements of Complete Forgiveness. This checklist is meant to be applied to each past conflict. Apply it to one painful event at a time:

1. acknowledging a wrong
2. expressing feelings about the instance with empathy

3. a deeper sharing of the stories connected to the act of harm (allowing both parties to speak, not just the person who was most harmed)
4. sincere apology
5. making amends
6. receiving the apology and cooperating with the amend-making
7. surrendering and accepting the current state of your life situation as a result of the past
8. releasing the wound, including all special attention that the wound brought with it, so that we are free to re-discover a greater sense of personal identity

When a little kid steals a toy from another child, he creates an emotionally charged situation. With some adult intervention, it becomes a teaching moment to acknowledge that something wrong has happened. Both children get to express themselves. Then amends are made by giving the toy back. Sharing is taught along with a spirit of abundance that everyone can play with the toy if they take turns. The offending child says he's sorry. The offended child then lets go of the painful experience and forgives his playmate when they learn to share and play together.

One of the biggest blocks to the forgiveness process is when an offender refuses to admit that they have done something wrong. They fear punishment or they have a strong belief about how their actions were justified, which usually has a long history of wounding that went into the formation of that limiting belief.

Even when an offender is willing to own what was done and participate in the healing process, the forgiveness process can still be interrupted by an uncooperative victim. Victims who haven't done enough catharsis around how they were harmed can become tyrants that block the forgiveness process. When all has been acknowledged and efforts are made by the offender to heal the past, the victim can still exploit the situation and try to punish the offender or attempt to get extra needs met by an offender who has become emotionally vulnerable by apologizing. This is a sign that there is an emotional debt that may pre-date this particular offense. Going through Realizations #4 and #5 can help clarify who else the victim is upset with and what past offenses may have been refreshed by the more recent wounding. Incomplete forgiveness keeps both people in limbo and can create additional suffering that may also need to be forgiven.

Exercise: Track the Progress of your Forgiveness

To help you actualize the elements of Complete Forgiveness, let's take you through a guided exercise to track how far along you are in forgiving past harm. Your greatest asset in assessing how far along you have come in the process of forgiveness is self-honesty. Focus on each of the following points of reference and earnestly answer the following questions. If you find that you are stuck on a particular question, take is as a sign that you need to rework the specific highlighted Realization(s).

Begin the exercise by putting your hand on your heart and breathing deeply. Rub your heart so that the energy comes out of your head and into your chest. When you feel a strong sense of connection to your heart, ask yourself the following questions:

Main Question: Do I need to forgive anyone? If so, who? Allow your heart to answer the question. You may have a feeling, a name, a face, or past memory that bubbles up when you ask the question. Let the response to the question bubble up from your chest area, paying attention to the tone of voice that is responding to the query. Do your best to trust the process.

Focusing on the person or situation that you need to forgive, ask the following questions. If you answer *yes* to any of them, return to the numbered Realization(s) associated with the questions and skim through the chapter until something catches your eye. Work on that piece in relation to the person who came up in the main question. Again, the heart can't lie so be sure to feel your heart with each question, not just the thoughts that are zooming through your brain. A genuine response will have a clear tone, a steady pass, and an air of truth to it.

1. Do I still have feelings about my past with this person or situation? Am I denying my feelings around a past betrayal? (#1)

2. Am I still carrying someone else's responsibility? If so, name it. (#2, #3)

3. Have I fully expressed my pain around this person or situation? Pause to really feel. (#4, #5)

4. Do I feel heard and empathically felt by the offender? (#4)

5. Do I have enough support?

6. Name what was taken from you. Did you reclaim it? (#5)

7. Acknowledge what benefits and gifts you received from this experience. (#6)

8. Did the challenge of the wound help you express your innate gifts? If so, how? If not, revisit (#6)

9. Am I carrying emotional debts around this struggle? (#8)

10. Was this the only person to take something from me or hurt me in this way? Are my emotional debts from other people being projected on the latest offender? (#7)

11. Do they owe me on behalf of all people who have offended me in a similar way? (#7, #8)

12. What is a fair reparation or amend? (#7)

13. Knowing that not all offenders make amends for their harms, what is the reality of my situation? (#7)
14. What do I need in order to trust life again? (#8)
15. Can I see who I am in the mirror without being the holder of this wound? (#7, #8)
16. Am I ready to let this wound go? (#8)
17. Say the words for forgiveness aloud from your heart. If you struggle, return to the beginning of (#8)

Be the Catalyst

The path of the Catalyst is not only a process of owning who you are as a unique being. It is also about forgiving those who do not own their power. When we deny our own sense of inner power, we can fail to step up at the right moments to protect younger people. We can devalue what we have to offer, and thus not try to help others, resulting in neglect of their needs.

Most of the people who have hurt you have done so unconsciously or with only partial awareness about the full impact that they've had on you. They haven't done enough work on themselves to recognize the cyclic wounding that they have inherited, so how could they be aware of how hurtful they are being to others by repeating that same harm again? The famous quote attributed to Christ, "Forgive them, for they know not what they do," can be heard by the most aware people who are witnessing how their loved ones act in unconscious ways. When a drowning swimmer pulls your head underwater, they are not in their normal state of being. They are not intentionally trying to drown you. They are intentionally trying to survive, however irrational their approach may be, and they will drown you if you let yourself become the next victim.

A Catalyst in action minimizes the impact on future generations. It's important that you embrace this truth even if those around you can't see or validate it. However harmful the unconscious patterns may have been to you, being a Catalyst means being part of the solution. Preventing the dumping of unfinished stories onto the next generation makes the painful acts that you endured more forgivable, because interrupting the cycle becomes a part of your purpose. Having that purpose challenges us to offer our gifts in a way that we normally would shy away from out of fear and shame. It pushes us into a corner and makes stand up for who we are and what we wish for the next generations. Being in the crucible of that generational conflict strips away all the images of who you thought you were, leaving behind the greatest gift that you could give yourself and the world: the true you.

Forgiveness is enhanced by personal empowerment. By now, you can see that you didn't just survive your upbringing. Through hard work, you found a way to transform those rough experiences into a way to thrive. You found a way to be you, no matter how intolerable or outrageous your past abuse may have been. A Catalyst recognizes that they are more powerful than the sum of that abuse.

One of the greatest benefits of having a child that you care about (children, grandchildren, nieces and nephews, the neighbor's child), is that you get to see them growing up without the toil and anguish that you endured. Knowing that you had a significant part in their healthy youth makes your earlier sacrifice seem more worth it. While many people find it difficult to celebrate their own life, it is much easier to celebrate the freedom of young ones playing on the beach or in the park. Their sense of play and celebration are still intact, uninterrupted by major wounding. There is a warm feeling that comes from knowing that you were part of what made that healthy moment possible.

Traps to Forgiveness

Trying to Will Forgiveness

Mentally affirming forgiveness in your head, when it hasn't happened yet in your heart, is the most common trap in the forgiveness process. Prematurely pushing yourself to move on when you have not released enough of the pain is more of an indication that you don't want to feel discomfort and less of a sign that you are ready to forgive someone. It doesn't matter how many years you have held onto the pain of the past; it only matters how much actual time you have focused on feeling and releasing the hurt.

By willing forgiveness without fully feeling your heart, you are essentially tricking yourself into believing that you are further along in the healing process than you actually are. You may, for example, oblige yourself to be a good daughter or son or spouse, so you return to that scripted role and convince yourself that the past is resolved. You may try to meet the expectations of other people in your spiritual or religious community and go back to the role of being a responsible Christian, Jew, Muslim, Hindu, Yogi, etc... in an attempt to emulate a spiritual teacher. But if you are actually feeling hurt and angry, pretending that you have forgiven a past hurt only delays the process. Pushing yourself in the wrong ways can all lead to a false representation of the actual forgiveness process.

Pushing yourself in the right way is not about rushing the process. Facing hard feelings and being courageous enough to have emotionally cathartic conversations is the best use of your will power. Forgiveness requires a clear willingness to see the process through to a resolution, even when the process is scary, fatiguing, or momentarily hopeless. To ensure that you are being honest with yourself, slow down enough to feel what is still left over from a past hurt. Once you are clear on what is still bothering you about the past, you can "push" yourself to speak your truth to the right people.

Pain-Based Identity

It is also possible to hold onto pain, even after all the other aspects of forgiveness have been addressed. When this happens, it is not about forgiving an individual for what they have done to you, rather it is about letting go of the residual pain at the end of the forgiveness process. In Realization #4, we spoke about how people identify so deeply with their victimhood that they derived a sense of identity from being the carrier of their wounds. In a similar way, we can hold onto our pain even after all the hard work has been done in the past Realizations, because pain is familiar. It's like an old friend who has always been there for you. You don't know who you will be without the pain, so you hold onto it out of fear of the unknown.

It's possible to stay attached to our pain, even when we are at the threshold of experiencing an uninterrupted state of peace. But after claiming your gifts, understanding your purpose, and embracing the inner direction provided by your Inner Voice of Truth, you actually have plenty of new discoveries that will help you become aware of yourself without the pain. Still, even with these potent rewards at your fingertips, they are still newer discoveries that will take time to trust. While you are learning to trust them, you can cling to old pain and the patterns of rehashing old fights that no longer hold meaning for who you have become, because you are still getting to know the current expression of your identity.

Hidden Demands

When the forgiveness process is halted, it can also be a sign that there is a hidden deep demand that has not yet been met. The wounded person will hold onto their abandonment or betrayal until that demand is met, even if it causes even more suffering to do so. They want validation from their inflictor that what they did was wrong. They want an apology and reparations. They may even want vindication, where the person who hurt them endures the same pain, or an even greater pain (revenge) than they caused.

Everybody deserves justice, validation, and reparations for past harms. But not all of our demands will be met from one offense, nor will the emotional debt from similar past offenses inflicted by other people, be fully satisfied in a single mediation.

Hidden demands keep us tied to our emotional debt. If a need isn't met by a mother or father, we will look to recruit other women and men into our story so that the debt owed can be paid by someone else. Giving up the wound can feel momentarily disempowering, because giving up the wound means giving up control of how an emotional debt will be paid. It takes trust in life to release someone from their emotional debt, including the trust that someday Life will give you what you truly need in another form.

Healing doesn't always happen in the way that we think it should and moving on can feel like you are surrendering the task of upholding justice. If the wounding has shaken your faith in life, then letting go and allowing life to handle the karmic settling of scores won't feel like a real option.

The Power Card

The Power Card is a last resort manipulation that can arise when we feel that life is not going in the direction that it should go. It's the ace up our sleeve that we save for our most desperate moments. While it's possible to pull the Power Card in a fight with another person, the core of the Power Card is most revealed when we are talking to Life. The Power Card is the most emotionally-charged demand that has the utmost consequences if the demand is not met.

For instance, if Life has not brought you the financial security, loving partnership, and supportive family that you feel you deserve, then one form the Power Card can take, is considering suicide. While this is not everybody's Power Card, many people encounter these thoughts to varying degrees when they are on the verge of feeling their deepest pain.

To help people clarify the demand around their Power Card, I ask them to speak directly to Life so that they can express their feelings and expectations. Here is an example of a dialogue that I have heard many times with my female clients, that illustrates both the strong emotions and hidden demands that prevent them from forgiving Life for the hardships that they endure.

Universe, I'm so disappointed that you haven't given me what I need in my life. I'm 41 years old and I've spent my life helping other people. I've done everything that was asked of me in my career. I've spent so much of life working on myself, and yet I'm still not financially secure and you still haven't brought me my soul mate. I'm running out of time to have a child and I really want to start a family of my own, especially since I had to leave so many toxic relationships from my bloodline family. This is not the life that I envisioned for myself and I don't know what else to do. I can't keep working this hard. How much more inner work do I have to do before I am healed enough to have a life-long partner?

If you don't give me a home, security, and a soul mate soon, then I'm not sure why I'm still living! I've waited long enough. I'm exhausted and I need this now! I can't wait much longer.

I've heard this desperation expressed from so many people coming from various cultural backgrounds, that I've come to see this as a very human script that tends to arise right around important milestone ages. The age at when this will be expressed differs between cultures, however, most women who have invested much of their time and energy into self-development and their careers will face this by the time they are 40 because of the pressures from their biological clocks. I've heard variations of this script with married women who have not been able to conceive a child and I have also heard this from married women who felt like they chose the wrong lifetime partner. However, this script may vary, the commonality is the Power Card issuing a demand to a Higher Power to deliver a deep need by a certain time in your life. If life doesn't deliver it, the Power Card manipulation in this case is using suicidal fantasies or attempts, as a way to express their wish to escape a painful life that hasn't given them what they truly needed to be in this world. It's like holding yourself hostage to see if life even cares about you, because if some benevolent force could feel what you are feeling, then it would surely intervene and stop you from harming yourself by giving you want you demand.

Men do this too. Here's another script that I have heard from many of my male clients.

Life, I've tried to be a good man my whole life. I've helped my family and set boundaries with harmful people in my life. I've dedicated myself to serving humanity through my work and by helping my friends. Yet I feel like I'm the one who is always trying to take care of others and no one is taking care of me in return.

I need a partner who can reciprocate. I need someone who sees that I'm a good man, someone who doesn't blame me for the way other men have abused them in the past. I don't see the point of working myself to death if I don't have someone to celebrate life with. I'm tired of feeling alone in my friendships and all my efforts to make my romantic relationships work have failed. I'm tired of blaming myself for this and I feel like you have failed to bring me the basic kindness and support that I give to other people. If I don't get this soon, then I will quit doing my charitable work in the world, stop taking care of other people, and just make a lot of money so that I can disappear from this empty life that I am now living.

I've heard both men and women use these two Power Cards, although women tend to face it earlier in life because of societal pressure being higher on women and because biologically, they have a shorter window during which they can have children. What is most important is to identify the unmet demand towards Life and the consequence (the way you will escape your Life because you feel like a Higher Power is not delivering their end of the contract).

In order to fully forgive Life, it is essential to grieve what hasn't come to be, and to release your manipulation towards Life for not taking care of you in the way you feel it should. Complete Forgiveness requires surrendering your Power Card(s).

The 8th Birthright

Shared Peace

Forgiveness makes room for trust to be re-established. When you surround yourself with enough trusted people, then the experience of Shared Peace is possible. I think of Shared Peace as the natural state of a healthy community. While it's true that war and cultural oppression are still prevalent around the world, these conflicts always have an unaddressed history of wounding that have few examples of forgiveness and reconciliation. If the future generations did not inherit the painful unfinished stories that start new conflicts and are behind each new war, then it would be easy to recognize Shared Peace as the natural state and war as the interruption to peace.

Peace is not the absence of war or interpersonal conflict. Peace is the state of arrival after forgiveness has happened and trust flows without interruption. Specifically, if we trust ourselves to make good choices, if we choose trustworthy people to be in our support network, and we trust the greater forces of Life, we can share a state of peace with each other.

Shared Peace requires constant inner awareness of how you are feeling and what wounds you are working on. It also requires that you bring your full presence to relationship conflicts, seeing them as learning experiences and opportunities to awaken our Innate Gifts. The work of forgiveness is a crucial part of the healing process where the wounds are allowed to close, and the gifts and lessons of the experience are appreciated.

Peace does not come from finishing all your inner work as fast as possible. It arrives in clear moments in between the catharsis, breakthroughs, and struggles. While some people may have had a spontaneous realization of peace that lasted for a long time, for most, these moments of peace flicker in and out of their awareness. At first, the moments of peace are brief. As the inner work clears the space for peace to happen, these experiences become more frequent and can even last for longer periods of time. Eventually, as we unburden the heaviness and forgive the past, we remember that peace is our natural state. Returning to a state of peace with our newly-realized strengths and gifts empowers the next expression of who you are, to be that much brighter and fulfilling than before.

A sustainable connection to peace comes from building enough trust with yourself, surrounding yourself with trustworthy supporters, and by developing enough acceptance about all the occurrences in Life that are out of your control. Residing in this spacious state of trust allows the peace inside of you to shine through and flourish. Through trusted relationships, the deep calm is reflected back to each other. This is shared peace.

The Triangle of Trust

The triangle of forgiveness guides us to Complete Forgiveness, the state of being that allows us to trust again. As we forgive each point of the triangle, namely yourself, other people, and Life, we clear the way for trust to flow again. When we have trust with each side of the Triangle of Trust, peace emanates freely.

The Triangle of Trust

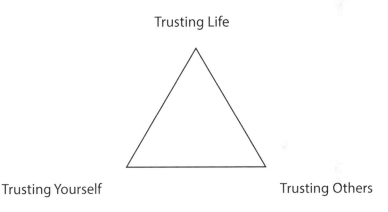

Figure 15. Triangle of Trust

One way to understand trust is that it's the open-hearted ability to receive the Innate Gifts from other people. If we are guarded from past hurts, then we block both beneficial aid as well as future harm. Essentially, we keep out the threats of being re-harmed again, but we also shut out the possibility of receiving life-enhancing goodness from Life and from other people.

Forgiveness is a life skill that builds trust. Imagine a plant that won't absorb the gentle rainwater, because the sky flooded it last spring and it almost drowned. This doesn't happen, because the plant knows, in its own instinctual way, that it needs water. Human beings also instinctively need contact with other people and with nature. We need to breathe in fresh air and need to receive appreciation, love, and care from other people. Sure, we can survive a long time without receiving these crucial streams of life force. We can be as independent as a lone cactus in the desert (and just as hug-able). But eventually, we will need that nourishment.

There comes a time to release the old thorny defenses of the past and take a chance at receiving some fresh support. We can do this by forgiving an old relationship where there was a hurtful conflict, or we can do this by opening up to a trustworthy stranger. Without trust, healing will be stifled, and life will feel unsatisfying, because we never receive the fresh water that helps our spirit blossom and completes our emotional maturation.

Trusting People

Much of our interpersonal tensions revolve around trusting people again after we have been hurt in the past. Unresolved hurt can make our hearts close in the present moment if we are faced with a present situation that reminds us of that painful period. In order to find trust again, we must be able to pass through that past pain that emerges from the similar circumstance and then see that the present situation in different. This part of the healing process often involves trusting a stranger, a new person who can help us see the situation with fresh eyes and offer renewed support.

In our Bloodline Healing workshops, we always strived to create a safe space that fostered a sense of trust. Each time a participant took a risk by sharing a personal moment, and was supported in that sharing, trust was built amongst members of the group. By honestly sharing about their struggles, participants were able to witness each other on a deeper level. This allowed people from very different walks of life to build trust in only a matter of a few days.

One such instance happened between Abby, a retired Native American elder, and Eliana, a young Jewish woman in her late 20's. These two participants were complete strangers before this workshop, yet their embrace was so endearing.

Though she was the youngest of her siblings, Abby was someone who carried herself with the authority of someone much older than her position as the "baby of the family." After several early deaths hit her family unexpectedly, she inherited multiple burdens from her grieving parents and elder siblings. Her family had come to lean on her for emotional support, making her an unconventionally young Elder among her extended family. Overwhelmed by the grief of family members who had died tragically, the family took Abby's support for granted. But it taught her how to summon her inner emotional fortitude and how to hold someone with empathy. Now, in her later years, Abby was a seasoned grandmother.

While sharing her family tree, Eliana revealed multiple betrayals in her family. Particularly, she shared that she didn't trust her parents. She described the elders in her family as self-absorbed, narcissistic, and manipulative. They often used guilt trips, ridicule, and threats to her inheritance as ways to control her. She moved away from them as soon as she could, after years of unspoken emotional neglect.

Even though Abby and Eliana came from vastly different worlds, they were both good-hearted women who knew the pain of deep family neglect. They both knew what it was like to feel alone in a room full of their kin.

Eliana wanted to do Ancestral Dialogue with the intention to speak to her deceased loved ones about her feelings of abandonment by her living elders. But as she shared the details of her family tree before beginning the dialogue with her ancestors, a mix of rage and deep disappointment surfaced. She erupted into tears. Overwhelmed by her emotions, she was unable to speak for a long time.

During her years of enduring this deep neglect, Eliana formed the belief that her family would never be there to support her. So, she changed her mind about doing the Ancestral Dialogue, because she also believed that contacting her ancestors as part of a cathartic process was pointless. She didn't believe that her family had any support for her, whether they were living or connected to her in spirit.

Instinctually, Eliana shielded herself, her arms hugging her knees, compressing her body for safety. As I stood next to her, I could feel a tense force field around her, as if she were trying to push away the family that had betrayed her out of her personal space. She needed support, but she declared that she would not receive anything from a lineage who had betrayed her too many times before. This is where we often need a trustworthy stranger to lend us their shoulder. When I asked her to choose a support from the group of participants, Eliana chose Abby.

"I understand what you are going through," Abby said. "I know what it's like to be left in an unspoken way. But you're not alone right now." Abby moved towards Eliana gently. Her inviting eyes put Eliana at ease. Eliana could feel Abby's powerful empathy as the tears fell down Eliana's face. That invisible wall which surrounded Eliana melted away when she stretched her arms out to Abby. Eliana looked like an orphan who was pleading for a hug. They embraced. Abby spoke softly into her ear, consoling and validating the younger woman. It was the female mentorship and guidance that Eliana did not get from the elders in her family.

Eliana cried hard, expressing how she had always needed this kind of support, sharing how her mother and grandmother failed to see how important this nurturing embrace truly was to her. But Abby knew exactly what Eliana needed. In her younger years, Abby carried the burdens of her grieving family without recognition. But now, Abby was being seen in her eldership by the group and was receiving the appreciation of Eliana who was the recipient of her empathy and support. Abby was also being healed, because she was finally being acknowledged for the service she had provided her family with for nearly her entire life.

Like a resonate symphony, the whole group respectfully moved closer to the two hugging women. Some of the participants cried, others smiled, as we all witnessed the courageous and intimate healing happening before our eyes. Eliana and Abby had become Catalysts to the rest of the room, as waves of healing energy rippled through all the supporters in the outer circle. The authentic sharing of their hearts along with the courageous sharing of struggle and Innate Gifts, had opened everybody's hearts. Trust flowed.

"I really needed this," Eliana said. "Thank you, Abby... Wow, this was intense! I knew I needed to be at this workshop, but I didn't expect this to happen." The group laughed, as many of them felt the same way.

By seeing these two strangers embrace with open hearts, my trust and faith in people was growing. Trust is contagious. Everyone in that room received something from this healing moment. It just further affirmed why we need such safe gatherings to remind people what it feels like to open their hearts and receive in a trusting way.

Self-Trust

When we surrender our wounds, we also release our former victimhood. By claiming our Inner Fire, our Innate Gifts that were awakened from our wounding, and we consistently speak our truth, we enter into a more empowered state of being. We are no longer powerless like when we were first wounded. Embracing that you are a powerful being and trusting how you will express your influence in your relationships becomes the focus of building self-trust. Because you are no longer susceptible to the same kind of wounding at this stage of the healing process, you can trust that you have the ability to keep yourself safe and to choose healthier relationships than in the past.

In order to trust other people, we must have a sense of trusting ourselves because we are the empowered selector of who will be part of our close community. Trusting our own senses, like our abilities to read people and to sense our gut instincts, is an essential milestone in building self-trust. We must choose the right people to confide in. We must be able to hear those subtle voices inside that tell us whether or not a person is safe to trust. So, trusting others is inseparable from a sense of self-trust, because we have the power to choose our supporters. In order to share the gift you have claimed, you must trust key members in the community who you know will receive the gift.

Trusting Life Again

People make up the communities that we live in. Beyond people, there are the greater forces of Life which affect our daily existence. These forces can be seen as luck. Good luck strikes when someone wins the lottery and bad luck hits when a home is destroyed during a hurricane. Whatever we call these greater forces of Life, what they all have in common is that they are beyond our direct control. So, when we refer to trusting Life, we are actually speaking about circumstances that we cannot directly influence (as we are able to do when we are in a relationship conflict or having an inner conversation with ourselves).

Life throws us a mixed bag: exciting new job opportunities, financial windfalls, and new fulfilling friendships that makes our hearts sing. But it

also deals out a fair share of challenges: job retrenchments, miscarriages, and chronic injuries being sustained in car crashes. The challenges and disappointments can harden our ability to receive life's rewards and can make us cynical about the trajectory of our lives. It essentially pinches off the ability to fully receive the greater flow of Life.

We often see individual people, such as our parents, teachers, Healers, and mentors, as representatives of Life and it is true that certain people are more connected to the benevolence of life. However, no one individual can represent the entirety of our needs. Being attached to certain individuals as your source of Life may be an indication of an innate distrust in the universe or God (or whichever term you prefer to use). Understanding our relationship with that great unknown power that created our universe goes beyond our human relationships. Having a robust trust in Life is a sign of great healing.

Interpersonal growth without celebration, without a necessary pause to feel the fruits of your labor, is sign of a deep mistrust in your life. I have noticed this so often in my clients who have done years of therapy or some other form of deep cathartic work, that I call it the Processing Trap. I've even witnessed whole intentional communities who stay in an agitated state of processing without ever fully finding resolution or stepping out of the catharsis and analysis long enough to feel the deeper rewards of this realization.

Exercise: Choosing a Peace Anchor

To help you shift your focus from the unburdening, catharsis and processing to a more peace-centric way of life, it can help to have a Peace Anchor. What anchors us in peace is different for each individual. There is no one right way to do it. Some people find peace in the security of their relationships with other people. Others find their serenity in nature, meditation, yoga, or martial arts.

Follow the next few steps to help you identify a peace anchor that may already be in your life, or to discover clues as to what may be an anchor for this phase of your life.

- Take a few deep breaths and feel your body.
- Ask the presence of peace inside of you to recall a memory of when you felt peaceful. This will be your point of reference for discovering your anchors. Trust the intuitive nature of this process, in that whatever information or memory may arise, it will be relevant to your current life. Ask your Inner Voice of Truth to give you wisdom.
- Open all your senses to feel for a response. Do you feel a sensation? Do you hear a calming or clear voice inside that is telling you something? Does a vision or memory appear inside your mind?
- If you feel a sensation, breathe into that area of your body and allow it to open up. This may be where your inner sense of peace resides. It may also be the feeling of wisdom that is slowly bubbling up and just needs more conscious attention to surface. Keep breathing and see what response comes out of the physical response.
- If you hear or see a response, allow the dialogue or movie in your head to speak to you.
- Feel how the response makes you feel in your body at this moment.
- Allow this experience to give you a gift. This may be a person in your vision walking up to you and handing you something. It could be a tree at a favorite place shining something into you. It may be a sound that seems to resonate throughout your body. Allow yourself to receive this gift.

- Journal about your experience to help you remember it. You can revisit it many times as a way of staying connected to your peace.
- Consider the following questions after you have received a response:
  1. Was your Peace Anchor a person from your past? Was it someone you know personally or is it a public figure or teacher that you have followed? Was it your partner or friend? Was it someone that you haven't met yet? Keep in mind that this exercise might also reveal a shift in peace anchors that is currently underway in your life.
  2. Was your Peace Anchor a place? If so, what is significant about this place for you?
  3. Was your Peace Anchor a part of nature such as an animal, a mountain, or a tree?
  4. Was your Peace Anchor a practice? Did you receive new information on how this practice is evolving for you currently?
  5. Was your peace anchor a historic figure or deceased person who you feel a connection to? How does it make your body feel to remember the person?

Keep in mind that your peace anchors could currently be in transition. If you didn't get a definitive response on your first try, repeat this exercise periodically. You may uncover important insights as to how your sense of peace is evolving and shifting.

Recognize if *you* have actually become your own peace anchor, meaning that you are so in touch with your own sense of stillness that you only need to bring your attention inwards to feel that sense of peace. If this is the case, your work is more about prioritizing your own access to yourself by scheduling in time to meditate, hike in nature, or do whatever practice gives you the most access to your own presence. You may even find that you must fend off the needs of other people to have your own turn at feeling your inner peace. This is a sign that you are doing too much and need to be with yourself more often. Your practice may be as simple as turning on the right music and feeling your own sense of inner calm.

A Story of a Peace Anchor

Before I served a reminder to others that a personal sense of peace is possible, I had people in my life that reflected this truth back to me. The most profound peace anchor in my life was my maternal great grandfather, who I called 'Pop.

Growing up, I spent many weekends at Grandma and Pop's house. Great Grandma was the matriarch who truly directed our family and served as the central authority figure. In short, Grandma was the undisputed boss. Pop was the joyous presence who emanated a calmness to the rest of the family. He rarely took center stage like my grandmother, but I always felt his presence. My cousin Christy, who often spent weekends at Grandma and Pop's with me, would fight me for the seat at the dinner table next to Pop. Christy always won and Grandma was very vocal about us kids not picking the seat next to her instead.

In many ways, Pop was a peace Wifi. When he was doing his "work" at family parties by broadcasting his calmness throughout the house, all was well. Much like internet Wifi, when it's working no one really consciously notices, it until it stops working. When the Wifi service is interrupted, everyone using it gets agitated and disturbed. In this way, peace is often taken for granted, as are our peace anchors. Yet their presence in our lives is essential.

Grandma and Pop became personal reminders as to why we live. When the going got tough and it was time to roll up our sleeves, Grandma showed us how it was done. She organized events, put people in their places when they were being nasty or selfish, and made sure everybody had a roof over their heads and food in their bellies. Pop represented the simple joy of drawing comics with his grandchildren and the celebration of each day of life without demanding that it drastically change. He resided in a consistent space of calmness and shared his presence generously. In the same way Grandma and Pop modeled from me the elements of a sound life, they also helped me to realize the importance of balancing what we do to make things better, with just being with what is already here in the moment. We need to be able to unburden and release the past through our personal efforts with the help of others. We also need to be able to be present with Life in an authentic way.

Sharing Peace

Sharing peace happens when we consciously connect to each other from our inner spaciousness. All the work leading up to forgiveness has cleared our insides to allow our peaceful essence to shine through to the surface. Our Inner Fire protects and clears this peace on a regular basis when we allow it to flow.

Peace can be shined to each other through our gifts. It is through the sharing of our gifts that our creativity takes form in a way that our intellect can recognize, and that our Essence can receive. Just like the beacon in the lighthouse, we shine on each other. The Essence itself is not work. It is experienced through surrender.

When we cannot see eye to eye during conflicts, it means that we have lost sight of our shared connection of peace. We get caught up on the more surface layers of our personality, from the most surface observations like the color of our skin to the emotional levels where we get stuck on somebody's "attitude." Our gifts, when brilliant displayed, are often the only things that can break the mental noise that keeps us in conflict. It's like getting into a fight with your spouse right before a great play. The actors move both of you through their song, dance, and dramatic prowess. By the end of the play, you are able to see each other again past the original conflict. The inspiration brought you back to the deep passions and calmness of your shared peace.

The expression of our gifts leads to the forging of bridges between cultures. It humanizes our transformation and conflict resolution, making the new shared peace a part of the grander human experience. As other people go through that shift, it no longer seems strange or foreign to leave the script of our ancestors in conflict. We discover that our transformation is not nearly as scary as we first made it out to be. We just simply arrive, and other people arrive with us, eventually.

No longer do we see ourselves locked in the contracts of desperately formed relationships that are initially forged in a state of shared survival. We no longer view ourselves as a rigid handful of archetypes. Those facets of the jewel are just the place where the bean of light bounces off before touching the heart of a fellow being. The jewel of our archetypes rotates freely, allowing us the ultimate freedom to be human. When the steady shine of our Essence is unearthed and realized, it becomes the constant. Shakespeare captured this human truth when Julius Caesar said, "I am constant as the northern star." Our inner star gives us a constant core by which the outer layers are given permission to morph as needed. This gives us a sense of play, that fluidity in our emotional and creative expression that makes us human. We no longer need to cling to rigid ideologies or beliefs as the core of who we are. We are not just "Mom" or the "Manager" in everything that we do. The more instinctual flows ring true.

I have seen the dismay of Catalysts when they try to share their new discovery with the people they love. If the people are not also working to discover themselves, they will not understand what you are sharing because words alone are not enough to embody these experiences.

Shared peace needs mutual spaciousness to beam and flow. It is generated from the reciprocation between two people who can relate to that shared experience of having connected to their own truth. This is why bringing the Catalysts of the world together is crucial. You sustain each other as each person you know moves at their own pace. There is no reason why you should be without people who understand the transformation that you are undergoing, nor should you stop trying to share your experience with people who have yet to have it. The happiest Catalysts whom I have met are those who share their inner experience with people who get it. That exchange feels like play. They also find a fulfilling way to share with people who are less attuned to their inner being. That exchange feels like worthwhile work.

The 8 Realizations are a Path to Peace

Each Realization leads to personal liberation. Liberation from each unfinished story happens by arriving at forgiveness for the actions and circumstances that caused the wound. Forgiveness clears the path for the peace to shine.

Let's revisit the previous steps to see how each of them inspires the forgiveness that makes space for the peace to shine through.

Realization #1: Leaving Survival Mode: While we are in the struggle and numbness of survival mode, we have tunnel vision. We're not unable to see how we have been wounded nor can we detect the pain of the how we've been hurt. We think that everything is ok, yet our Inner Voice of Truth knows that we are not well. How do we forgive our wounds when we are not even in touch with them?

In survival mode, we reside in a very efficient and focused part of our mind. But that level of focus requires denial of any feelings that need to flow in order to forgive. We may try to force our forgiveness and pretend that we have healed the wound, however without feeling the deeper impact and cathartically releasing the emotions inside of the wound, all we have is the illusion of forgiveness.

We rarely have access to feeling our hearts when we are in survival mode. Coming out of that focused, adrenaline-fueled state of mind, gives us some initial relief that gives us more space for forgiveness to happen. As we become more aware of how deeply we have been affected by our past, emotions may begin to rise up, which is a beneficial movement from the wound.

Realization #2: Recognizing the Invisible Burden: Once we realize that we are carrying a heavy story, we begin to feel validated. When we detect the burden, it is no longer invisible, and we can begin to address the responsibilities and unexpressed emotions that we are carrying. As we identify the story that we are carrying, we can even begin to see how other people in our family may be carrying the same story, or perhaps they too had something dumped on them. When the dumping is real, we have a right to feel how we feel about it.

Until we recognize that we've been carrying hardship on behalf of others, we don't realize how much we have been doing behind the scenes all the time. The wounds begin to become a little less personal when we realize that we are not the only ones in the family to carry them. The forgiveness process usually tends to get messier as we move forward, before it gets cleaner.

Realization #3: Unburdening brings us Freedom: It's rare to forgive your captors if you were to be kidnapped while you are still captivity. All you can think about is escaping. Perhaps you might also think about how you would like to satisfy your rage in vengeful ways. The same is true when the cyclic abuse keeps repeating and we are still holding onto the painful burdens that were dumped on us. Because we are still feeling the after-effects of the imposed suffering, and because the same abuse may still be happening, our forgiveness may be caught. This is especially so if the abused person was pressured into keeping the abuse secret, even after fact. That secret is a form of burden that can be internally damaging if held onto indefinitely.

Most people need for the abuse to stop and to unburden the secrets of how they were harmed before they can forgive. To forgive a hurtful act that is still repeating itself means that fresh wounding is actively being re-inflicted. It makes more sense to stop the abuse before opening the heart to the deeper levels of healing. Part of unburdening is breaking the scripted behavior that would allow the abuse to repeat. This is often required so that the person can go to safety and then allow the deeper, more vulnerable catharsis to happen.

By releasing the burden, you are dissolving your previous agreement that required you to put the other person's demands before your own core needs. When you give yourself permission for self-care, you reclaim the space, energy, and inner permission necessary for the next steps of forgiveness.

Realization #4: Reclaiming Empathy of Self and Others: Self-empathy gives us permission to feel. It's necessary to delve into the emotional sludge and expunge the festering feelings in order to clean out the wound. While initially, as feelings of hate, rage, and disgust may make it seem like the forgiveness process is going backwards, the process is, in fact, just getting deeper. The movement of pain helps forgiveness to flow.

Empathy provided to you from supporters creates a field of warmth and support which comforts the Catalyst during release. Just having that support available can be an enormously liberating experience. When we cry, we feel the hurt, but something about the crying feels good. We may even feel gratitude that the people around us care enough about us to give us that warmth and attention. It helps us to value ourselves and our feelings again. Because betrayal and abuse can be so demoralizing, having that level of attention and care can give us a sense of self-value again. Once the hurt has been fully expressed, we are more likely to be forgiving of other people, because we are no longer suffering.

Realization #5: Claiming our Inner Fire: Our Inner Fire is essential to melting the glue to the unfinished stories that have been stuck on us. By separating from the stories that are holding us back, we also awaken our passion. It's a healing force that most are taught to fear, but the liberation that it brings can be very encouraging and empowering. The Inner Fire clears a path for the truth to be expressed, setting the record straight and standing up for our rights. When we claim that empowering moment, we lose our victimhood and former fragility to claim new-found strength. No longer in a compromised position, it is easier to reaffirm our self-worth and to be the "bigger person" in matters of conflict. When we are safe, valued, and in a position of power, then we are more likely to forgive the wounds that helped us find our empowerment.

Realization #6: Claiming an Innate Gift: If the hardships of our lives were just exercises that caused us meaningless agony, it would be hard to trust Life. Without that trust, our hearts would be closed, and empathy would stop completely. In this trustless state, forgiveness would be hindered. Some degree of trust is required for meaningful forgiveness to happen. As forgiveness happens, trust can be rebuilt.

Gifts and wounds are linked. The connection between them are not random, rather the wounds usually give us deep awareness of ourselves, bring our consciousness deeper inside of ourselves to discover a sense of purpose. When we start to claim the Innate Gifts that were awakened from the wounding, it gives meaning to the hardship. An Innate Gift can help us recognize "why" the painful wounding happened to us.

Before an artist can paint a beautiful piece showing heart break, they must first experience a broken heart. Before a young woman discovers her intelligence and sense of integrity as a lawyer, she must first have endured or observed some type of injustice where accountability was not upheld, to inspire her quest for justice. Many of our best doctors have lost some one dear to them to some type of disease, so they become physicians to help keep people alive in an effort to prevent early death in other families.

Finding a sense of purpose that is informed by your Innate Gifts can enhance our fulfillment of our lives. A life worth living can be hindered by the unresolved past. Our gifts help us transform our pain into something inspiring for others. Expressing them makes the world a better place. By recognizing how our lives have become better as a result of those gifts, we may even experience a sense of gratitude for the hard experiences that helped us get there. The clear sense of identity that comes from knowing our Innate Gifts thus helps us to honor the struggle it took to find them, which in turn makes forgiveness easier to attain, because so much growth came out of a hurtful situation.

Realization #7: Speaking Your Truth: Our Inner Fire clears a path for our truth to be expressed. It melts away the guilt, fear, and hesitations that would otherwise prevent us from saying what needs to be said. That truth can be expressed in words, art, theater, writing, and many other forms of personal and creative expression. They are all expressions of our Truth.

However, there is something very specific about needing to share our truth with the world by speaking it directly. In our personal relationships, this can mean sharing with a friend, partner, or family member what you have always wanted to tell them. It can also mean standing up to a bully or speaking out about a form of abuse that you had to endure. It is not enough to hear the inner voice; we must also speak it.

There is no one way to share that Truth. For some, that moment of truth may come from serving as witness or plaintiff in a trial. For another it may be singing a song on stage. Another person may need to become a teacher to help the next generations face the challenges before them. Someone else may need to be the leader where they are heard very often, like a politician who gives public speeches.

Speaking our Truth begins in direct ways much earlier in the process, starting with the moment when we first chose to share our stories with another person. It's our Inner Voice of Truth that tells us to tell our story and who to tell it to. As we are unburdening, as we create empathy for the catharsis, as we shout and cry, our inner Truth is becoming more refined, clearer as we grow to know it. The past hardships inspired our truth to start shaking inside of us, pushing its way to the surface so that we could hear it.

Gratitude grows as we recognize how we needed certain experiences to discover who we needed to become. Nelson Mandela spent 27 years in prison for his opposition to apartheid in South Africa. Later, he became president of South Africa, a position that gave him many opportunities to speak his Truth about human equality.[26] At the celebration of his 20th

---

26 https://www.nelsonmandela.org/content/page/biography

anniversary commemorating his release from prison, he invited Christo Brand who had been his jailer at both Robben Island and Pollsmoor Prison. While someone who was unjustly imprisoned could grow to hate their captors, Mandela said that his interactions with his former jailer "reinforced my belief in the essential humanity of even those who had kept me behind bars."

When we are in the empowered state where we can speak our truth, it helps us to celebrate being in the present moment when our life circumstances are better than they previously were and where our strengths are recognized. The more deeply we are able to live in our Truth, the less influence the hurts of our past have on us. Speaking his Truth, Mandela was able to see that he had forgiven his jailer. He was able to see past the role of jailer and see the human being in front of him, even when he suffered the ordeal of imprisonment. A whole nation, in fact the entire watching world, benefited from the honest exchange of those two men in a prison cell.

Realization #8: Embodying Shared Peace: The modern English word 'forgive' comes from the Old English word *forgiefan*, which means to 'give up' punishment, to 'give in' or to 'allow'[27]. Forgiveness means we give up the need to punish, to hold accountable and to allow the natural state of Peace to resume. We acknowledge internally that we have learned all that we can learn from the wounding and that we have done all that we could do to serve justice. When that happens, and we truly give up the wound, we no longer hold ourselves back from sinking into the vibrant presence of Peace. We no longer hold onto a mission of revenge. Finally, the evidence of our past hurt is surrendered. Forgiveness means giving up the lament,

---

27 https://www.etymonline.com/word/forgive

the grief, and the hatred that had formerly tied our identity to the cyclic suffering. When we give those things up, we are finally free.

Not everyone is ready to embody peace. Very often, the courage and endurance to do this inner work is too much for those who are not ready to look inwards. But when you have made it through all the work of the previous Realizations, resisting forgiveness when we are so close to being healed doesn't honor all the sacrifice that was made to change your life for the better. Why stop just before the finish line and walk away from the end of the journey?

Peace in Action

Personal liberation leads to the liberation of others when direct service is made. It is essential to be with yourself in retreat to firmly anchor into your own stillness. That is the inhale of peace. But we are also built to live in some kind of community and once we have anchored in our peace, we can share it directly with whoever else is ready to receive it. That is our exhale of peace. As our relationships continue to evolve, we exchange peace, mutually inhaling and exhaling peace to each other in reciprocity.

In practice, families who are doing the inner work, would be giving their children the direct nurturing, encouragement, and attention that they need in order for them to mature into well-adjusted and whole adults. Loving your children from afar, thinking about them often, and praying for them every night are good practices, however they are a insufficient substitutes for the hands-on time together.

Being a Catalyst engaged with the world is essential to the shifts that lead to shared peace. With a growing confidence in your gifts and your ability to center your life within a peaceful presence, your actions have more impact than they did in the past. Anchoring in peace makes sure that your efforts are sustainable and that you are not over-reaching in your efforts. Sharing your gifts brings fulfillment and a sense of passion for your Inner Fire to flow through. A flowing Fire means a vital life.

When it comes to Speaking your Truth, non-violent protests are only one example of necessary efforts to change society. Speaking your Truth in your daily life without necessarily fulfilling an agenda can have an enormous impact. A more practical example is when a member of your family speaks up against family abuse. It sends a ripple effect through the extended family as well, because each family member shares some elements of the same story. When a cousin breaks the family rule of never leaving home to go away to college, this has an impact on the other cousins. That bravery inspires them, showing them that it is possible. We all have people whom we have compared ourselves to at some point in our lives. They are our peers, someone who is in the same vocation as us, or are the same age as us. When they move into a new phase of life or get a promotion of some kind, it impacts us more deeply than when it happens to a public figure on TV who we don't personally know.

Our personal liberation impacts other members of our community. It may trigger envy or resentment, but these are the emotions that are stuck in the Emotional Body that need to be cleared for that friend or family member to move forward in their own lives. That is their work. We, as the Catalysts, are not to blame for other people's feelings. By following the most authentic impulses coming from our Essence, we shake the world up in the right ways. The shared peace comes after the ruffled feathers, not instead of it.

Peace and our Inner Fire work together when they are clear and synchronized. Truth comes from that deep peace inside of us and is ushered into the world by our Inner Fire. The Inner Fire is the will and motivation to share our voice passionately into the world. It ensures that our Truth makes it out into the world. We need not forsake our Inner Fire to have our inner peace. That Fire is the guardian of our peace. It protects from the invasive burdens and blame of others, if we let the Inner Fire do its job. It is the source of passion when we cry out about injustice, to clear a space for that peace to expand. The Inner Fire blazes the trail and our Inner Voice of Truth directs us forward.

Final Chapter

What Happens Next?

What's the grand benefit from embodying these Eight Realizations? Besides the gradual rewards that come with reclaiming your birthrights, these realizations facilitate a greater transformation when practiced repeatedly. It's not a state of being that you achieve or a challenge that you conquer. For most people, this transition into self-awareness is not a one-off shift into enlightenment. Far more people experience their growth as flickering moments of expansion in empowerment and self-acceptance. Gradually, that flicker becomes more consistent, with moments of clarity and aliveness occurring more frequently until that shift becomes the new constant. The Eight Realizations clean out the vessel that is your mind/body, so that there is room for Peace to be your natural state of being.

While having that one moment of epiphany or that one great meditation retreat are important indicators of your inner development, these moments alone are not the total measurement of how much you have grown. Arriving into who you are is not about hitting one spiritual grand slam. As much as you admire the luminaries who have spontaneous moments of enlightenment, consider that your process may happen in a way that is unique to you. Your self-awareness may come from several waves of peace that overcome you, over and over again, until that becomes your new norm.

The more you let go of the unhealthy scripts, the more you give yourself permission to be the true you. The spaciousness of your liberation allows an intense sense of inner acceptance to grow. In time, you will meet the emotional conflicts and real-life crises from a peaceful center that is constantly guided by your Inner Voice of truth. Those conflicts and crises will no longer be able to knock you out of connection with yourself anymore, because the birthrights nourish your sense of true identity, solidifying your relationship with yourself. In short, you will no longer care what people think of you and your focus will be on sharing yourself with those who receive you.

This process often feels like you are walking the unknown path. But it only remains unknown until you become familiar with the essence of who you are, that deepest part of your being that has been there all along. Get to know it. Make it the priority in your life. Doing so activates it, awakens it, and gradually the truth of who you are takes over each area of your life. Let it happen.

These Eight Realizations essentially help you to strip away all the things that are not you. The Eight Birthrights feed your true identity so that it becomes more powerful than any undertow that could pull you back to your old ways. When the weight of the unfinished stories has been lifted, and the wounds have been cleaned, your Inner Voice of Truth speaks to you without interruption. When this happens, being yourself is remarkably simple and astoundingly direct.

The Difference Between Storytelling and Dumping

The challenge of raising children and mentoring the younger generations is teaching them about the family and culture they came from, without dumping your unresolved experiences onto them. Children need to know enough of their family history to identify the ancestral patterns that will be a part of their life's work later on. They also need it to appreciate the progress made in the family by all the Catalysts who stood up for what was right. Without that appreciation, they will take the goodness of their lineage for granted. Without that context, they will struggle to develop empathy for others, because if they don't understand the hardships of their lineage, how will they be able to have compassion for someone else going through rough experiences? They need to know the story of their lineage.

As a child, growing up on Long Island, NY, many of my friends at school were from Jewish lineages that migrated to the United States during World War 2. They were the families escaping the Holocaust. I remember walking to the deli one day with my father. I was probably ten years old at the time. We passed by two of our neighbors, a 5-year-old boy and his grandmother, who had set up a table in front of their house to sell flowers. My father asked me to pick some of the flowers as he passed a crisp dollar bill to the young boy, teaching him how to do business. The grandmother smiled, extending her hand to teach her grandson how to accept the money. That's when I saw the numbers tattooed onto her forearm. When we walked away from the booth, in a quiet voice, my father explained to me that those were concentration camp numbers tattooed onto her arm. "That's what the Nazis did to the Jews," he said in a hoarse whisper.

Despite having so many friends and neighbors that came from Holocaust survivor lineages, no one ever spoke about it. Instead, I went to lavish Bar Mitzvas and Bat Mitvas at fancy catering halls. While the teenagers were trying to slip away from the reception area to experience their first kiss, there was at least one person from the older generation wiping back a tear, whispering their gratitude to a deceased family member who couldn't be there in body. But those deceased family members were remembered for their spirit, their laughter, their sacrifices, and their courageous acts which ensured that the family could live on. These gatherings didn't just celebrate the transition of a young child into their adulthood. It also celebrated that the child would have a better life than the previous generations. But none of my Jewish friends spoke about this after their Bar Mitzva was over. They were too busy talking about how they got to second base with the cute girl sitting behind us.

Sharing the story of your family with the younger generations is important. It can be done at any time, though memorials and rites of passage are ideal moments to be courageous and share these stories. It need not always be somber. Sometimes a pure celebration is all that is needed to inspire the younger generations. Celebration helps us thrive.

The difference between dumping your heavy emotions onto someone else and storytelling is conscious intention. If you are aware of why you are sharing the stories -- for instance, to ensure that your grandchildren realize the benefits that they have in their lives compared to what you and your elders endured -- then share enough to help them recognize the story of their lineage. If the stories are just too raw, then share them with a friend or therapist first, so that your need to be heard and emotionally supported can be met first. Then when you share the stories with the younger generations, you will know that it is primarily for their benefit. You can trust that if you are consciously participating in the Realizations of this path, you will not be dumping onto the younger generations when you share the family stories. You will be actually be empowering them to the story of their lineage, which helps them both recognize the scripts that they inherited, and also appreciate the progress and benefits gained in their family.

Likewise, if you are of a younger generation and still have living elders in your family, ask them to unearth the old photographs or to help you update a family tree. Sometimes being a Catalyst happens just by simply showing interest in knowing more about your family and sparking an occasion for sharing between generations. Both storytelling and listening to someone else tell a story can lead to new awareness and heartfelt exchange.

Applying the 8 Realizations to a Crisis

Throughout the time you have been working this program, you may very well have gone through a crisis. Embrace the crisis as an opportunity to practice the Realizations to glean the most from this catalyst event. Some of the Realizations you may progress through quickly without even thinking about them. Other steps may feel like sticking points. Use the following guide to see where you are stuck, then follow the guidance to help you move through the sticking points. It may help to go back to the specific Realizations that the process below reveals as the roadblock, and rework the exercises provided.

Crisis is our friend because it can be a liberator. It interrupts our complacency and brings us to our limits. When we hit those limits, we can do things that we'd never thought we would do and choose a different path that we never thought we'd choose.

The Eight Realizations gives us a guiding handrail through the unsettling catharsis that comes with an interruption to our expected flow of life.

Let us recap the Eight Realizations and their corresponding Rewards.

- Recognizing our Survival Mode leads to Relief and slowing down.
- Identifying the Invisible Burdens leads to Greater Awareness that the issues did not begin with us, rather it was inherited.
- Unburdening is how we release the Invisible Burdens and create room for new choices
- By sharing our wounds with others, we receive heart nourishing Empathy and invite in more support
- Each Crisis helps us to see our Unique gifts which leads to a new sense of purpose, a powerful avenue to rewrite the script of our life.
- Sharing our gifts ignites our Inner Fire, the source of our passion that dissolves limiting self-beliefs.
- By Speaking Our Truth, we set the record straight and build trust in the inner wisdom that comes from our Inner Voice of Truth.
- By Forgiving, we release our attachment to the pain of our wounds, we release the evidence of our victimhood and allow shared peace to emerge.

When a crisis hits, use this Self-Enquiry Exercise to assess where you are getting stuck in the healing process. The number of the question corresponds directly to the Realization connected to the response.

FINAL CHAPTER

Self-Enquiry Exercise:

1. Am I experiencing numbness or haste?
2. What burden am I carrying for others?
3. How do I give the burden back to the other person?
4. How do I feel for myself? How do I feel towards others involved?
5. What gift is emerging from this conflict?
6. What's the most invigorating way to share that gift?
7. What wisdom does my Inner Voice of Truth offer me?
8. Who do I need to forgive?

As you write down the answer each question, do a Gut Check to see if the response fits. If your gut feels like there is something off or incomplete in your response, ask yourself the question again and try to respond as honestly as possible. When you feel resistance, clinching in your stomach or chest, anxiety, spontaneous fatigue, or even boredom, it is a sign that you are resisting that particular step of the process.

When you identify a sticking point, go back and skim the chapter on that particular Realization until you find a particular passage that can help you through your resistance. Re-work the exercises to see if they can help you move through whatever block you are experiencing.

It's possible that more than one step shows up with resistance as you go through each question. Each Realization is connected to the others somehow. Trust your visceral reaction to which Realizations have more of a charge on them than the others. Work those Realizations first.

Once you feel the forgiveness process flowing, consider celebrating a job well done. Celebrate with the people who see the truth of your life and can appreciate the importance of having a personal breakthrough in self-awareness. Not every accomplishment will have a tangible outer product that you can hold in your hands. Many of our most productive life steps happen internally, without external acknowledgement or celebration. This is why it's so important that you mark the occasion of a breakthrough or piece of significant work (like finishing this program) for yourself.

Riding the Waves

I rediscovered my passion for surfing when I moved to Oahu, Hawaii. The mountains of this island are green, strong, and dramatic. The crystal teal waters are cleansing and inviting. The beauty of the nature here constantly calls me back to the present moment, reminding me to receive the goodness of life. Here, in the place where surfing was born among Hawaiian Royalty, I embrace surfing not only as a fun pastime, but as a metaphor for how I now live my life.

We all must ride the emotional waves that life brings us. Some days will be a calm, flat ocean that glistens in the sun. Other times, the storms will come, and the waves will rage. Surfing reminds me of what is in my hands to control and what is out of my power to influence.

When I paddle out into the ocean, I don't know what Life will bring me. A calm ocean can bring waves twice my height in a matter of moments. It's for this reason that I still have a respectful fear of the ocean, especially since I almost drowned as a teenager years ago. But I don't let that fear stop me from paddling out and practicing the craft that helps me to feel refreshed and expressed. I face my fear and I accept what nature gives me in the moment.

Instead of treading water, I now glide above the ocean, deftly maneuvering through forces greater than I. The huge waves are by far stronger than I am, however, if I choose the right wave, if I paddle hard to get into the wave, and stand up on my surfboard, I have the chance to redirect that massive force behind me in a way that allow me to use my skill and will to make art. Every wave ridden becomes a unique work of art using forces of incredible magnitude as my canvas. The lines drawn by the fins of my surfboard are a momentary painting, until the canvas of the wave's face ruptures and explodes onto the shore. I emerge from the white water in salted glory.

As I continue to learn how to more skillfully surf the waves that life sends me, I feel a greater sense of trust in myself and my abilities, as well as a deeper appreciation for all that life has given me. As I slide across the ocean surface, the closest experience I'll have to walking on water, I'm grateful for my challenging past because it taught me to honor who I am.

You are not doing this work alone!

Join the growing community of Catalysts at
GKHunter.com

This is your portal to:
Weekly Blogs & Vlogs about inspiration healing topics
GK Global Tour schedule for in-person
Talks, Book Signings & Workshops
Information and Trailers for my upcoming Documentaries

Learn more about my
Upcoming Online Catalyst Program

Stay connected through social media:
FB: GK Hunter
Youtube: GK Hunter
IG: Authorgkhunter
Twitter: Authorgkhunter

To invite G. K. Hunter to speak at your event, visit:
gkhunter.com/globaltour/

References

1. Rafferty, J.P. (2019). Hurricane Andrew. *Encyclopædia Britannica.* Retrieved from https://www.britannica.com/event/Hurricane-Andrew

2. Wallace, P. (1946). *White roots of peace.* Santa Fe, NM: Clear Light Publishers.

3. Sogyal, R. (2002). *The Tibetan book of living and dying.* New York, NY: Harper One.

4. *Boeree, C. (2006). Abraham Maslow: 1908-1970. In Personality theories. Retrieved from* http://www.social-psychology.de/do/pt_maslow.pdf

5. Maslow, A. H. (1943). *A theory of human motivation.* Originally published: *Psychological Review, 50*(4), 370-396.

6. Rilke, R. M. (1946). *Letters to a young poet.* London, England: Sidgwick & Jackson.

7. Collective unconscious. (n.d.). *Encyclopædia Britannica.* Retrieved from https://www.britannica.com/science/collective-unconscious

8. Wagner-Moore, L. (2004). Gestalt therapy: Past, present, theory and research. *Psychotherapy: Theory, Research, Practice, Training, 41*(2), 180-189.Retreived from https://www.counseling.org/docs/david-kaplan's-files/wagner-moore.pdf

9. Good Therapy. (2016). Family constellations. Retrieved from https://www.goodtherapy.org/learn-about-therapy/types/family-constellations

10. Jung, C.G. (1971). Volume 6: Psychological types. In *Collected Works of C.G. Jung* (2nd ed.).
Retrieved from https://pdfs.semanticscholar.org/c6ee/e67ee75c47ff05cb1535d4d51d1b911dafd4.pdf

11. Skeat, W.W. (2013). *An etymological dictionary of the English language.* Mineola, NY: Dover Publications.

12. Nummenmaa, L., Glerean, E., Hari, R. & Hietanen, J.K. (2014). Bodily maps of emotions. *Proceedings of the National Academy of Sciences of the United States of America, 111*(2), 646-651.

13. Keller, M.S. (2013). Expressing, communicating, sharing and representing grief and sorrow with organized sound (Musings in eight short sentences). In S. Wild, D. Roy, A. Corn & R.L. Martin (eds.), *Humanities Research: One Common Thread the Musical World of Lament, XIX*(3), 3-14.

14. Pukui, M.K., Haertig, E.W. & Lee, C. (1972). **Nānā** I Ke Kumu: Look to the Source Vol. 1. Honolulu, HI: Hui Hānai.

15. Stroebe, M., Schut, H., Stroebe, W. (2007). Health outcomes in bereavement. *The Lancet, 370* (9603), 1960-1973.

16. Mental Health America (MHA) (2018). Co-Dependency. Retrieved from https://www.mentalhealthamerica.net/co-dependency

17. Pierrakos, J. (2005). *Core energetics: Developing the capacity to love and heal.* New York, NY: Core Evolution Publishing.

18. Northern Illinois University. (n.d.). Howard Gardner's theory of multiple intelligences. Retrieved from https://www.niu.edu/facdev/_pdf/guide/learning/howard_gardner_theory_multiple_intelligences.pdf

19. McCrea, S.M. (2010). Intuition, insight, and the right hemisphere. *Psychology Research and Behavior Management, 3,* 1-39.

20. Gandhi, M.K. (1983). *An autobiography or the story of my experiments with truth* (M. Desai, Trans.). New York, NY: Dover Publications, Inc.

21. Bach, R. (2012). *Illusions: The adventures of a reluctant messiah* (Reprint Ed.). London, UK: Delta.

22. Wing, N. (2013). September 11 timeline: A chronology of the key events that shaped 9/11.

Huffington Post. Retrieved from https://www.huffpost.com/entry/september-11-timeline_n_3901837

23. McCaleb, I.C. (2001). Bush tours ground zero in lower Manhattan. *Cable News Network.* Retrieved from http://edition.cnn.com/2001/US/09/14/bush.terrorism/

24. Goodstein, L. (2008). Serenity prayer stirs up doubt: Who wrote it? *The New York Times.* Retrieved from https://www.nytimes.com/2008/07/11/us/11prayer.html

25. Nelson Mandela Foundation. (n.d.). Biography of Nelson Mandela. https://www.nelsonmandela.org/content/page/biography

26. Forgive. (n.d.). *Online Etymology Dictionary.* Retrieved from https://www.etymonline.com/word/forgive

27. Gandhi, Arun (2017) *The Gift of Anger: And Other Lessons from My Grandfather* Mahatma Gandhi Publisher:Gallery/Jeter Publishing

Tables and Figures

Table List

Figure List

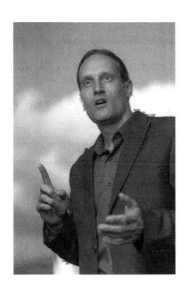

About the Author

After 15 years of working as an Intuitive Healer with Jewish Holocaust Survivors, Native Americans, the homeless, veterans, and physicians, G. K. Hunter developed a step by step process to unburdening the heavy history that we all inherit from our ancestors. The Bloodline Healing Method TM was born. By releasing our invisible burdens, we can claim our innate gifts and expand to meet our most purposeful and liberated life.

Hunter is the director of **Sakura & Pearls**: *Healing from World War 2*, a documentary about Japanese Atomic Bomb Survivors meeting the American Survivors of Pearl Harbor. **It's the first time that the approach of Bloodline Healing was captured on camera, resulting in deeply emotional exchanges between people who had survived some of the most monumental events in history.** **Sakura & Pearls** premiered at the Pearl Harbor Visitor Center and continues to be shared by educators throughout the world.

G. K. Hunter is known as an electric speaker and has appeared on several television shows, radio programs, and in university classrooms, including his alma mater Cornell University.